REHABILITATION COUNSELOR
PREPARATION AND
DEVELOPMENT

REHABILITATION COUNSELOR PREPARATION AND DEVELOPMENT

SELECTED CRITICAL ISSUES

Edited by

WILLIAM G. EMENER

Professor
Department of Rehabilitation Counseling
University of South Florida
Tampa, Florida

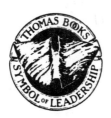

CHARLES C THOMAS • PUBLISHER
Springfield • Illinois • U.S.A.

Published and Distributed Throughout the World by
CHARLES C THOMAS • PUBLISHER
2600 South First Street
Springfield, Illinois 62717

© *1986 by* CHARLES C THOMAS • PUBLISHER
ISBN 0-398-05173-9
Library of Congress Catalog Card Number: 85-16849

With **THOMAS BOOKS** *careful attention is given to all details of manufacturing and design. It is the Publisher's desire to present books that are satisfactory as to their physical qualities and artistic possibilities and appropriate for their particular use.* THOMAS BOOKS *will be true to those laws of quality that assure a good name and good will.*

Printed in the United States of America
Q-R-3

Library of Congress Cataloging in Publication Data
Main entry under title:

Rehabilitation counselor preparation and development.

Includes bibliographies and indexes.
1. Rehabilitation counseling—Study and teaching
(Graduate)—United States.   2. Rehabilitation
counselors—Training of—United States.
3. Rehabilitation counseling—Study and teaching
(Continuing educations)—United States.
4. Rehabilitation counselors—Supervision of—Study
and teaching—United States.   I. Emener,
William G. (William George)
HD7256.U5R424   1985   362'.0425   85-16849
ISBN 0-398-05173-9

To

DR. THOMAS L. PORTER

The rehabilitation educator
who shaped my career,
The rehabilitation leader
who shaped a profession,
The friend
so many of us rely upon.

For all you do
For being you

Bill Emener

ABOUT THE EDITOR

WILLIAM G. EMENER is currently a professor of rehabilitation counseling and the associate dean of the College of Social and Behavioral Sciences at the University of South Florida. He received his M.A. degree from New York University and his Ph.D. from the University of Georgia. He has been a high school English teacher, rehabilitation counselor and supervisor, program director of rehabilitation education at Murray State University, program coordinator of rehabilitation services education at Florida State University, and director of the rehabilitation counseling program at the University of Kentucky.

His honors and awards include eight biographical personalities and *Who's Who* listings, four Outstanding Service Awards from professional associations, and two National Research Awards (from the American Rehabilitation Counseling Association and the National Rehabilitation Administration Association). His professional activities include membership in 14 national and state professional associations and in addition to other leadership positions was the 1983-84 president of the National Rehabilitation Administration Association.

Over the past several years, Doctor Emener has been an editor and co-editor of over 14 special publications, was co-editor of the *Journal of Applied Rehabilitation Counseling* from 1978-1982, and served as a member of the Policy Board for the *Journal of Rehabilitation Administration* from 1983-1985. His publications and writings include three research monographs, three other books (since 1981), book chapters in five different texts, over 18 non-published professional papers, 65 authored/co-authored articles in 16 different professional refereed journals, and over 55 professional papers presented at professional association meetings.

CONTRIBUTORS

ATKINS, B.J.
Associate Professor and Coordinator of the Rehabilitation Counselor Education Program at the University of Wisconsin, Milwaukee, WI

BAKER, R.J.
(Deceased) former Editor of the Vocational Evaluation and Work Adjustment Bulletin and a Professor in the Rehabilitation Institute, Southern Illinois University, Carbondale, IL

BALLOU, M.
Assistant Professor, Department of Counseling and Human Services, State University of New York, NY

BLUM, C.R.
Clinical Associate in the Department of Counseling and Human Services, State University of New York, Buffalo, NY

BRITTON, J.O.
Professor in the Department of Counseling and Educational Psychology at Pennsylvania State University, University Park, PA

CARTER, S.A.
Case Manager, Goodwill Industries, Inc., Madison, WI

CRIMANDO, W.
Assistant Professor in the Rehabilitation Institute, Southern Illinois University, Carbondale, IL

CRYSTAL, R.M.
Associate Professor and Director of the Graduate Program in Rehabilitation Counseling, University of Kentucky, Lexington, KY

DIAMONTI, M.C.
Associate Professor of Education, University of New Hampshire, Durham, MA

EMENER, W.G.
Professor of Rehabilitation Counseling and the Associate Dean of the College of Social and Behavioral Sciences, University of South Florida, Tampa, FL

FREEMAN, J.B.

(Currently J.B. Patterson) Associate Professor and Coordinator of the Rehabilitation Services Education Program, Florida State University, Tallahassee, FL

GEIST, G.O.

Professor and Director of the Rehabilitation Education Program, Illinois Institute of Technology, Chicago, IL

GUALTIER, J.J.

Clinical Associate in the Department of Counseling and Human Services, State University of New York, Buffalo, NY

HINMAN, S.

Research Scientist at the Arkansas Rehabilitation Research and Training Center, Fayetteville, AR

HOLLINGSWORTH, D.K.

Assistant Professor in the Department of Rehabilitation Counseling, Louisiana State University Medical Center, New Orleans, LA

JAQUES, M.E.

Professor and Chairperson of the Department of the Counseling and Human Services, State University of New York, Buffalo, NY

KAUPPI, D.W.

Associate Professor and Director of the Rehabilitation Counselor Training Program in the Department of Counseling and Human Services, State University of New York, Buffalo, NY

KUNCE, J.T.

Professor of Educational Psychology and Counseling at the University of Missouri, Columbia, MO

LORENZ, J.R.

(Deceased) former Editor of the Journal of Rehabilitation Administration and a Professor and the Director of the Rehabilitation Institute, Southern Illinois University, Carbondale, IL

LYNCH, R.K.

President of Professional Rehabilitation Services, Ltd., Madison, WI

MARR, J.N.

Professor and Research Scientist at the Arkansas Rehabilitation Research Training Center, University of Arkansas, Fayetteville, AR

MARS, M.G.

Program Analyst for Vocational Rehabilitation, Office of Vocational Rehabilitation—HRS, Lakeland, FL

MARTIN, T.

Coordinator of the Job Seeking Skills Program for the Virginia Department of Rehabilitation Services, Mt. Vernon, VA

MATKIN, R.E.

President of Vocational Management Systems, Inc., Murphysboro, IL

MCFARLANE, F.R.

Professor and the Director of the Region IX Rehabilitation Continuing Education Program, San Diego State University, San Diego, CA

MCMAHON, B.T.

Program Developer, New Medico Head Injury Rehabilitation System, Boston, MA

MURPHY, S.T.

Associate Professor in the Division of Special Education and Rehabilitation, Syracuse University, Syracuse, NY

NADOLSKY, J.M.

Editor of the Journal of Rehabilitation and an Associate Professor in the Department of Rehabilitation Counselor Education, University of Tennessee, Knoxville, TN

PANKOWSKI, J.M.

Assistant Program Staff Director of the Florida Office of Vocational Rehabilitation, Department of Health and Rehabilitative Services, Tallahassee, FL

PANKOWSKI, M.L.

Associate Vice President for Academic Affairs and Director of the Center for Professional Development and Public Services, Florida State University, Tallahassee, FL

PARKER, R.M.

Editor of the Rehabilitation Counseling Bulletin and a Professor of Rehabilitation Counseling at the University of Texas, Austin, TX

PUCKETT, F.D.

Doctoral Candidate in the Doctor of Rehabilitation Program, Rehabilitation Institute, Southern Illinois University, Carbondale, IL

RASCH, J.D.

Associate Professor of Rehabilitation Counseling in the College of Social and Behavioral Sciences, University of South Florida, Tampa, FL

ROESSLER, R.T.

Senior Research Associate and a Professor of Rehabilitation Education at the University of Arkansas, Fayetteville, AR

RUBIN, S.E.

Professor and Director of the Doctoral Program, Rehabilitation Institute, Southern Illinois University, Carbondale, IL

SAWYER, H.W.

Professor and Chairperson of the Department of Rehabilitation Counseling, University of Florida, Gainesville, FL

SAXON, J.P.

Associate Professor, Department of Rehabilitation Counseling, University of Florida, Gainesville, FL

SCALIA, V.A.

Associate Professor and Director of the Region VIII Rehabilitation Continuing Education Program, University of Northern Colorado, Greeley, CO

SCHMIDT, J.F.

Graduated Summa Cum Laude with a B.S. degree in Psychology from Florida Southern College, Lakeland, FL

SCORZELLI, J.F.

Associate Professor and Director of the Rehabilitation Counseling Program, Northeastern University, Boston, MA

SPECTOR, P.E.

Associate Professor, Psychology Department, College of Social and Behavioral Sciences, University of South Florida, Tampa, FL

SULLIVAN, M.

Training and Evaluation Specialist for Region IX Rehabilitation Continuing Education Program, San Diego State University, San Diego, CA

THOMAS, K.R.

Professor, Department of Studies in Behavioral Disabilities, University of Wisconsin, Madison, WI

THORESON, R.W.

Professor and Director of the Graduate Program in Rehabilitation Counseling and Personnel Services, University of Missouri, Columbia, MO

USDANE, W.M.

(Deceased) former Assistant Commissioner of the Rehabilitation Services Administration, Social and Welfare Service, Department of Health, Education and Welfare, Washington, D.C.

WOLFE, R.R.

Professor and Coordinator of the Graduate Program in Rehabilitation Counseling, University of Northern Colorado, Greeley, CO

WRIGHT, G.N.

Professor, Department of Studies in Behavioral Disabilities, University of Wisconsin, Madison, WI

FOREWORD

DESPITE REHABILITATION counseling's relatively long history, numerous questions still are being raised by consumers, related professionals, employers, and funding agencies regarding the profession. For example, varied definitions of rehabilitation counseling still exist, several different professional organizations representing rehabilitation counselors have somewhat different goals and constituences, Congress and federal agencies continue to raise questions regarding the need for persons trained as rehabilitation counselors, and additional research projects have been designed to address concerns facing the profession.

In April, 1985 the National Council on Rehabilitation Education (NCRE) sponsored a symposium at the American Association for Counseling and Development annual conference in New York City entitled "Critical Issues in Rehabilitation Education." Three past presidents of NCRE, Kenneth Reagles, William Jenkins, and William Graves accepted the responsibility of defining current concerns and issues. To provide the reader with a perspective on these concerns, several of the thought provoking observations by Graves (1985) are summarized as follows: Despite the fact that Congress in 1984 finally recognized the need for trained professionals and inserted the phrase "qualified personnel" in the Rehabilitation Act, educators still are being asked to prove that education makes a difference in the counselor performance. Although ample evidence exists that educational programs have an impact on the kind and quality of rehabilitation services provided to severely disabled persons, federal decision makers demand even more evidence to justify federal funds for training and research. Unless Congress can be convinced of the need for and benefits of trained professionals, it appears likely that training funds will be reduced even further. Eliminating preservice programs would mean that in fiscal year 1986 people with severe disabilities, who would be served by newly hired rehabilitation counselors, would have only one chance in four of being served by a qualified professional. Opportunities for inservice and continuing education would similarly be decreased, reducing the potential of rehabilitation agencies to upgrade the skills of current employees.

These issues are not new. In fact, the history of rehabilitation counselor education can be characterized by such terms as ambiguity, change, conflict, and uncertainty. In part, these characteristics can be ascribed to the complexity of the profession and the many variables impinging on it. (Dr. Emener provides an overview of historical developments in his Introduction to Part I: Historical Perspectives.)

The development of the profession of rehabilitation counseling was stimulated in 1954 by the passage of Public Law 565 which authorized federal training monies for rehabilitation counselor preparation. With the establishment of university programs, educators began to recognize the need for enhanced communication to develop common standards in educational programing and to have a greater voice in determining their own destinies. By 1956 approximately 25 universities had received federal funds to establish rehabilitation counseling programs. The first meeting of coordinators was held in Washington, D.C. in the Spring of that year (Miller, 1980). Recognizing the need to bring together educators to address the problems and operations of their training programs, the Office of Vocational Rehabilitation (now the Rehabilitation Services Administration) provided Michigan State University a grant to conduct the first annual Rehabilitation Counseling Trainer Workshop. The first Workshop was held in April, 1957. In addition to the Workshops, educators met informally at conferences such as the National Rehabilitation Association and the American Personnel and Guidance Association and ultimately began meeting periodically with state directors of vocational rehabilitation agencies. A Coordinators Liaison Committee was established as a counterpart of the Personnel Development and Training Committee of the Council of State Administrators of Vocational Rehabilitation (CSAVR) as educators recognized the necessity of close communication with the then largest employer of program graduates. It is particularly interesting to note the major topics of concern expressed at the 1960 joint meeting of educators and state directors (many of which still are being addressed today):

1. Follow-up studies of rehabilitation counseling program graduates hired by state agencies;
2. Problems, methods, and standards in recruitment and selection of students for rehabilitation counseling programs;
3. Curriculum development;
4. Field instruction or internship for students in rehabilitation counseling programs (Miller, 1980).

Despite the cooperative meetings between educators and state directors and the establishment of the American Rehabilitation Counseling Association as an APGA division, which meaningfully addressed some of the developmental needs of rehabilitation counselor education, many leaders expressed the concern that no specific organization existed which truly represented educators on such matters as educational policy and standards, relations with the federal government and coordination with state and private rehabilitation agencies. In 1967 several leading educators including Robert Warnken, John Muthard, Bob Johnson, and Greg Miller polled educators regarding their desire to establish a separate organization. Receiving a highly favorable response, these leaders formed the Council of Rehabilitation Counselor Educators (CRCE), the predecessor of the National Council on Rehabilitation Education (NCRE) (see Szuhay, 1980 for a comprehensive history of NCRE). The early years of CRCE were focused on curricular development and programmatic issues and the profession moved forward rapidly (see Part II of this text: Developmental Issues in Rehabilitation Counselor Education).

In 1971, however, the startling announcement by Mr. Harold Shay on behalf of the Rehabilitation Services Administration that the federal government was planning to eliminate grants to training programs, dramatically altered the goals, composition, and posture of CRCE. The leaders agreed that the organization must become politically active, must take an active posture regarding the future of rehabilitation counselor education rather than merely reacting to federal and state mandates, and must expand its membership to include all constituencies involved in the continuum of rehabilitation education from preservice to inservice to continuing education. In 1976 CRCE voted to change the name of the organization to the National Council on Rehabilitation Education (NCRE) and to expand institutional membership to include all graduate and undergraduate rehabilitation training, research, and educational programs in universities and agencies. Not only was this organizational expansion viewed as a way to increase the potential impact of NCRE, but it was believed that curricular improvements and coordination could result from bringing together rehabilitation counseling educators with those from such closely related professions as workshop administration and vocational evaluation. Today NCRE represents 517 individual members located in 79 institutions. The stated goals of the organization are:

1. To determine the skills necessary for effective rehabilitation services and the most effective training for developing these skills.
2. To assist in documentation of the impact of rehabilitation education in improving the quality of services to handicapped citizens.
3. To develop and implement a continuous process for determining personnel needs in rehabilitation and future priorities of personnel needs.
4. To work toward the identification of basic competencies for rehabilitation personnel as a basis for professional standards in service, education, and research.
5. To involve and interact with consumers of rehabilitation services and rehabilitation education and research in all major planning and policy matters that relate to them.
6. To assist in the development of clearly defined role and function models

for rehabilitation personnel, a methodology for assessment of role performance, and work toward application of such models throughout the nation.

7. To interact and collaborate with other related professional associations in matters of common concern and in achieving shared goals.

8. To work toward integration of federal, state, and private sector standards in the development of uniform licensure and certification requirements for rehabilitation personnel at all levels.

9. To work conjointly with the Council on Rehabilitation Education (CORE), Commission on Rehabilitation Counselor Certification (CRCC), Commission of Accreditation of Rehabilitation Facilities (CARF), and other accrediting or certifying resources to insure consistency in rehabilitation education direction.

10. To provide a unified forum that will represent the needs, the assets, and the direction of all facets of rehabilitation education.

11. To impact on public and private sector policies and practices that relate to rehabilitation education and research.

12. To identify and recommend individuals and institutions having particular expertise to policymakers and administrators needing such expertise in rehabilitation education and research.

13. To keep its members abreast of relevant developments and their implications for the profession of rehabilitation education and research (Szuhay, 1980, p. 32).

Rehabilitation counseling still represents the largest constituency of NCRE and as such the Board of Directors enthusiastically reviewed the proposal of Dr. William G. Emener to prepare this book of selected readings. It is our hope and belief that this important work will not only enhance rehabilitation counselor education as well as education in related rehabilitation disciplines, but that it also will serve as a resource to counter the voices of many of our critics. As the many important and crucial articles contained in this text are reviewed, the oft cited criticism that a professional literature does not exist finally should be put to rest. Despite the breadth and variety of writings regarding rehabilitation counseling, one must note the variety and number of sources in which they are found. Perhaps the existence of so many diverse and high quality journals including the *Rehabilitation Counseling Bulletin,* the *Journal of Applied Rehabilitation Counseling,* and *The Journal of Rehabilitation* constitute both a blessing and a curse. The retrieval of much of our literature until today has not been an easy task for either professionals or students. Now references delineating the development of the profession, key contents and constructs of rehabilitation counselor education, and student/trainee issues are available in *one* resource.

Although the Master's degree in Rehabilitation Counseling generally is accepted as the necessary entry level preparation for the profession, it certainly is not complete in itself. As a long-time rehabilitation counselor and educator, the rapid changes in our profession have always excited and stimulated me. Nevertheless, keeping abreast of the needs of emerging client groups and the developments of rapidly expanding technology places an extreme burden on the already busy practitioner. Hence, the vital impact of both inservice and continuing education and developments in these arenas will provide a more complete picture of the "total" field. As rehabilitation moves forward into the 1990s, professionals will meet many new challenges. Persons who are even more severely disabled will seek and require services, the transition of disabled youth from school to work must be facilitated, the rapidly emerging technologies of rehabilitation engineering and computers must be incorporated into service opportunities for clients, and independent living must become a reality for disabled persons. Rehabilitation workers will need to expand their knowledges and this text will provide an important basis for prospective employees. It also will be useful in updating the understanding of currently employed practitioners. Finally, the many writings contained in this volume will provide Congress and federal officials with many of the answers to their questions and concerns regarding rehabilitation professions.

The National Council on Rehabilitation Education thus is proud to cooperate with Dr. Emener in this worthwhile endeavor. On behalf of our membership, I wish to convey our appreciation to him for his comprehensive and timely work.

Ann Beck Meyer

President, National Council on Rehabilitation Education
Professor and Associate Dean, The Graduate School
University of Wisconsin-Milwaukee
July, 1985

References

Graves, W.H. (1985). Rehabilitation training, services to people with severe disabilities, and the funding crisis. *NCRE Report* 11 (3), 1.

Miller, G.A. (1980). Early years. In J.A. Szuhay (Ed.) *The History of the National Council on Rehabilitation Education*, (pp. 5-9) Washington, D.C.: The National Council on Rehabilitation Education.

Szuhay, J.A. (Ed.)(1980). *The History of the National Council on Rehabilitation Education*. Washington, D.C.: The National Council on Rehabilitation Education.

PREFACE

IN THE PROCESS of preparing books, book chapters, research monographs, and journal articles over the past three years, I have reviewed and studied numerous journal articles relevant to rehabilitation counselor preparation and development. Moreover, I have shared my collection of materials with practitioners, students, and colleagues — not only in the Tampa Bay area and at the University of South Florida but at many other locales and universities as well. Repeatedly, it was offered that these amassed materials collectively provided an important historical and developmental appreciation for rehabilitation counselor preparation and development, and an articulation and concretion of numerous critical issues in the area of professionalism in rehabilitation. Practitioners, students, and educators have stated to me that this collection of published writings from rehabilitation journals offered valuable knowledge and insights. They also expressed that "it is unfortunate that these works are not available in one volume." Experiences such as these over the past few years provided the initial impetus, rationale, and purpose for me to engage in this undertaking.

Based on the assumption that it is important to genuinely appreciate a "lifelong learning model" of professional preparation, this book was designed to provide a carefully selected and synthesized distillation of published works for the specific purpose of enhancing students', practioners', educators', human resource development specialists', and other rehabilitation professionals' conscious awareness of historical, developmental, and temporal critical issues in the area of rehabilitation counselor preparation and development. While I was rather quickly convinced of the need for this book, I also concluded that the level of professionalism in the field of rehabilitation counseling would render a demand for a volume such as this one. The ultimate litmus test of this latter conclusion, obviously, will be revealed by the use, influence, and impact of the book over the next three to five years. *Practicing rehabilitation counselors,* as part of their professional reading, and *students* in rehabilitation counselor education programs, ideally as part of their required reading and study early in their coursework, should find this book helpful to their understanding and appreciation of the profession of rehabilitation counseling, its roots, its continuing developments, and their own "lifelong development" as professional rehabilitation counselors. *Human resource development specialists* and *rehabilitation educators* should find this book helpful in their planning, implementation, and evaluation of education, training, and development programs. I also suggest that supervisors, managers, administrators, researchers, and policy developers will value this work and consider it a meaningful addition to their personal and professional libraries. In a variety of ways, this book has some unique features.

The limitations imposed by the realities of space and publication costs made the decisions of which published journal articles to include and not include very difficult. This aspect of the book's development was heightened due to the availability of many excellent works worthy of a place in this book. My initial review of approximately 250 journal articles produced a selected, categorical list of 104 journal articles worthy of consideration for reproduction. Three prominent rehabilitation counselor educators, representing a blend of valuable experience across many areas pertinent to rehabilitation counselor preparation and development, provided exceptionally valuable assistance to me. Each of these three experts independently rated the 104 proposed journal articles on a five point scale (1 = definitely not include; 5 = definitely include). Moreover, they offered individual comments and recommended other articles (ones I had not suggested) as well. Their individual and group ratings and mean ratings on the 104 articles were then used in determining the final list of articles which comprise the 31 chapters of the book.

The book has six parts. **Part I** offers an important appreciation of the historical and current distinction(s) between baccalaureate and masters level preparation; **Part II** focuses on rehabilitation counselor education with special attention to fundamental aspects and issues, educational models, evaluation, and other relevant critical issues—developmental, contemporary, and continuing; **Part III** addresses key constructs and contents of rehabilitation counselor education: content determination and development, clinical components, selected construct areas, and brief attention to the growing emphasis on computerization issues; **Part IV** discusses, among others, three major aspects of students/trainees: recruitment and selection, their characteristics and attributes, and critical issues relevant to graduates of rehabilitation counselor education programs; **Part V** articulates issues relevant to inservice training and continuing education: historical perspectives, needs assessment, and evaluation; and, **Part VI** focuses on four critical aspects of related professional development components: administration and supervision, facilities, vocational evaluation, and private sector rehabilitation.

These six Parts contain 20 subparts, the 31 chapters, and 44 selected abstracts of professional journal articles (articles which could not be reprinted as chapters but yet were determined to be important in terms of their contributions to the body of knowledge). The references for these 44 abstracts are included in the references at the end of each of the six Parts. To assist the reader in appreciating the magnitude and rich integration of contructs within rehabilitation's professional literature, in my "Introduction Commentaries" to each of the six Parts, I refer to a total of 286 different references and suggested additional readings. These intro's were designed to assist the reader in appreciating the importance of each chapter, their relevance to each other and as a group, and continuing issues for the future that the chapters directly and indirectly offer as challenges to us all.

There are many individuals to whom I would like to express sincerest appreciation and gratitude for their unselfish assistance and encouragement throughout the numerous processes of the book's development. While running the risk of not thanking and acknowledging everyone to whom I am appreciative, I do want to thank some special people for their special meaning to this book. The National Council on Rehabilitation Education (NCRE) not only endorsed the concept of this book and encouraged its development, NCRE also put up almost all of the upfront permission fees for the reproduction of the published journal articles. It is an honor to work with the Council in this collaborative way. Dr. Ann Beck Meyer, who graciously wrote the Foreword, was extremely encouraging throughout — among her important contributions, Ann was the facilitative energizer who kept me going. The selection of articles to reprint was not easy, to say the least, and my three rehabilitation education experts (raters) gave me the guidance, feedback, and suggestions I needed to make decisions I feel good about. A hearty thanks to Dr. Jeanne M. Patterson, Florida State University, Dr. Richard T. Roessler, University of Arkansas, and Dr. John Thompson, Seattle University. The 47 authors/coauthors of the 31 chapters unselfishly and enthusiastically granted permission to reprint their published articles. The five journal editors of the journals in which the 31 articles were originally published, were encouraging all along the way, and they spiritedly and with "no charge" granted permission to reprint the 31 articles. For their operationalized commitment to the mission and purposes of this book, I offer my genuine appreciation to: Dr. Richard W. Bradley, Editor, *Counselor Education and Supervision;* Dr. Julian M. Nadolsky, Editor, *Journal of Rehabilitation;* Dr. John F. Newman, Editor, *Journal of Rehabilitation Administration;* Dr. Randall M. Parker, Editor, *Rehabilitation Counseling Bulletin;* and Dr. Arnold Wolfe, Editor, *Journal of Applied Rehabilitation Counseling.* The Media Committee of the American Association for Counseling and Development (AACD), however, reviewed the prospectus materials of the book and decided that even though the book's contributors and Editor were contributing all of the book's royalties to the National Council on Rehabilitation Education, AACD's regular permission fees had to be paid. Mr. Michael G. Copeland, Supervisor of the Information Processing Center, College of Social and Behavioral Sciences, University of South Florida, relentlessly provided the technical brilliance which pulled things together; to Nita C. Desai, Cecile L. Pulin, and Peter A. Selle, Word Processing Operators, I extend my appreciation to their refreshing blend of competence and patience. My sincerest appreciation also is extended to Ms. Leslie Lavender, a colleague and friend, who rated the 104 proposed articles from a private sector/practitioner's perspective and also critically critiqued the drafts of the six "Introduction Commentaries." Two very special people in my office graciously helped with this book in many ways, and understandingly and patiently tolerated my aberrant behavior around due dates — a warm thanks to Linda L. Pickrell and Carol I. Clark. To my wife, Rae, who not only is my number one proofreader and critic, but compassionately tolerates compulsiveness and situational workaholism, I owe my deepest gratitude!

The greatest reward for me, and the most worthy payoff for the contributors of this book, would be for the future to reveal that rehabilitation counselor education and development programs were maximizing their potential contributions to the provision of high quality, professional rehabilitation counseling services. Our operationalized compassion for our fellow Americans with disabilities compels us to expect nothing less than the best.

William G. Emener

CONTENTS

Page

About the Editor vii

Contributors ix

Foreword — Ann Beck Meyer xiii

Preface xix

PART I. HISTORICAL PERSPECTIVES 3

Introduction Commentary 5

    1. Why a Master's Degree in Rehabilitation Counseling? 9
       Mary L. Pankowski and Joseph M. Pankowski

Selected Abstracts 15

References and Suggested Additional Readings for Part I 17

PART II. DEVELOPMENTAL ISSUES IN REHABILITATION
COUNSELOR EDUCATION 21

Introduction Commentary 23

    2. Rehabilitation Counselor Education 27
       Vincent A. Scalia and Richard R. Wolfe

    3. Behavioral Objectives and Rehabilitation Counselor Education:
       A Critique 37
       Michael C. Diamonti and Stephen T. Murphy

    4. An Integrative Model for Rehabilitation Training and Practice 45
       Ralph M. Crystal

    5. A Futuristic Model of Rehabilitation Education 53
       William G. Emener and Fred R. McFarlane

    6. Knowledge Adequacies and Training Needs of
       Rehabilitation Educators 65
       William G. Emener, John D. Rasch, and Paul E. Spector

    7. Contemporary Rehabilitation Counselor Education 73
       George N. Wright

8. The Changing Role and Function of the Rehabilitation
Counselor 77
Stanford E. Rubin and Frank D. Puckett

9. A Critique of Trends in Rehabilitation Counselor Education
Toward Specialization 85
Kenneth R. Thomas

10. Training Independent Living Rehabilitation Specialists 93
Richard T. Roessler

11. Placement Personnel — A Graduate Program Concept 101
William M. Usdane

Selected Abstracts 106
References and Suggested Additional Readings for Part II 109

PART III. REHABILITATION COUNSELOR EDUCATION:
KEY CONTENTS AND CONSTRUCTS 113

Introduction Commentary.. 115

12. Assessing the Content of a Rehabilitation Counseling Program 119
James F. Scorzelli

13. Actual and Preferred Instructional Areas in Rehabilitation
Education Programs... 125
William G. Emener and John D. Rasch

14. Clinical Practice in Master's Level Rehabilitation Counselor
Education... 137
Bobbie J. Atkins

15. Internships for Rehabilitation Counselors: On the Way to
a Professional Career 145
Glen O. Geist

16. Training Counselors to Write Behavior-Based Client Objectives..... 147
Suki Hinman and John N. Marr

17. Computer-Assisted Instruction in Rehabilitation Education 159
William Crimando and Richard Baker

Selected Abstracts 164
References and Suggested Additional Readings for Part III.............. 167

PART IV. STUDENT/TRAINEE ISSUES 171

Introduction Commentary.. 173

18. The Educator Counselor: Responsibilities in a Service Society...... 177
Julian M. Nadolsky

19. Student Recruitment Issues in the 1980s........................ 183
*John D. Rasch, David K. Hollingsworth, John P. Saxon,
and Kenneth R. Thomas*

20. The Rehabilitation Counselor: A Student of Life 187
   William G. Emener
21. The Protestant Work Ethic, Disability, and the Rehabilitation
   Student.. 193
   Kenneth R. Thomas, Sue A. Carter, and Jean O. Britton
22. Rehabilitation Counselor Education Trainee Selection Factors
   and Subsequent Occupational Outcomes 199
   Joseph T. Kunce, Richard W. Thoreson, and Randall M. Parker
23. Job Satisfaction Predictors of Rehabilitation Counseling
   Graduates 205
   Dwight R. Kauppi, Mary Ballou, Marceline E. Jaques,
   John J. Gualtieri, and Craig R. Blum
Selected Abstracts.. 211
References and Suggested Additional Readings for Part IV.............. 214

PART V. INSERVICE TRAINING AND CONTINUING EDUCATION ... 217

Introduction Commentary.. 219
24. Educational and Training Needs of Rehabilitation Counselors:
   Implications for Training..................................... 223
   Fred R. McFarlane and Michael Sullivan
25. Rehabilitation Counselor and Supervisor Perceptions of Counselor
   Training Needs and Continuing Education 229
   Jeanne B. Freeman
26. Client Feedback in Rehabilitation Counselor Evaluation:
   A Field-Based, Professional Development Application 237
   William G. Emener, Mary G. Mars, and Joan F. Schmidt
27. Rehabilitation Counseling in the Private Sector: A Training
   Needs Survey 251
   Ross K. Lynch and Terrence Martin
Selected Abstracts.. 258
References and Suggested Additional Readings for Part V 259

PART VI. ADMINISTRATIVE, SUPERVISORY,
AND SETTING-BASED ISSUES 263

Introduction Commentary.. 265
28. Rehabilitation Administrators and Supervisors: Their Work
   Assignments, Training Needs, and Suggestions for Preparation 271
   Ralph E. Matkin, Horace W. Sawyer, Jerome R. Lorenz,
   and Stanford E. Rubin
29. Convergence and Divergence in Rehabilitation Counseling and
   Vocational Evaluation: Implications for Rehabilitation Education ... 295
   Richard J. Baker and Jerome R. Lorenz

Page

30. Private Sector Rehabilitation: Benefits, Dangers, and
    Implications for Education 299
       Brian T. McMahon
31. Preservice Graduate Education for Private Sector
    Rehabilitation Counselors 307
       Brian T. McMahon and Ralph E. Matkin
   Selected Abstracts 315
   References and Suggested Additional Readings for Part VI 318

Author Index 323
Subject Index 331

REHABILITATION COUNSELOR
PREPARATION AND
DEVELOPMENT

PART I
HISTORICAL PERSPECTIVES

PART I. HISTORICAL PERSPECTIVES

Introduction Commentary

THE HISTORY of rehabilitation counseling reveals many important perspectives relevant to the numerous critical issues surrounding it today. For example, while the first time the term "rehabilitation counselor" appeared in formal documents was five decades ago (Finch, 1937), up until the 1950s the practice of rehabilitation counseling primarily entailed the provision of vocational guidance services to previously employed, industrial and wartime injured individuals (Hamilton, 1950; McGowan & Porter, 1967). With Public Law 565s federal support initiatives for professional preparation and research programs by the mid-1950s (Eighty-Third Congress, 1954), coupled with the simultaneous advancements of cognate human service disciplines (especially counseling psychology), rehabilitation counseling started moving toward becoming a professional human service. It is important to note, however, that to a great extent the history of rehabilitation counseling mirrors the history of rehabilitation in the United States. Interested students and professionals are encouraged to appreciate rehabilitation's historical, personal account, writings (Garrett, 1969; Lassiter, 1972; McGowan & Porter, 1967; Obermann, 1965; Rusalem, 1951) as well as rehabilitation's historian's synthesized writings (Bitter, 1979; Rubin & Roessler, 1978; Rusalem, 1976; Smits, Emener & Luck, 1981; Wright, 1980). Historical and developmental antecedents of the practice of rehabilitation counseling are available (e.g., Parker & Hansen, 1981); the history of rehabilitation counseling as it reflects the history of rehabilitation is also available (e.g., Emener, 1984). The study of works such as these is sine qua non to establishing a rich appreciation of the roots of rehabilitation counseling. There are, nonetheless, some key historical antecedents which deserve specific address in this Introduction Commentary.

Around the turn of the century, the Industrial Revolution and the resulting societal shifts from being a rural, agrarian society to an urban, industrialized society meaningfully influenced the history of rehabilitation and the delivery of rehabilitation services. Medical advancements during the 1940s and 1950s, the Technological Revolution of the 1950s, and other societal phenomena, such as

5

upswings in the economy, shocked the field of rehabilitation counseling with a burgeoning manpower development concern (Hosie, 1979; Hylbert & Kelz, 1970; McGowan & Porter, 1967; Wright, 1980). By the 1960s, professional literature was replete with statements such as: "Today we are so pressed from all sides to produce large numbers of practitoners of all services relating to health, education, and welfare, that one is probably quite safe in assuming the difference between the professional cream and the professional skim milk is rapidly becoming minute" (Seidenfeld, 1962, p. 11). Training and education programs were at full throttle to meet manpower development needs. Pivotal to the provision of rehabilitation services is the rehabilitation counselor, and rehabilitation services programs were in dire need for trained, educated, competent rehabilitation counselors. Concerns regarding the need for standardization of training and education programs for rehabilitation counselors abounded (Hamilton, 1950; National Rehabilitation Association, 1951; Ninth Annual Workshop on Guidance, Training and Placement, 1956; Olshansky, 1967; Patterson, 1969). Fittingly, Seidenfeld (1962) captured this standardization issue: "Of one thing we may be sure: the variations in training are still far too great for any proper identification with a profession" (p. 12). The operationalized concern of individual professionals, professional associations, and state-federal vocational rehabilitation programs, nonetheless, eventually did establish standards for the professional preparation of rehabilitation counselors (see American Rehabilitation Counseling Association, 1978; Council on Rehabilitation Education, 1978; Hansen, 1971).

When Seidenfeld (1962) stated, "Any profession truly worthy of the name is more likely to be known by what its practitioners do than by what they say" (p. 11), he addressed an exceptionally critical issue in the preparation and development of professional rehabilitation counselors. Inspection and study of empirical evidence regarding what rehabilitation counselors do (viz., their roles and functions) from a historical perspective reveals continuous *change* (Berven, 1979; Emener & Rubin, 1980; Fraser & Clowers, 1978; Muthard & Salomone, 1969; Parham & Harris, 1978; Rubin & Emener, 1979). In spite of many changes in society, in the field of rehabilitation, and in the practice of rehabilitation counseling (see Smits, Emener & Luck, 1981), there has always been a genuine focus on the preparation and development of rehabilitation counseling *as a profession* — during the earlier years (Salomone, 1972; Seidenfeld, 1962) and during more recent times (Brubaker, 1977, 1981; Emener, 1981; Hershenson, 1982; Lynch & McSweeney, 1981; Parker & Thomas, 1981). Thus, while history bears witness to understandable, constant and spiralling *change* affecting the practice of rehabilitation counseling, there has always existed an authentic concern for standardization and professionalism in the preparation and development of the rehabilitation counselor.

Pre-service preparation of the rehabilitation counselor is predominately at the master's degree level. Nonetheless, the development of bachelor's and doctoral programs are meaningfully related to rehabilitation counselor education and therefore deserve consideration. The history of rehabilitation education would be glaringly incomplete without appreciation of the landmark work of Ken Hylbert (1963) and the first undergraduate curriculum he established at The Pennsylvania State University. His initiative was predominately designed to meet "a lack of professional manpower" (p. 23) in state vocational rehabilitation agencies. Curriculum refinements of growing numbers of undergraduate rehabilitation education programs have continued (see Culberson, Alcorn & Daniels, 1982; Feinberg, Sunblad & Glick, 1974; Redkey, 1971), and employers' perceptions of their graduates and employment trends of their graduates also have been studied (Culberson, 1979; Gandy, 1983; Geist & McMahon, 1981; Witten, 1980). Doctoral programs in rehabilitation emerged over forty years ago. Maki, Berven and Allen's (1985) study of thirty-eight current doctoral programs found that "According to the data collected at least 919 doctoral degrees have been awarded since New York University's first graduate in 1944" (p. 148), and "Graduates find positions in rehabilitation education, research, training, administration, and direct service" (p. 154). Thus, while bachelor's and doctoral programs are clearly relevant to the preparation and development of rehabilitation counselors, "The master's degree is generally considered the terminal degree for the professional practice of rehabilitation counseling" (Maki, Berven & Allen, 1985, p. 146). Energized by the PL 565 federal initiative in 1954, by 1955 twenty-six master's degree programs were either established or under development (Wright, 1980), and today there are more than seventy-five master's degree programs in existence (Council on Rehabilitation Education, 1983).

The preparation of rehabilitation counselors at the master's degree level encompasses a major thrust of this book. The role of federal funding, from a historical perspective, has been pivotal and extensively compelling. The funding and programmatic influences of the federal government in the 1950s (Eighty-Third Congress, 1954; Hall & Warren, 1956), and the resulting negative effects of recent funding reductions and shifting programmatic emphases of federal funding, cannot be ignored (Arnold, 1982; Emener, Lauth, Renick & Smits, 1985; Graves, 1979). These latter funding and programmatic influences have been documented (see Jaques, Kauppi, Steger & Lafaro, 1979; Parker & Hansen, 1981), and Emener, Lauth, Renick and Smits (1985, p. 11) recently and alarmingly stated:

> Rehabilitation counseling's development as an autonomous profession will be an arduous one as a result of the deep-rooted "shaping" on behalf of the state-federal program over the past three decades. Now that these shaping contingencies are being cut, reduced, and/or changed, the continued emergence of rehabilitation counseling's symbols of professionalism are in

jeopardy — research and development, active professional associations, self-policing, professional culture, social sanctions and exclusive practice domains, and public recognition, among others.

Thus, the influence of funding cannot be underestimated.

A recurring question regarding the preparation of rehabilitation counselors has been, "Why a master's degree?" From a historical perspective, the influences of cognate human services developments (e.g., counseling psychology — see Division of Counseling Psychology, 1963; social work — see Geist & Emener, 1981), documented manpower development needs issues, and preferred personal (e.g., maturity), as well as professional (e.g., competencies) attributes of the rehabilitation counselor, have loomed large in the response to this question. For example, work-study programs were developed to prepare and enhance the employed rehabilitation counselor (who already had a bachelor's degree) through cooperative programming efforts between state-federal vocational rehabilitation programs and colleges and universities (consult Porter & Settles, 1967; Wright, 1980). Pankowski and Pankowski (1974) articulated the multidimensional responses to the question, "Why a master's degree?", and the reader is urged to carefully study their considerations (see Chapter 1).

In conclusion, the preparation and development of the professional rehabilitation counselor circa 1985 entails numerous considerations and issues which have not emerged in a vacuum. Appreciating current state-of-the-art perspectives is pivotal to the purpose and thrust of this book.* Full appreciation and rich understanding of such perspectives, however, become much more meaningful if they are viewed with deep awareness of the historical antecedents which directed, guided, and tempered them.

W. G. Emener

---

*See Emener (1984) for detailed discourse on relevant developmental antecedents and current issues.

CHAPTER 1

WHY A MASTER'S DEGREE IN REHABILITATION COUNSELING?

MARY L. PANKOWSKI AND JOSEPH M. PANKOWSKI

Abstract

In the last year or so state rehabilitation agencies have been under attack by various administrative branches of state government relative to the specified need for a master's degree requirement for job applicants. This article explores the potential implications of the removal of the requirement for the advanced degree, how it will affect the delivery of rehabilitation services and argues in favor of retaining it.

THE QUESTION of whether or not it is advisable for counselor applicants to have a master's degree has been discussed off and on for several years. In some cases administrative departments in state government have said that the requirement for the advanced degree should be eliminated for it is a specific requirement that is "not absolutely necessary for satisfactory performance of the job."

The key word in the last phrase appears to be "satisfactory." The word implies marginal acceptability and that good or even excellent performance is not necessary or worth striving for in working with handicapped people. Mediocre performance appears acceptable.

Furthermore there is advanced the argument that this satisfactory level could be achieved by employees possessing several years work experience in vocational rehabilitation, counseling, guidance, psychology or a related field. This implies that on-the-job experience can substitute for graduate coursework and study.

Reprinted by permission from Volume 5 (1974), *Journal of Applied Rehabilitation Counseling*, pp. 147-152.

Implicit in this argument is the supposition that by watching and working with handicapped people over a period of years a counselor will be able to understand motivation and based upon this understanding will be able to work effectively with the clients in his caseload to lead them through the rehabilitation process. It supposes that:

By placing disabled persons the counselor will learn proper placement techniques. That by doing he will learn extended evaluation, medical evaluation, educational evaluation, economic evaluation and vocational evaluation.

After working with a few clients he will learn which services are needed and the sequence in which the services should be provided. He will learn which services are not needed.

After a few trial and error measures he will learn to anticipate costs (using the agency's fee schedule) and will learn when and if amendments of a rehabilitation plan are needed.

He will pick up ideas on how to arrange physical restoration services, will know when the client needs counseling and will know what kind of training (college, junior college, business school, trade school, rehabilitation facility, on-the-job, correspondence, tutorial, personal adjustment, etc.) is indicated. He will learn the importance of involving the client's family in the selection of a vocational goal and school. He will learn when training is not indicated.

When faced with unusual problems he will know when and where to get reader services, interpreter services, etc. and will eventually acquire the necessary knowledge of the world of work (licenses, tools, etc.). He will eventually learn about wage and hour rules and regulations. He will learn about statewide contracts and prior approval regulations.

Somewhere during his first few years of employment he will broaden his knowledge of medical and psychological aspects and will learn how to not overlook secondary and hidden disabilities. After working with a few clients he will not stumble through the easier medical terms and will be able to understand at least a part of the medical information presented to him.

He will learn the technique of walking through the community he serves in order to gain an understanding of its jobs, industries, people and organizations.

By practicing on a few clients he will learn how to jointly formulate a rehabilitation plan with client participation based upon sound rehabilitation principles. He will learn which handicaps can be lessened or removed and which resources can be used.

He will begin to learn the differences between physical therapy, occupational therapy, etc. as well as will begin to become familiar with lower extremity prosthetics and orthotics vs. upper extremity prosthetics and orthotics. He will learn about walking braces, wheelchairs, transfer boards, ramps, whirlpool baths, catheters and lifts.

It may be awhile before he knows the difference between an optometrist and ophthalmologist but he will soon learn the difference between a psychiatrist and a urologist. His first meeting with the district medical consultant will be traumatic but perhaps after a few years he will learn the rationale for medical consultation and the role of the consultant.

He will become competent to handle the typical medical problems he will face as well as the one or two very unusual cases in his caseload for the rest of his life. At coffee break he will hear about the theories of counseling and will soon pick an eclectic approach for he will hear that approach is "sound," especially when one has not studied counseling theories and does not understand them. He will hear names of people like Rogers, Patterson and Thomason and may even read about Olshansky in one of his rehabilitation journals but may never understand who they are and what they can offer him in his everyday encounter with clients.

Over the years he will pick up approaches on how to handle a client who is reluctant to admit need for help, what to do when the client disagrees with everything that is presented, what to do with the client who agrees with everything that is presented, what to do with the client who breaks down and cries. He will soon decide to structure the interview to establish rapport and will begin to refrain from making snap judgments.

After awhile he will learn of the special needs the spinal cord injured have in the course of their rehabilitation. Over the years he may pick up the skills of observing, listening, questioning, informing, guiding, recording, analyzing and synthesizing.

He will know what is confidential and when he can release it. He will know how to handle occupational information with clients along with reinforcement therapy techniques.

He will not panic facing the special problems in rehabilitation before his first lunch break and which will later include schizophrenia, paranoia and neurosis. He will see heredity, acquired and birth trauma mental retardation along with the bewildered parents who come to him as their last hope. He will think about them that same evening and wonder why he even went into rehabilitation.

He will learn to use comprehensive rehabilitation facilities and centers with the wealth of admission procedures, general requirements and center regulations and services. Eventually he will learn those who specialize in vocational vs. evaluative services; which are therapeutic vs. educational and which offer work adjustment vs. personal adjustment services. He will learn the meaning of teamwork and consultation. As a member of the team he will know what is meant by pre-vocational evaluation, work tolerance, job training, job try-out, interim employment, terminal or sheltered employment, transitional employment, etc. He will learn to decide when to use extended evaluation in workshops and facilities and will begin to understand what constitutes a good psychological report, which tests are valid and reliable, how to interpret psychological examinations and test scores and how to follow recommendations made.

Eventually the new counselor will realize that he is not alone in his work and that, to rehabilitate any individual, he will need to call upon the resources of his community. He will develop the necessary skills to work with other professionals in the employment services, the public health offices, social security offices, voluntary associations, professional associations, workshops, etc.

He will learn how to work with the physicians and small hospitals in rural communities as well as the vast medical centers in the large cities. He will recognize their needs and will satisfy them to help his clients.

He will become knowledgeable of the school system, the dropout problems, the slow learners, the retarded, the maladjusted mean kids, etc.

He will be ready when his supervisor calls upon him to do his part in public relations and he will make the speeches to civic clubs, will learn to get the rehabilitation message out via the broadcasting facilities in his area and will learn how to get good press coverage.

He will soon learn the benefits of proper involvement of the client's family and how the social worker and his skills should be used. The similarities and differences of the two professions will evolve over the years and he will eventually begin to foster communication and cooperation to engender teamwork for the client's benefit.

As time progresses the new rehabilitation counselor will come to understand the complexities of the social security system and its relationships with the DVR agency. The process of disability claims will become apparent. Perhaps it will not take too long for him to understand the evaluation system and the current evaluation issues in determination. He will come to learn how to work with the specialized problems inherent in the client whose determination has not been reached and how to work with him once the determination is known.

He will learn all about workmen's compensation, will receive court subpoenas for appearance with his client's file, will testify for and perhaps against his client and will wonder often if he will ever completely understand this particular rehabilitation system.

When faced with a low achieving deaf person who cannot read or write he will realize the value of manual communication skills and will learn them.

He will soon realize that every other agency in his country will refer him clients who they have trouble with and who could "certainly straighten out if they had rehabilitation."

He will come to learn much more than has been presented in this short discussion of what awaits the new counselor.

So what does this have to do with the question of whether or not a person needs a master's degree? A review of the content of the rehabilitation related coursework required in the master's degree programs reveals that most, if not all, of the areas covered will be used by the new rehabilitation counselor within the first year of his practice dependent upon the assignment given him. Unfortunately not even the master's degree programs can fully prepare the individual to work within all assignments and should he specialize with a certain field (for example mental health) it will be necessary for that individual to take part in a very comprehensive in-service training program sponsored by the rehabilitation agency.

Rehabilitation agencies could not have made the progress they have achieved over the years without the trained counselors provided by the master's degree programs. Often the case is made that the agency could be responsible for training its staff once they are on board. If we take the necessary time to examine the multitude of skills necessary for satisfactory performance it is apparent that no agency staff development program could be expected to duplicate the knowledge provided by a two year graduate program. There just is not the time unless they are willing to release all new staff counselors for the period that would be required to impart this knowledge base.

Therefore if rehabilitation agencies are to remove the need for a master's degree it appears that they will have only one of two choices:

1. The agency will need to provide the necessary training in order to impart the skills and knowledge necessary to serve disabled citizens effectively, or
2. The agency is willing to offer third rate services to these same disabled individuals.

The second alternative is entirely unacceptable and rehabilitation programs are therefore faced with the first. This will not only be most time consuming but very expensive. Right now the master's degree job applicant has a firm base of knowledge and understanding upon which agencies can build in their own agency staff development program. He may not be a completely polished stone but he is far from an uncut one. He has demonstrated competence via the internship route and has committed himself to the field. His investment has been made and there is a fairly good chance that he will be able to handle a full caseload from the moment he is employed. He is ready to work.

It is inconceivable to believe that the ABC accounting firm would be willing to hire a college graduate in business who did not have strong coursework in accounting. They would not feel it is the responsibility of their firm to provide the necessary inservice training to teach these skills. Hart, Hart and Smith, a local law firm, would never hire an individual without a law degree and plan to teach him law. The point is that employers want, and should expect, to get trained people. If that training is only offered in an advanced degree program the employer should require that training. This is the case in rehabilitation. If a bachelor's degree program was available that would provide this same type and degree of training there would be no reservation whatsoever for requiring that degree. There are no undergraduate programs available that offer this and until there are rehabilitation agencies should have no reservation whatsoever for requiring the type and degree of training necessary to serve the people they are legally charged to serve. To do less is not only irresponsible but immoral.

Selected Abstracts

Bachelor of Rehabilitation
K.W. Hylbert (1963)

This article describes the new, experimental undergraduate rehabilitation curriculum at The Pennsylvania State University. Specific course work and its rationale are offered along with an articulation of important considerations of this bachelor's degree program.

A Bachelor's in Rehabilitation — Revisited
K.W. Hylbert and J.W. Kelz (1972)

The Pennsylvania State University bachelor's degree program in rehabilitation is conceptually evaluated in its tenth year of existence. Course content, recruitment of students, advising, graduates' employment, and program impact are presented along with continuing developments and aspirations.

Undergraduate Curriculum: A Success
H. Redkey (1971)

Following discussion of a manpower development initiative behind the rehabilitation education movement, this article describes the B.S. degree program at Stout State University. The forty semester credit program is discussed along with indications of general work areas for which students are prepared.

The Need-Oriented Profession of Rehabilitation Counseling
M.A. Seidenfeld (1962)

The need for professionally trained rehabilitation counselors is discussed with foci on determinants of successful counseling. Critical aspects of rehabilitation counselor training are presented; specific services offered by the professional rehabilitation counselor are articulated with a concluding comment regarding ethics.

Preparing Counselors to Meet the Needs of the Handicapped
T.W. Hosie (1979, p. 271)

The Education for All Handicapped Children Act (PL 94-142) mandates a number of counseling and allied services for the handicapped and their parents. In many cases counselors will need to acquire additional information and training to meet the needs of this special population. This article outlines many competencies that need to be considered in developing pre-service and in-service programs for counselors serving the handicapped. Hosie discusses several professional development areas relating to these competencies, and provides resources and training materials.

*The Impact of Government Retrenchment on Professionalism: The Cases
of Rehabilitation Counseling and Social Work*

W.G. Emener, T.P. Lauth, J.C. Renick, and S.J. Smits (1985, p. 1)

There is a dramatic change occurring in the federal government's role in the
provision of human services. Under the Reagan Administration's version of
federalism, a greater responsibility for human services is shifting to the
states. Using Rehabilitation Counseling and Social Work as examples, the
authors examine the question, "What happens to human service professions
if the federal government suddenly reduces its reliance upon their services
and substanially withdraws its support for their growth and development?"
The examination concludes that the quality of these professions is likely to
diminish and that their numbers will be less inclined toward a public service
ethic and more concerned with job security and survival.

Doctoral Study in Rehabilitation Counseling: Current Status

D.R. Maki, N.L. Berven, and H.A. Allen (1985, p. 146)

The purpose of this study was to identify and describe all doctoral programs
in rehabilitation counseling. Information is presented describing the thirty-
eight identified programs, faculty curriculum admission policies, and employment of graduates. A discussion of the information compiled concludes
this report.

References and Suggested Additional Readings for Part I

American Rehabilitation Counseling Association (1978). A statement of policy on the professional preparation of rehabilitation counselors. In B. Bolton & M.E. Jaques (Eds.), *Rehabilitation counseling: Theory and practice.* Baltimore: University Park Press.

Arnold, C.K. (Spring, 1982). The federal role in funding education. *Change, 39-34,* 54.

Berven, N.L. (1979). The roles and functions of the rehabilitation counselor revisited. *Rehabilitation Counseling Bulletin, 23,* 84-88.

Bitter, J.A. (1979). *Introduction to rehabilitation.* St. Louis: C.V. Mosby.

Brubaker, D.R. (1977). Professionalization and rehabilitation counseling. *Journal of Applied Rehabilitation Counseling, 8*(4), 208-217.

Brubaker, D.R. (1981). Identify and organizational problems in professional rehabilitation. *Journal of Rehabilitation, 47*(1), 54-58.

Council on Rehabilitation Education, Inc. (1983). *Recognized master's degree programs in rehabilitation counselor education.* Chicago: Author.

Culberson, J.O. (1979). Undergraduate education for rehabilitation: Agency perceptions of training and characteristics preferred of job applicants. *Journal of Rehabilitation, 45*(2), 39-43, 88.

Culberson, J.O., Alcorn, J.D., & Daniels, J.L. (1982). Making undergraduate rehabilitation education relevant: A cooperative project. *Rehabilitation Counseling Bulletin, 25*(4), 228-230.

Division of Counseling Psychology (1963). *The role of psychology in the preparation of rehabilitation counselors.* Washington, D.C.: American Psychological Association.

Eighty-Third Congress (1954). S. 2759. *Amendments to the Vocational Rehabilitation Act, Public Law 565.* Washington, D.C.: U.S. Government Printing Office.

Emener, W.G. (1981). A consolidation of professional rehabilitation counseling: Reality, reluctance, and (re-)action. *Journal of Applied Rehabilitation Counseling, 12*(2), 93-94.

Emener, W.G. (1984). Rehabilitation counselor education: A state of the art perspective. In E. Pan, T.E. Backer, & C.L. Vash. *1984 annual review of rehabilitation.* New York: Springer, (in press).

Emener, W.G., & Rubin, S.E. (1980). Rehabilitation counselor roles and functions and sources of role strain. *Journal of Applied Rehabilitation Counseling, 11*(2), 57-69.

Emener, W.G., Lauth, T.P., Renick, J.C., & Smits, S.J. (in press). Impact of government retrenchment on professionalism: The cases of rehabilitation counseling and social work. *Journal of Rehabilitation Administration.*

Feinberg, L.B., Sunblad, L.M., & Glick, L.J. (1974). *Education for the rehabilitation services: Planning undergraduate curricula.* Syracuse, N.Y.: Syracuse University, School of Education.

Finch, F.H. (1937). Qualifications for rehabilitation counselors. *Occupations, 36,* 382-387.

Fraser, R.T., & Clowers, M.R. (1978). Rehabilitation counselor functions: Perceptions of time spent and complexity. *Journal of Applied Rehabilitation Counseling, 9*(2), 31-35.

Gandy, G.L. (1983). Graduates of an undergraduate rehabilitation curriculum. *Rehabilitation Counseling Bulletin, 26*(5), 357-359.

Garrett, J.F. (1969). Historical background. In D. Malikin & H. Rusalem (Eds.), *Vocational rehabilitation of the disabled.* New York: New York University Press.

Geist, G.O., & Emener, W.G. (1981). Rehabilitation counseling and rehabilitation counselor education: Implications for social work and social work education. In Browne, J.A., Kivlin, B.A., & Watt, S. *Rehabilitation services and the social work role: Challenge for change.* Baltimore: Williams & Wilkins.

Geist, G.O., & McMahon, B.T. (1981). Pre-service rehabilitation education: Where graduates are employed. *Journal of Rehabilitation, 47*(3), 45-47.

Graves, W. (1979). The impact of federal legislation for handicapped people on the rehabilitation counselor. *Journal of Applied Rehabilitation Counseling, 10*(2), 67-71.

Hall, J.H., & Warren, S.L. (Eds.) (1956). *Rehabilitation counselor preparation.* Washington, D.C.: National Rehabilitation Association and National Vocational Guidance Association.

Hamilton, K. (1950). *Counseling the handicapped in the rehabilitation process.* New York: Ronald Press.

Hansen, C.E. (1971). The rehabilitation counselor training and employment. *Journal of Rehabilitation, 37*(3), 39-42.

Hershenson, D.B. (1982). Rehabilitation counseling is a profession. *Rehabilitation Counseling Bulletin, 25*(4), 251-253.

Hosie, T.W. (1979). Preparing counselors to meet the needs of the handicapped. *Personnel and Guidance Journal, 58*(4), 271-275.

Hylbert, K.W. (1963). Bachelor of rehabilitation: Experiment at Penn State. *Journal of Rehabilitation, 29*(2), 23-24.

Hylbert, K.W., & Kelz, J.K. (1972). A bachelor's in rehabilitation—revisited. *Journal of Applied Rehabilitation Counseling, 3*(2), 44-52.

Hylbert, K.W., & Kelz, J.W. (1970). Combating rehabilitation counselor shortages in the public agencies. *Journal of Applied Rehabilitation Counseling, 1*(2), 13-26.

Jaques, M.E. (1959). *Critical counseling behavior in rehabilitation settings.* Iowa City: State University of Iowa.

Jaques, M.E., Kauppi, D.R., Steger, J.M., & Lafaro, G.A. (1979). The education and training of rehabilitation counselors. In J. Hamburg (Ed.), *Review of allied health education: 3.* Lexington: The University Press of Kentucky.

Lassiter, R.A. (1972). History of the rehabilitation movement in America. In J.G. Cull & R.E. Hardy (Eds.), *Vocational rehabilitation: Profession and process.* Springfield, Illinois: Charles C Thomas.

Lynch, R.K., & McSweeney, K. (1981). The professional status of rehabilitation counseling in the state/federal vocational rehabilitation agencies. *Journal of Applied Rehabilitation Counseling, 12*(4), 186-190.

Maki, D.R., Berven, N.L., & Allen, H.A. (1985). Doctoral study in rehabilitation counseling. *Rehabilitation Counseling Bulletin, 28*(3), 146-154.

McGowan, J.F., & Porter, T.L. (1967). *An introduction to the vocational rehabilitation process.* Washington, D.C.: Department of Health, Education, and Welfare, Vocational Rehabilitation Administration.

Muthard, J.E., & Salomone, P.R. (1969). The roles and functions of the rehabilitation counselor. *Rehabilitation Counseling Bulletin, 13*(1-SP), 81-168.

National Rehabilitation Association, Committee on Training (1951). Personnel standards and training. *Journal of Rehabilitation, 17*(3), 26.

Ninth Annual Workshop on Guidance, Training and Placement (1956). *Utilization of counselor's services in state VR agencies.* Report of Proceedings. Washington, D.C.: Office of Vocational Rehabilitation, United States Department of Health, Education and Welfare.

Obermann, C.E. (1965). *A History of vocational rehabilitation in America.* Minneapolis: The Dennison Company.

Olshansky, S. (1967). An evaluation of rehabilitation counselor training. *Vocational Guidance Quarterly, 5,* 164-167.

Pankowski, M.L., & Pankowski, J.M. (1974). Why a master's degree in rehabilitation counseling? *Journal of Applied Rehabilitation Counseling, 5*(3), 147-152.

Parham, J.D., & Harris, W.M. (1978). *State agency rehabilitation counselor functions and the mentally retarded.* Lubbock, Texas: Texas Tech University, Resource and Training Center in Mental Retardation.

Parker, R.M. & Hansen, C.E. (1981). *Rehabilitation counseling.* Boston: Allyn and Bacon, Inc.

Parker, R.M., & Thomas, K.R. (1981). Rehabilitation at the crossroads: Is professional rehabilitation experiencing growth pains or death throes? *Journal of Applied Rehabilitation Counseling, 12*(2), 85-86.

Patterson, C.H. (1969). *Rehabilitation counseling: Collected papers.* Champaign, IL: Stipes Publishing Co.

Porter, T.L., & Settles, R.B. (1968). *Post-entry training programs for rehabilitation counselors.* Preliminary Report of Workshop Proceedings, Atlanta, April 24-26.

Redkey, H. (1971). Undergraduate curriculum: A success. *Journal of Rehabilitation, 37*(6), 15-17.

Rubin, S.E., & Emener, W.G. (1979). Recent rehabilitation counselor role changes and role strain: A pilot investigation. *Journal of Applied Rehabilitation Counseling, 10*(3), 142-147.

Rubin, S.E., & Roessler, R.T. (1978). *Foundations of the vocational rehabilitation process.* Baltimore: University Park Press.

Rusalem, H. (1951). *An analysis of the functions of state vocational rehabilitation counselors for the development of a training course at teachers college.* Doctoral dissertation, Teachers College, Columbia University.

Rusalem, H. (1976). A personalized recent history of vocational rehabilitation in America. In H. Rusalem & D. Malikin (Eds.), *Contemporary vocational rehabilitation.* New York: New York University Press.

Salomone, P.R. (1972). Professionalism and unionism in rehabilitation counseling. *Rehabilitation Counseling Bulletin, 15* 137-146.

Seidenfeld, M.A. (1962). The need-oriented profession of rehabilitation counseling. *Journal of Rehabilitation, 18*(4), 11-13.

Smits, S.J., Emener, W.G., & Luck, R.S. (1981). Prologue to the present. In W.G.

Emener, R.S. Luck, & S.J. Smits, (Eds.), *Rehabilitation administration and supervision*. Baltimore: University Park Press.

Whitehouse, F.A. (1969). Professional concepts. In D. Malikin and H. Rusalem (Eds.), *Vocational rehabilitation of the disabled: An overview*. New York: New York University Press.

Witten, B.J. (1980). *Preparation and utilization of undergraduate workers in rehabilitation: Comparative perceptions of respondents*. Unpublished doctoral dissertation, Syracuse University.

Wright, G.N. (1980). *Total Rehabilitation*. Boston: Little, Brown, and Company.

PART II

DEVELOPMENTAL ISSUES
IN REHABILITATION
COUNSELOR EDUCATION

PART II. DEVELOPMENTAL ISSUES IN REHABILITATION COUNSELOR EDUCATION

Introduction Commentary

REHABILIATION COUNSELOR education, since its inception, has continuously attended to numerous issues relevant to its mission(s). Such issues have been and still are representative of the continuous, spiralling rate of change in society and the field of rehabilitation; moreover, such issues are developmental in nature. For example, earlier rehabilitation counselor education programs were predominately public sector oriented (viz., they operationalized their manpower development mission in coordination with the state-federal vocational rehabilitation program) (McGowan & Porter, 1967; Mosher, 1978; Rubin & Roessler, 1978). In the past few years, however, the field has had to be responsive to manpower development needs within the private sector (Matkin, 1980; McMahon, 1979; McMahon & Matkin, 1983). Other developmental issues, considered critical to the field, include: (a) the impact of certification (Livingston, 1979; Wright & Reagles, 1973) and accreditation (Council on Rehabilitation Education, 1978; McMahon, Geist, Geist & Berry, 1981); (b) the ostensible uniqueness of the rehabilitation counselor (McFarland & Diapola, 1979); (c) the view of the rehabilitation counselor as a counselor or a coordinator (Patterson, 1957); (d) the relevance of the work setting in which the rehabilitation counselor works (Feinberg & McFarland, 1979; Sussman & Haug, 1967); and (e) the issue of the rehabilitation counselor as a generalist versus a specialist (Patterson, 1965, 1967; Thomas, 1982). Appropriately responding to developmental issues such as these, while not sacrificing or losing the fundamentals of rehabilitation counselor preparation, has been in and of itself a key issue for the field. For example, Scalia and Wolfe (1984), in Chapter 2, address the need for specialization within rehabilitation counselor education (in this case in response to the influence of mainstreaming), and yet maintaining the basic, necessary ingredients of an "accredited" rehabilitation counselor education program. Their discussion of the nature and limitations of preservice rehabilitation counselor education (and continuing education) are extremely relevant.

23

From the earlier influences of cognate educational disciplines such as social work education (Geist & Emener, 1981), counselor education (Lofaro, 1982) and counseling psychology education (Division of Counseling Psychology, 1963) to the current influences of special education trends (Scalia & Wolfe, 1984), rehabilitation counselor education has witnessed continued development of alternative "models of rehabilitation counselor education." For example, numerous "models" have been offered over the past decade and a half, such as: (a) *the experiential model* (Holbert & Miller, 1970); (b) *the reality-based model* (Thomason & Saxon, 1973); (c) *the behavioral model* (see Chapter 3, Diamonti & Murphy's, 1977a "Critique," and Anthony, Dell Orto, Lasky Power, Shrey & Spaniol's 1977 "Response" and Diamonti & Murphy's 1977b "Reply"); (d) *the training model* (Anthony, Dell Orto, Lasky, Marinelli, Power & Spaniol, 1977); (e) *the integrative model* (Chapter 4, Crystal, 1981); (f) *the competency-based model* (Chiko, Tolsma, Kahn & Marks, 1980); Harrison, 1980; Jones & Dayton, 1977; Porter, Rubin & Sink, 1979); (g) *the systems approach model* (Rimmer, 1981); (h) *the human resource development — continuing education model* (Bitter, 1978; Bruyere & Elliot, 1979; Stephens & Kneipp, 1981); and (i) *the service delivery model* (Clowers & Belcher, 1978). The extent to which these are nine models or simply approaches is yet another interesting issue. In Chapter 5, however, Emener and McFarland (1985) suggest a "Futuristic Model" and conclude with what could be a very important aspect of any model of rehabilitation counselor education:

> The rehabilitationist in the present and in the future is and should be required to utilize a multiplicity of skills, knowledges and attitudes which historically were nonexistent. The current rehabilitation education curriculum ultimately needs to develop a future-responsive model by modifying courses, changing curriculum, and offering an integrated approach which provides students in rehabilitation a continuum of learning in an effective, efficient, and stimulating manner.

While Emener and McFarland were addressing the generic field of rehabilitation, their observations would appear equally relevant to rehabilitation counselor education.

The evaluation of rehabilitation counselor education programs has been an important component of rehabilitation counselor education (Dellario, 1980; Geist, Hershenson & Hafer, 1975; Olshansky, 1967). The developmental and synergistic aspect of this phenomenon was aptly stated by Dellario (1980): "The current demand for accountability in the field of rehabilitation has resulted in major efforts to evaluate the effectiveness of rehabilitation interventions. . . . These accountability pressures are no less evident in rehabilitation counselor education (RCE) programs" (p. 128). As rehabilitation counseling has struggled with finding acceptable, relevant bases for the evaluation of counselor performance (e.g., see Downes, McFarland & Alston, 1974), rehabilitation counselor education has challenged the classical barriers to meaningful program evaluation in rehabilitation (Hollingsworth & Reagles, 1980) and diligently worked hard to measure the effectiveness of rehabilitation counselor education programs even in view of their understandable variability (Wright, Reagles & Scorzelli, 1973). Evaluation of rehabilitation counselor education issues also include: (a) the utilization of advisory committees and groups (Berven, McCracker, Jellinek & Doran, 1983); (b) the use of standardized simulations (Berven & Scofield, 1980) and the measurement of learned competencies (Harrison, 1980); (c) the interrelatedness of program evaluation and program accreditation (Berven & Wright, 1978); (d) the role of systematic client feedback (Emener & Placido, 1982a, 1982b); and (e) the role of a program's graduates in its own program evaluation (Geist & McMahon, 1981). Based upon the assumption that a rehabilitation counselor education program's most critical variable is its faculty, in Chapter 6 Emener, Rasch and Spector (1983) report the findings of a national survey of rehabilitation educator's perceptions of their knowledge adequacies and training needs. The evaluation of rehabilitation counselor preparation and development programs is critical to their viability and impact. The reader, nonetheless, should carefully review these suggested writings: knowing *what* to evaluate and *how* to evaluate it are only two of the many critical issues in need of continuous address, investigation, and exploration.

Numerous contemporary issues within rehabilitation counselor education are continuing unresolved issues (e.g. consult those identified ten years ago by the Arkansas Rehabilitation Research and Training Center, 1975), and some are relative avant-garde in nature. George Wright (1982), in Chapter 7, articulates the critical, contemporary issues facing the field. For example, rehabilitation counselor educators rely on professional literature to provide the knowledge base for student learning (Emener, 1980, Emener & Koonce, 1978). The availability and accessibility of such materials therefore represents an important aspect of rehabilitation counselor education (Emener & Rasch, 1982). As observed throughout this book, the notion of change incorporates a multitude of issues relevant to rehabilitation counselor education. And in Chapter 8, Rubin and Puckett (1984) demonstrate the changing role and function of the rehabilitation counselor and state: "It may very well be that any observable changes in rehabilitation education curriculums during the 1970s demonstrate more of an attempt to become consistent with an already established RC job role than to be responsive to changes in that role." One set of issues the reader may choose to consider may be represented in the following question: "What is the role of rehabilitation counselor education with regard to 'change' in the practice of rehabilitation counseling — to respond to change, to accommodate change, or to influence change?" Be careful in your response though, because it may be relatively easy to suggest "adding on" to rehabilitation counselor education programming in the face of change; but as Pipes, Buckhalt and Merrill (1983) suggest in their discussion of the "psychology of more," bigger (or more) is not necessarily better!

One of the critical, continuing developmental issues of rehabilitation counseling that is extremely relevant to rehabilitation counselor preparation and development is aptly articulated by Thomas (1982) in Chapter 9: "Throughout the relatively brief history of rehabilitation counseling it has been debated whether counselors should be generalists, specialists, or both." Patterson (1965, 1967) discussed this issue at length and the interested reader is urged to read his earlier works in this area. The rubric, "Specialization," however, can be considered from a variety of viewpoints. For example, it could be looked at from a job task perspective: the independent living specialist (Geist, 1980; and, Roessler, 1981 in Chapter 10), the placement specialist (Hutchinson & Cogan, 1974; Smits & Emener, 1980; Usdane, 1974 in Chapter 11), and the medical/nursing oriented specialist (Hanna, Mulinax & Sadler, 1983). Second, it could be viewed from a clientele perspective such as the rehabilitation counselor who works with black clients (Townsend, 1970), Mexican Americans (Kunce & Vales, 1984), older clients (Engram, 1981), or rehabilitation constituency groups in a leadership capacity (Browning, 1982). Third, specialization could be setting-based (Feinberg & McFarlane, 1979). And fourth, specialization within a rehabilitation counselor education program could represent an educational content orientation (e.g., philosophy—Dowd & Emener, 1978; Emener & Ferrandino, 1983; sexuality—Ames & Boyle, 1980; or human rights—Atkinson, 1981).

In conclusion, it is entrusted that the reader will *not* approach this part of the book with the sense that the developmental issues included herein are all inclusive. On the contrary, those included, while in the opinion of the editor are the more critical, are merely but a few of those already acknowledged and those constantly emerging. Hopefully, the interested reader will understand and appreciate these issues; hopefully, the energetic reader will find them challenging and assist in the continuing search for reconciliation and resolution.

W.G. Emener

CHAPTER 2

REHABILITATION COUNSELOR EDUCATION

VINCENT A. SCALIA AND RICHARD R. WOLFE

Abstract

A chronology of Rehabilitation Counselor Education, including the evolution of
the basic core curriculum is provided. The authors focus upon the core curriculum and its relationship to the recognition of rehabilitation counseling as a profession. Rehabilitation Counselor Education, treated as pre-service training, is
viewed as preparing the student for a profession, whereas the Continuing Education programs provide skills training for a specific job. These two kinds of programs are considered complementary, not competitive.

Introduction

REHABILITATION as a definable body of knowledge and practices entered the field of human services sixty-plus years ago. Early practitioners
had the general goal of returning the disabled individual to functioning as effectively as possible toward the goal of becoming self-supporting.

In the ensuing sixty years, the country's rapid technological and medical advancements made working with the disabled more complex. Not only do the
disabled populations served by vocational rehabilitation require specialized
services, but the combined effect of these advancements mandated the development of more highly trained rehabilitation counselors.

The professional rehabilitation counselor is finally coming of age. The professional rehabilitation counselor is responsible for aiding disabled individuals,
appraising their abilities and interests, understanding their needs, adjusting to
their handicaps and obtaining employment consistent with their capacities and
capabilities. "Professional" is the key word. Professional indicates the counselor

Reprinted by permission from Volume 15, 1984, *Journal of Applied Rehabilitation Counseling,* pp. 34-39.

is performing a needed function, knowledgeable and skillful, trained, ethical and involved in Continuing Education to keep abreast of the most recent advancements in service delivery. The professional counselor must possess special knowledges and skills. These knowledges and skills are acquired through specialized training and continuing education.

A complementary relationship among research, pre-service training, continuing education and service has gradually developed since rehabilitation education was authorized by Congress in 1954. The result has been an impressive network of pre-service and continuing education programs based in colleges and universities throughout the nation.

Rehabilitation Counselor Education as described in this article is limited to the pre-service education — University Degree Program — and Continuing Education — the continuing education provided through the various Regional Rehabilitation Continuing Education Programs. No attempt is made to focus upon the agency in-service training programs or the short term training programs once funded through federal resources. These areas may be mentioned as they aid in developing the Rehabilitation Counselor Education theme.

Historical Perspective

Although states had concern about trained personnel to provide services, the Rehabilitation Act of 1920 provided no federal funds to meet this need. Through the VR Amendment Act of 1943 (PL 78-113) administrators of state programs were authorized to train or pay for training of personnel. No specific federal dollars were funded for this purpose. As the rehabilitation program grew it became evident that qualified personnel were needed if the program were to reach its potential.

Through the VR Amendment Act of 1954 (PL 83-565) federal monies were made available for training. Funding included, but was not limited to, training grants for physicians, nurses, occupational therapists, physical therapists, and rehabilitation counselors. As of August 15, 1955, about a year after the 1954 Amendment was signed into law, 91 teaching institutions had arranged their curricula and had received grants to help expand their teaching programs in rehabilitation. To aid students, 104 traineeship grants were made available to institutions, aiding nearly 600 students in physical therapy, occupational therapy, rehabilitation counseling, social work, and other fields closely allied to vocational rehabilitation (Switzer, 1956).

Patterson, introducing Part III of his Readings in Rehabilitation Counseling (1960) discussed the concept of the counselor as a generalist or jack-of-all trades. His contention was that this approach leads to a training program which is broad based but one with little depth and no core.

Hahn (1954) suggested dividing skill materials into four broad areas which he labeled as *Psychology, Social Casework, Medicine,* and *Contributing Areas.* He suggested forty to fifty percent of the training in the psychology area, thirty to forty percent in social casework, as much as ten percent in medicine, and five to ten percent from the contributing area. (This contributing area included tests and measurements, occupational information, etc.)

Levine and Pence (1953) discussed the action of the Education and Research Committee of the San Francisco Chapter of the National Rehabilitation Association. The curriculum recommended covered a two academic year preparation, to be presented at the graduate level, and to terminate in a Masters Degree in Rehabilitation Counseling. This program was seen as one that could be built upon an undergraduate major in any of the social sciences fields. In this proposal, the student would have one didactic academic year and one clinical internship year — three months each in three different agencies — for the second year. Topical headings for the didactic part of the program included: rehabilitation counseling; medical survey of rehabilitation aspects in illness and injury; psychodynamics of personal, social, and occupational adjustment; communication organizations; assessment of individual differences — a survey of psychological testing — legal, financial, and administrative aspects of rehabilitation including public assistance and welfare legislation, social casework, and vocational and occupational counseling.

Cantrell (1958) researched what state rehabilitation counselors and privately employed rehabilitation counselors as well as the Veterans' Administration's rehabilitation psychologist believed to be the important knowledges and skills. In rank order, those topical areas identified included: counseling and interviewing, professional activities of the counselor, field work and supervised practice, psychological and related areas, testing, occupational information, casework, rehabilitation, social, community and related areas, research and statistics.

Patterson (1960) discussed the interdisciplinary nature of rehabilitation counselor training. In his summary he stated that the training is basically psychological and the rehabilitation counselor is fundamentally a psychological/vocational counselor working with handicapped clients.

Patterson (1969) presented "The University as a Producer of Rehabilitation Counselors" to the Joint Liaison Committee of the Council of State Directors of Vocational Rehabilitation and Rehabilitation Counselor Educators (JLC) in 1967. He stated this was essentially the same topic discussed between those two groups (directors and educators) some ten years earlier. Patterson cautioned that all suggestions for change should not be blindly accepted, that we should think twice before abandoning current practice for untried innovations. Patterson gave three principles which he felt should be understood by both the counselor educators and the employers of counselors.

    1. A first and basic principle of professional education is that such education is *directed toward preparation for a profession.*

2. A second principle is that it is *theoretically oriented*.
3. A third principle of professional education is that it is oriented toward *preparing persons not simply for the present, or for an existing profession, but for the future.*

In a statement policy, American Rehabilitation Counseling Association, August 1968 (cited in Moses, H.A., & Patterson, C.H., 1971) it is stated that the objective of graduate education is to prepare the individual for entering upon a lifelong profession, not for a specific job or position (p. 91). To be included in the curricular content, according to the policy statement, are an understanding of the philosophy, the theory, and the psychological, sociological, and economic principles that constitute the foundations of counseling; a two year course of study; curriculum elements which are shared with all counselors; curriculum elements specific to rehabilitation counseling; supervised experiences; and an internship.

The Preamble to the Ethical Standards of the American Personnel and Guidance Association (1961) (cited in Moses, H.A., & Patterson, C.H., 1971) focuses upon the marks of a profession and a professional organization. Highly emphasized in this preamble is the need for knowledge and skills and how these knowledges and skills might be gained. It is important that we as educators review our philosophical belief.

The Joint Liaison Committee (JLC) cited above was instrumental in developing some guidelines to be used in rehabilitation counselor training programs. Although these documents are now relatively old, much of what is seen in our current rehabilitation counselor education curricula can be traced to these philosophical positions. A series of pamphlets entitled Studies in Rehabilitation Counselor Training were produced and/or commissioned through the JLC. Seven publications in this series include:

No. 1   Guidelines for Supervised Clinical Practice
No. 2   Experience of State Agencies in Hiring VRA Trainees
No. 3   Agency-University Communication, Coordination and Cooperation in Rehabilitation Education
No. 4   Medical Information in the Rehabilitation Counseling Curriculum
No. 5   Communication Dissemination and Utilization of Rehabilitation Research Information
No. 6   The Rehabilitation Counselor Rating Scale
No. 7   The Utilization of Support Personnel in Rehabilitation Counseling.

As one reviews these documents the joint effort of college/university educators and state rehabilitation administrators in solving mutual problems and impacting on curriculum is evident.

CONTEMPORARY PRACTICE

Pre-Service Education

A study of the Region IX Task Force on Graduate Preparation in Rehabilitation Counseling was published in October 1973. This task force was chaired by F.R. McFarlane and the report was compiled and edited by McFarlane, Hillis, Johnson and Meadows.

The objective of the study was two fold (1) to assess and report the present functioning of graduate education in rehabilitation counseling in Region IX, and (2) to identify and develop a model and recommendations which could be used by graduate programs in rehabilitation counseling. Included in the present curriculum were principles of rehabilitation, organization of rehabilitation services, medical aspects of disabilities, psychological and social aspects of disability, psychosocial and medical aspects of disability, career and life style development, appraisal in school/agency counseling, evaluation in rehabilitation, transitional work programs in rehabilitation counseling, clinical procedures in rehabilitation counseling, counseling practicum, internship and rehabilitation counseling.

The task force developed a curriculum model. The elements of the model included: education in supervisory and administrative skills, ability to effectively use local community resources, understanding of the medical/psychological/societal aspects of all major disabilities, in-depth command of techniques of individual and group counseling. Ability to analyze past, present, future trends in the profession, ability to assess human behavior, study career development process, psychology of the work-factors influencing adjustment to specific work settings, ability to engage in program development, consultation skills.

Wrenn and Darley (1949) (cited in Patterson, 1969) discussed the movement of rehabilitation counseling towards becoming a profession. In their discussion they compared the progress of rehabilitation toward accepted criteria. The criteria of a profession, as described by Wrenn and Darley includes the following:

A. Is the performance of a socially needed function.
B. The definition of job titles and functions.
C. Existence of a body of knowledge and skills.
D. Application of standards of training.
E. The self-imposition of standards of admission to practice and of professional performance.
F. Development of a professional consciousness and professional groups.
G. Development of a Code of Ethics.
H. Legal recognition—by certification or licensing of practitioners.

The goal of rehabilitation leaders has been to establish rehabilitation as a profession. That goal has now been attained.

The Council on Rehabilitation Education, the accrediting body for masters degree programs in rehabilitation counseling has designated a required curriculum content for graduate study. The stated goal of that curriculum is "to provide for obtaining essential knowledge, skills and attitudes necessary to function effectively as a professional rehabilitation counselor" (p. 3). The curricular areas of study include: (1) history, philosophy and legislation related to rehabilitation; (2) organizational structure of the vocational rehabilitation system; (3) counseling theories, issues, and practices (individual and group); (4) case management process; (5) theories, methods and practices of career vocational development; (6) medical aspects of disability; (7) psychological aspects of disability; (8) planning client vocational rehabilitation services; (9) utilizing occupational information; (10) knowledge of community resources; (11) understanding requirement and characteristics of a variety of jobs; (12) vocational placement; (13) rehabilitation research; (14) trends, issues, legal, ethical tenets of practice; and (15) supervised clinical experience.

In a recent (undated) memorandum, the Board for Rehabilitation Certification issued guidelines for criteria for CRC eligibility effective July 1, 1985. Subjects areas which were included encompass those requirements for college/university accreditation, and also reflect the current needs of the field. These were categorized into five rehabilitation counseling job functioning areas, (1) job development and placement; (2) case management; (3) professional development and administrative planning; (4) vocational counseling and assessment; and (5) affective counseling.

In this review of the progression of rehabilitation counselor education, it is evident that the didactic material deemed critical for rehabilitation counselors has not significantly changed from the 1953 recommendations of the San Francisco Chapter of the National Rehabilitation Association. There have been significant changes in technology and in delivery systems, but the basic curricular core remains intact. This reinforces the concept that rehabilitation is a profession. Certification of rehabilitation counselor standards reflect both the body of knowledge and the current state of the art.

Through the supervision of interns and interactions with agency personnel rehabilitation programs are aware of current needs and these are incorporated into the various courses in the curriculum. The core, however, remains intact.

Rehabilitation education programs have incorporated more emphasis on vocational evaluation, job development and job placement into the curriculum. Independent living rehabilitation, private for profit rehabilitation, workers' compensation rehabilitation, legal aspects are just a few of the concerns of the practitioner that have been addressed in the curriculum. Some universities have developed complete masters degrees in special unique areas, i.e., vocational evaluation, job placement, administration, etc. Other programs have included the concepts in existing masters degree programs. Recent studies (Matkin, 1983; Rubin, Matkin, Ashley, Beardsley, May, Onstott & Puckett,

1984) consistently confirm the efficacy of the basic core curriculum. Additional research indicates that counselors, vocational evaluators and work adjustment personnel bring a common knowledge base to the rehabilitation process (McFarlane & DiPaola, 1979), and that many counselors rise quickly to administrative roles (Matkin, Sawyer, Lorenz & Rubin, 1982; Riggar & Matkin, 1984) basing their performance on their counseling education.

Curricular offerings are reviewed and modified on a regular, continuing basis, yet the long-term rehabilitation training programs (pre-service programs) cannot respond to the immediate needs and concerns of all agencies, organizations and facilities. In the past much of this attention to the mission and goals of the agency was accomplished through short-term training and/or in-service training. Rehabilitation education staff of the various rehabilitation counselor programs were called upon to aid in the delivery of the training.

Nature and Limitations of Pre-Service Education

Pre-service education is limited to preparing individuals for professional counseling activities which must be performed. Pre-service education emphasizes basic theory and general principles of practice. It is directed toward preparation for a profession, not for a specific job. There is a general perception among many educations that rehabilitation counselor training be directed specifically or wholly toward preparing counselors to work in state agencies. Traditionally, state agencies have been a large employer of rehabilitation counselors. However, they are not the only employer of rehabilitation counselors nor for many programs the largest employer of graduates. Thus the profession of rehabilitation counseling goes beyond a particular setting. The preparation, then, through pre-service education emphasizes the development of understanding and the acquisition of some general principles which will guide a rehabilitation counselor in general practice and not a given setting. Since rehabilitation counseling is practiced in many different settings it is not possible for pre-service training programs to prepare people specifically or completely for any particular setting. Pre-service education offers training in a theoretical base. Once in practice, rehabilitation counselors will have ample opportunity to learn from experience. The short time of a counselor's professional life in pre-service education may be the only opportunity to obtain a theoretical foundation for practice.

Finally pre-service is viewed as a beginning, not an end, of professional training. It is designed to orient the new counselor to the present condition and prepare the counselor for the future and change.

Continuing Education

The primary emphasis on rehabilitation training during the 1950s and 1960s was in pre-service education. The general objective of pre-service education was then, and remains today to prepare counselors for the duties and responsibilities of the profession. As a profession, rehabilitation counseling is not static but rather a rapidly changing and developing field and a truly professional rehabilitation counselor must be prepared to change. The very nature of a profession dictates that professional education must continue during a person's entire professional life. A profession, then, carries the responsibiliy for supplementing and extending the preparation obtained in the pre-service (academic) setting.

In 1974 the Regional Rehabilitation Continuing Education Programs (RRCEP's) were established by the Rehabilitation Services Administration (RSA) as primary resources for continuing education of rehabilitation personnel in public and private rehabilitation agencies and facilities. The RRCEP's were developed as a means to complement existing RSA training efforts (pre-service, short-term) with an emphasis on multi-state recurrent training needs of rehabilitation personnel at all levels. Predominately training was directed toward rehabilitation counselors. The emphasis on "multi-state recurrent training needs" differentiated this training effort from other continuing education efforts, such as the state agency in-service program and RSA's short-term training program. The four goals established for the RRCEP's by the Rehabilitation Services Administration are:

1. To deliver continuing education programming to rehabilitation personnel.
2. To provide assistance in post-employment training program development within rehabilitation agencies.
3. To coordinate continuing education resources and serve as a resource center for a variety of training materials and information data.
4. To develop continuing education instructional content for meeting identified manpower training needs.

The training provided by RRCEP's is based on a broad integrated sequence of training activities and focuses on meeting recurrent training needs common throughout a multi-state geographic area. There are eleven RRCEP's with at least one in every federal region. Each RRCEP determines, in collaboration with its advisory board, the content and manner in which the RSA objectives will be met.

The continuing education efforts provided by RRCEP are financed with federal funds through RSA. The major thrust of the continuing education efforts is directed at state vocational rehabilitation agencies and rehabilitation facilities. The general approach of the continuing education efforts is toward the specific aspects of functioning in a particular setting.

RRCEP's provide continuing education from a framework of Human Resources Development (HRD) (Nadler, 1978). The HRD model incorporates training, education and developmental activities. Training is defined as that set of activities which is geared to increasing skill in one's present job. As such, training activities are skills based and job/role centered. Education can be defined as that set of activities which is geared toward informing and enlarging the individual's repertoire responses in a given situation. Education activities are designed to enhance the responses the individual can bring to bear when faced with any issue or problem. Developmental activities can be defined as that set of learning activities which help prepare individuals for an uncertain future. They are often process centered and designed to bring about a change over long periods of time.

Pre-service education is directed at training individuals for the field of vocational rehabilitation. Continuing education is directed at training rehabilitation counselors for a specific job or position. Pre-service education is more than the inculcation of skills and techniques. It is more than imparting information and knowledge. Pre-service education aims at developing the student to think critically, analyze, synthesize and exercise judgment. Continuing education takes the counselor in the work setting and provide the means, or upgrades the ability of that person, to function effectively in his/her specific job. Pre-service education addresses identified shortages of rehabilitation personnel, while continuing education serves to upgrade knowledges and skills of current personnel.

The professionalization of rehabilitation is dependent to a large degree on the availability and maintenance of competent professionals. Rehabilitation education (pre-service) and continuing education meet all the criteria to identify rehabilitation counseling as a profession. Rehabilitation education and continuing education are the underpinnings of the profession. As the two areas become more sophisticated and grow so will the profession of rehabilitation counseling. Rehabilitation education and continuing education taken together create a synergistic product, professional rehabilitation counselors, and demonstrate that the whole is greater than the sum of its parts.

REFERENCES

American Personnel and Guidance Association, A State Policy (1968). In Moses, H.A. & Patterson, C.H. 1971. *Readings in Rehabilitation Counseling,* (2nd Ed.), Stipes Publishing Co., Champaign, IL.

American Personnel and Guidance Association, Ethical Standards (1961). In Moses, H.A. & Patterson, C.H. 1971. *Readings in Rehabilitation Counseling,* (2nd Ed.), Stipes Publishing Co., Champaign, IL.

Cantrell, D. (1958). Training the rehabilitation counselor. *Personnel and Guidance Journal,* 36, 246-248.

Criteria for CRE Eligibility effective July 1, 1985, undated memorandum, Board for Rehabilitation Certification, Chicago, IL.

Hahn, M.E. (1954). The training of rehabilitation counselors. *Journal of Counseling Psychology,* 1, 246-248.

Levine, L.S. & Pence, J.W. (1953). A training program for rehabilitation counselors. *Journal of Rehabilitation, 19*(1), 16-20.

Matkin, R.E. (1983). The roles and functions of rehabilitation specialists in the private sector. *Journal of Applied Rehabilitation Counseling, 14*(1), 14-27.

Matkin, R.E., Sawyer, H.W., Lorenz, J.R., & Rubin, S.E. (1982). Rehabilitation administrators and supervisors: Their work assignments, training needs, and suggestions for preparation. *Journal of Rehabilitation Administration, 6*(4), 170-183.

McFarlane, F.R. (October, 1973). A study of the region IX task force on graduate preparation in rehabilitation counseling. San Diego State University, San Diego, CA.

McFarlane, F.R. & Di Paola, S.M. (1979). Rehabilitation counselor, vocational evaluator and work adjustment specialist: Are these professionals different? *Journal of Applied Rehabilitation Counseling, 10*(3), 148-153.

Nadler, L. (1979). *Developing Human Resources,* Learning Concepts, Austin, Texas.

Patterson, C.H. (1960). *Readings in Rehabilitation Counseling.* Stipes Publishing Co., Champaign, IL.

Patterson, C.H. (1969). Rehabilitation counseling: Collected papers. Stipes Publishing Co., Champaign, IL.

Riggar, T.F. & Matkin, R.E. (1984). Rehabilitation counselors working as administrators: A pilot investigation. *Journal of Applied Rehabilitation Counseling, 15*(1), 9-13.

Rubin, S.E., Matkin, R.E., Ashley, J., Beardsley, M.M., May, V.R., Onstott, K. & Puckett, F.D. (1984). Roles and functions of certified rehabilitation counselors. *Rehabilitation Counseling Bulletin, 27*(4), 199-224.

Switzer, M.E. (1955). Role of the federal government in vocational rehabilitation. *Archives of Physical Medicine and Rehabilitation,* 37, 542-546.

Wrenn, C.G. & Darley, J.G. (1979). An appraisal on the professional status of personnel work. In Williamson, E.G. (Ed.). Trends in Student Personal Work. Minneapolis; University of Minnesota Press.

CHAPTER 3

BEHAVIORAL OBJECTIVES AND REHABILITATION COUNSELOR EDUCATION: A CRITIQUE

Michael C. Diamonti and Stephen T. Murphy

Abstract

Recently, there has been a heightened interest among rehabilitation educators in using behavioral objectives for the training of rehabilitation counselors. In this article, it is argued that such an approach to graduate training has glaring inadequacies as an educational strategy. It is noted that such an orientation represents a distorted view of science, promotes conceptual narrow-mindedness, undermines the meaning of evaluation and objectivity, and fosters student passivity. Alternative strategies are also discussed.

IN A RECENT issue of this journal, an investigation was reported by Anthony, Slowkowski, and Bendix (1976) that advocated the increased use of behavioral objectives for the training of rehabilitation counselors. This viewpoint reflects a growing enthusiasm by educators for competency-based, behaviorally oriented programs in rehabilitation counseling. Contrary to the views of the authors, however, this strategy holds few advantages for the profession. The proposals set forth in such an educational model distort the scientific process, foster conceptual narrow-mindedness, undermine the meaning of evaluation and objectivity, and encourage student passivity.

MISUSE OF SCIENCE

Usually, one engages in a competency-based, behaviorally oriented approach to obtain a more exact and scientific analysis. However, the view of

Reprinted by permission from Volume 21 (1977), *Rehabilitation Counseling Bulletin*, pp. 51-57.

scientific activity underpinning the use of behavioral strategies in teaching and curriculum design is based less upon an accurate view of scientific processes than it is upon an after-the-fact examination of scientific products. A distinction that is helpful here is one between the logic-in-use of a science and its reconstructed logic (Kaplan, 1964, pp. 3-11). Logic-in-use connotes what scientists actually do. This does not entail necessarily the linear progression of stating absolutely clear goals of hypothesis testing, and of verification or falsification through statistical or other analyses. The reconstructed logic of science connotes what observers, philosophers of science, and others say that the logic of scientific inquiry looks like. There has been an exceptionally long history in the social sciences of borrowing the reconstructed logic of scientific activity and expecting it to be sufficient for treating the complex problems of the times.

Unlike the unceasing quest for sureness among educators, scientific activity has *not* been characterized either by a preference for certainty, or by a slow and steady accumulation of technical data. What most members of the scientific community would label good science is a process that is constituted upon the leap of faith, an aesthetic sensitivity, a personal commitment, and of great importance, an ability to accept ambiguity and uncertainty (Polanyi, 1964). Without such qualities, which maintain the scientific enterprise as an essentially human and changing artifact, science becomes mere technology.

The view of science used to give legitimacy to the behaviorally oriented model of graduate training in rehabilitation counseling is similar to the reconstructed logic of science rather than the logic-in-use of science. In this respect, it is more reminiscent of a nineteenth century brand of positivism than it is of current scientific and philosophical discourse. Although the trend toward naive reductionism in approaching human action was stemmed in philosophy by 1930s (Urmson, 1956, p. 146), much of rehabilitation counseling's rationality today has apparently progressed no further.

This behavioral orientation has usually developed in order to guarantee certainty and to rationalize and make explicit as many aspects of people's activity as possible, be it the researcher, the instructor, or the student/counselor. This approach has been described as "technological" (Ellul, 1964) in that it seeks to use strict forms of means-ends or process-product reasoning. Such an orientation, however, seems primarily interested in efficiency, thus tending to exclude other modes of valuing. The behavioral objectives model has sought to reduce student action to specifiable forms of overt behavior, so that the rehabilitation educator can have certitude of outcome. Although the need for certainty is understandable, given the large sums of money spent on education, the perspective on behavioral objectives as facilitating a more scientific approach to graduate training can be both superficial and misleading.

CONCEPTUAL NARROW-MINDEDNESS

There is an assumption in the behavioral model of training that the atomized behavioral elements of knowledge are addictive. That is, by merely presenting elements in "bite-sized pieces," the task of mastery of higher order operations is simplified. Unfortunately, a distinction must be made between knowing the component parts of a skill and the artful performance of the skill itself. Polanyi (1964) has pointed out that "human experiences and feelings are more than the sum of their several components" (p. 94). In more commonsense terms, one may be able to successfully fulfill all the subroutines of bicycle riding—steering, pedaling, balancing correctly on a seat, etc.—yet, the coherence of all these component parts into a working "gestalt" is not guaranteed. One may, in fact, not be able to put them all together and may fail miserably at riding a bicycle. This is a very real problem when applied to the area of professional training and practice.

The behavioral objective approach to rehabilitation education also promoted conceptual narrow-mindedness by presenting a limited, and therefore simplistic, definition of the proper activities of the rehabilitation counselor. For example, in the Anthony et al. (1976) investigation it is implied that there exists universal agreement regarding the roles and functions of the rehabilitation counselor. However, even a cursory examination of the literature (Jaques, 1970; Lamb & Mackota, 1975; Malikin & Rusalem, 1976; Muthard & Salamone, 1969; Patterson, 1957; Whitehouse, 1975) reveals that the proper role of the rehabilitation counselor has been an ongoing subject of controversy for many years. It would seem that before a competency-based rehabilitation counseling curriculum may even be considered, a more universally accepted definition of what constitutes the proper roles and functions of the rehabilitation counselor must be achieved.

Since there is diversity of opinion surrounding the issue of graduate training in rehabilitation counseling, it seems important to expose students to these varied viewpoints regarding the roles and functions of the rehabilitation counselor. This should be promoted in order that students be able to examine critically the relative merits of these views. Under a behavioral model, however, course instructors are apparently encouraged to implement their philosophical and theoretical biases for the sake of more accurate measurement. This approach severely limits the latitude of student exposure and inquiry.

Using the course described by Anthony et al., as an example, it is difficult to imagine students being able to examine critically the basic assumptions of the Rogerian/Carkhuffian model of helping. This sort of inquiry is certainly a legitimate area of intellectual and professional inquiry, especially for students who are in the process of developing a framework for counseling practice in the field of rehabilitation. Inquisitive behavior is critical to student development. An approach that contributes to the minimizing of such student behavior cannot, except within the narrowest context, claim to facilitate the definition of what constitutes the specific skills and knowledge of the rehabilitation counselor.

EVALUATION AND BEHAVIORAL OBJECTIVES

Anthony et al. (1976) propose that all required courses in the rehabilitation counseling curriculum include "specific, observable goals that can be used to measure effectively whether the course changed any of the student's physical, intellectual, and emotional skills" (p. 456). They contend that such goal setting "allows objective assessment of the value of the course . . . facilitates more systematic programming . . . to ensure the achievement of these observable course goals," and aids in "the definition of what constitutes the specific skills and knowledge of the rehabilitation counselor" (p. 461).

The notion of course evaluation employed in this context is described as an "objective assessment" procedure that is designed to measure the extent to which the predesignated course goals were achieved. However, the authors expose their own lack of objectivity with regard to the selection of course content by stating that the course work was structured "to the best of the instructor's ability" (p. 458). Therefore, such an approach provides no more than a flimsy facade of objectivity. An evaluation procedure in any model of training that consists of the instructors' determining and administering the measuring instrument and controlling the flow of information between such measurement periods, hardly seems objective in any sense of that term.

The entire concept of observable goals advocated by the behavioral objective approach obscures the pernicious relationship that exists between the evaluation process and course content. There is an attempt by proponents of goal setting to claim the mutual exclusivity of evaluation and course content. Such an argument should not be allowed to minimize the danger of allowing the process of evaluation to shape the course's character and content. This danger appears to be imminent when a primary function of goal setting is viewed as facilitating "more systematic programming of the course to ensure the achievement of these observable course goals" (Anthony et al. 1976, p. 457).

Another example that illustrates the degree to which evaluation procedures may be misused by such "programming" occurs when Anthony et al. (1976) note that "where enrollment in a course is restricted, selection can be based in part on the student's pretest scores." They justify this practice by noting that numerous training studies "have found significant correlations between students' pre and posttest levels of functioning" (p. 461). Although the authors employ the qualifying phrase "in part," it is not distortion to point out that such a screening practice is so arbitrary as to border on the unethical. What these investigators seem to suggest by such a proposal is that one good method of achieving the desired course objectives is to select students who are already functioning at high levels of these objectives. Further, if the authors were not so preoccupied with the successful achievement of course goals, they might recognize the merit of selecting people with low pretest scores in order to raise student functioning to minimally effective levels.

STUDENT PASSIVITY AND SOCIALIZATION

Although the role of the student in a behavioral model of education has only been implied thus far, it seems evident that the student has been relegated to the role of passive recipient. The teacher is essentially viewed as a presenter and controller. Without getting into a long-standing debate concerning the advocacy of discovery versus other approaches, it would seem as if this view tacitly accepts as a fundamental premise that the teacher is to preselect content that is set out to be "acquired" by the students. Content seems to include not only "cognitive" knowledge, but also thought processes, skills, attitudes, propensities, dispositions, etc. This has as its basis a model of the human mind as a container. That is, knowledge is reified into things that are known before acts are engaged in. These things can then be appropriated by students, and they will demonstrate that they now have these things inside them by believing according to preestablished criteria.

This is one of the most disturbing aspects of the behavioral approach to graduate training because of the implications such a subtle socializing attempt holds for the entire concept of graduate study in rehabilitation counseling. The influence of curriculum on the process of student socialization is well documented in the literature. The manner in which students are taught and the roles assigned to them during such training are certainly important factors that affect how they perceive their eventual occupational roles. The message being provided by advocates of a behavioral approach to training seems fairly clear: passivity and uncritical thought are important ingredients for success in the agencies and facilities in which counselors will be employed. Although this message may be essentially correct, the insertion of this socializing function into the curriculum characterizes the program of graduate study as merely an instrument for maintaining the *status quo* in rehabilitation agencies and facilities. As such, the field's claim to intellectual legitimacy is all but eliminated.

ALTERNATIVE MODEL

A behavioral objectives approach to training may be useful only when it is not allowed to dominate the curriculum. Further, such an approach should be employed after students have been exposed to a broad range of diversified opinion existing within the field regarding counselor practice. Competency-based practicums, field work courses and advanced specialized courses could have merit, if such offerings functioned to implement student preferences for practice rather than to provide students with a prepackaged model which they would be required to accent. The former approach allows students the necessary latitude to more autonomously engage in professional decisionmaking.

SUMMARY

Proponents of a behavioral objectives approach to training conclude that the setting of observable course goals will be a major stimulant to the growth and development of the rehabilitation counseling field. Anthony et al. (1976) state that "the practice of rehabilitation counseling must be identified with something more than just degrees and certificates. . . . That something more may be training in a unique combination of physical, intellectual, and emotional skills that are presently duplicated by no other profession" (p. 461). Proponents of this view would have educators and students believe that these skills may best be achieved through the setting of observable goals.

Nevertheless, there are certain problematic concerns related to the setting of observable goals which appear to stifle rather than to stimulate the field's growth and development. Consequently, such an orientation fails to recognize the real issues surrounding rehabilitation counselor competencies that must be addressed before meaningful course or program goals may be initiated. Historically, the field of rehabilitation counseling has depended heavily upon the work of professionals from related disciplines for its conceptual growth and development. Rehabilitation counseling still needs the diversified input of peripheral disciplines in order to continue its intellectual growth. Thus, the quest for professional identity based upon criterion-referenced competencies at this stage in the field's development is misguided and premature. Such a quest would only serve to narrow the scope of professional focus and further distort the source of intellectual roots.

REFERENCES

Anthony, W.A.; Slowkowski, P.; & Bendix, L. Developing the specific skills and knowledge of the rehabilitation counselor. *Rehabilitation Counseling Bulletin,* 1976, *19,* 456-462.

Ellul, J. *The technological society.* New York: Random House, 1964.

Jaques, M.E. *Rehabilitation counseling: Scope and services.* Boston: Houghton-Mifflin, 1970.

Kaplan, A. *The conduct of inquiry.* San Francisco: Chandler, 1964.

Lamb, H.R., & Mackota, C. Vocational rehabilitation counseling: A second class profession? *Journal of Rehabilitation*, 1975, *41*.

Malikin, D., & Rusalem, H. *Contemporary vocational rehabilitation*. New York: New York University Press, 1976.

Muthard, J.E., & Salamone, P.R. The roles and functions of the rehabilitation counselor. *Rehabilitation Counseling Bulletin*, 1969. Special Issue, *13*.

Patterson, C.H. Counselor or coordinator? *Journal of Rehabilitation*, 1957, *23*(3), 13-15.

Polanyi, M. *Personal knowledge*. New York: Harper & Row, 1964.

Urmson, J.O. *Philosophical analysis*. London: Oxford University Press, 1956.

Whitehouse, F.A. The rehabilitation clinician: An emerging role. *Journal of Rehabilitation*, 1975, *41*.

... ...
... ...

CHAPTER 4

AN INTEGRATIVE MODEL FOR
REHABILITATION TRAINING
AND PRACTICE

RALPH M. CRYSTAL

Abstract

A model for the integration of rehabilitation counselor training and practice is proposed. The emphasis is placed on examination of training and practice variables from a systems analysis competency-based perspective. Particular consideration is placed on the inter-relationship between a core curriculum for the training of rehabilitation counselors and knowledge and skill requirements necessary for practice. The proposed model incorporates client, rehabilitation counselor, and external and internal rehabilitation environment variables. In this respect rehabilitation counselor educators and practitioners will have a model for training and practice which is responsive to clients' needs while maintaining traditional academic standards. The proposed framework can be used for the training of rehabilitation counselors to work in state agencies, as well as rehabilitation facilities, and private (profit and nonprofit) rehabilitation organizations.

THE RELATIONSHIP of rehabilitation counselor functioning to client change and outcomes is a concern of clients, families of clients, counselors, program administrators, and employers. From the ethical perspective of providing clients with the most appropriate rehabilitation services to alleviate their handicapping conditions, and from the standpoint of program accountability, it is necessary that counselor, service, and monetary resources be utilized in as effective and efficient a manner as possible. To accomplish this, an approach for integrating rehabilitation training and practice will be suggested that emphasizes a systems analysis competency-based perspective. The framework can be used for the training of rehabilitation facilities, and other rehabilitation organizations (profit and nonprofit).

Reprinted by permission from Volume 12 (1981), *Journal of Applied Rehabilitation Counseling,* pp. 191-194.

The literature related to rehabilitation counselor training focuses on two areas: (a) recommendations for a core curriculum for rehabilitation counselor education (RCE) programs (Hall & Warren, 1956; NRCA, 1962; Joint Liaison Committee, 1963; APA Division of Counseling Psychology, 1963; APGA, 1964; McGowan & Porter, 1967; ARCA, 1974; and Tripp, 1975); and (b) what rehabilitation counselors actually are doing (Muthard & Salomone, 1969; Scorzelli, 1975; and Wright & Frazer, 1975). The foci of the core curriculum approach has been to suggest general curriculum and course areas for RCE programs. The emphasis has been placed on defining the role of the rehabilitation counselor from the perspective of rehabilitation counselor education. The second approach has concentrated on knowledge and skill requirements of rehabilitation counselors from the perspective of the practitioner. This has resulted in a great amount of specificity regarding the tasks performed by rehabilitation counselors.

From the framework of rehabilitation practice, Maki, McCracken, Pope, and Scofield (1978) argue for a theoretical model of vocational rehabilitation that provides a base from which programmatic, fiscal, legislative, educational, and professional decisions can be made. An attempt to combine approaches was undertaken by Harrison and Lee (1979). These investigators reported a study in which ninety competencies for rehabilitation counselors were identified, field tested, and assigned to eleven categories. The results were used to form the competency-based Rehabilitation Counselor Education program at The University of Michigan.

The conceptual approach to be suggested views the training of rehabilitation counselor from a systems analysis, competency-based perspective. This provides a framework integrating rehabilitation counselor training with practice. Essentially a systems analysis perspective means that the rehabilitation counselor is trained to be cognizant of all variables impacting on the rehabilitation process: the client, the counselor, the rehabilitation agency and associated facilities, and the external environment—society, the family, the workplace. For each client, the counselor is aware of the interrelationships occurring among these variables and the impact and influence they have on one another. A competency-based approach is an accountability system in which individual client goals and objectives (based on client needs) are developed and clearly specified, a service plan implemented which is related to the identified goals and objectives, and a procedure available to document client gains achieved through participation in the rehabilitation process.

It is not intended that the proposed model be viewed as a replacement for the core rehabilitation counselor education curriculum. It is assumed that the components of the paradigm are already part of such programs. The proposed model can be used to bridge the gap between the way courses are taught and the way practitioners function. The components of the model transcend specific courses and a specific sequence for the delivery of rehabilitation services.

For example, the evaluation of client needs usually taught as part of one academic course and occurring primarily at the initiation of the rehabilitation process, is in fact on-going throughout the process as new circumstances arise. In addition, the needs that are identified and served through rehabilitation services have an impact on other aspects of the rehabilitation process for the client. Providing different services or using different service providers might have a different impact on the client.

The components of the paradigm are: (a) Assessment of Client Needs; (b) Development of Counseling Competencies; (c) Understanding of the Rehabilitation Process; (d) Understanding the Environment; (e) Development of Caseload Management Skills; and (f) Development of Self-monitoring and Evaluation Skills. In this model, rehabilitation counseling students would develop these components within the framework of the traditional core rehabilitation counseling curriculum including the practicum and internship experiences. A description of these areas follows.

ASSESSMENT OF CLIENT NEEDS

A major goal of the rehabilitation process is the satisfactory placement of clients in employment. To achieve this vocational objective, rehabilitation counselors may need to assist clients in other areas of functioning, including psychological, physical, social, economic, and family life. This has taken on added importance for counselors employed in the state-federal program with recent legislative emphases on giving service priority to severely handicapped individuals, providing rehabilitation services to clients who may not have a vocational objective, and providing rehabilitation services for independent living.

A counselor may possess excellent interpersonal and facilitative counseling skills, but if the counselor does not understand the needs of his/her clients and cannot differentially apply counseling skills to meet those needs, then the likelihood increases that the rehabilitation process will not succeed. Rehabilitation counselor trainees need to develop observation and listening skills which enable them to identify individual client needs related to the previously mentioned disability, demographic, social, and family factors.

The critical factor, however, is not just to determine client needs. This can be done through interviews, diagnostic, and evaluation procedures traditionally used in rehabilitation. The important element is for the rehabilitation counselor to use the assessment of needs as a framework to work with the client to develop rehabilitation goals and objectives. Client goals and objectives should be systematically related to client needs. Client rehabilitation goals and objectives are established in light of the client's abilities, the services that can be provided by the rehabilitation program, and the competencies possessed by the rehabilitation counselor.

DEVELOPMENT OF COUNSELING COMPETENCIES·

It is essential that rehabilitation counselor trainees have a thorough knowledge of, and be able to demonstrate the application of interpersonal and counseling skills in a counseling situation. It is important that students be familiar with a variety of counseling approaches. The ultimate choice of a counseling approach is dependent on the nature of the counselor's employment situation and the individual's personal characteristics. Beyond exposure to counseling approaches, there are counseling skills that need to be taught which transcend any specific counseling theory. These include the interpersonal dimensions which have been demonstrated to correlate with counseling success regardless of theoretical approach — empathy, positive regard, genuineness, and concreteness (Traux & Carkhuff, 1964, 1966).

It is important for the rehabilitation counselor to be able to know (through an understanding of the impact the disability has on a client) how to assess client needs, and through a facilitative counseling process, help the client establish goals and objectives. Through the use of the counseling relationship, the rehabilitation counselor helps the client develop a rehabilitation program which meets the client's needs. In this way, the counseling process is directly related to client needs and the established rehabilitation goals and objectives. This in turn will facilitate the identification and documentation of the relationship between rehabilitation counselor functioning and the achievement of client outcomes.

UNDERSTANDING THE REHABILITATION PROCESS

The rehabilitation process can be a barrier or a facilitator to client success. As a barrier, rehabilitation programs can encourage dependency by not allowing the client to take responsibility for his/her program and even not allowing the client the chance to fail or to learn through his/her mistakes. As a facilitator, rehabilitation programs can serve as a catalyst to the client enabling him/her to develop and test new skills and behaviors and to take responsibility for the outcome of the rehabilitation program.

The rehabilitation process is unique among counseling and human service professions in that the rehabilitation counselor can provide services to clients and can use the rehabilitation environment (rehabilitation facilities, training programs, sheltered workshops) as part of the counseling rehabilitation process. Rehabilitation counselors can use these resources to establish a program which (a) meets individual client and (b) provides an opportunity and a challenge for clients to develop their skills through the successive attainment of vocational and related objectives. In rehabilitation facilities, workshops, and vocational training programs, experiences can be established on an individual basis to meet client needs.

Counseling in rehabilitation extends beyond the counselor's office. As part of the rehabilitation process, for example, the counselor doesn't only need to depend on the client's verbal account of what is occurring in the program. The rehabilitation counselor can observe the client in the actual rehabilitation setting. Such observation can be used as part of the feedback process. Through counseling, clients can explore any variance between their perceptions and those of the counselor and facility personnel. In addition, in sheltered workshops and other facilities, the counselor is often viewed by the client as a part of the rehabilitation environment. These are unique aspects of rehabilitation counseling. Rehabilitation counseling students need to develop counseling skills which enable them to incorporate and utilize these resources as part of the rehabilitation counseling process.

This also presents a challenge to rehabilitation educators and practitioners. For the most part, the counseling theories taught in rehabilitation counselor education programs and practiced in rehabilitation settings were developed for use within traditional counseling settings, e.g., the counselor's office. What is called for is either the modification of existing theories or the development of new counseling approaches that integrates the use of the rehabilitation environment into the counseling process.

UNDERSTANDING THE ENVIRONMENT

The ultimate goal of the rehabilitation program is to enable the client to live and function in the environment outside of a hospital or other institution. For this reason, rehabilitation counselors need to be aware of factors in the environment that may impact on the client. These encompass, but are not limited to attitudes and accessibility. The above issues are often viewed as components of independent living.

Attitudes toward clients include employers, family members, the general public, and clients themselves. Counselor sensitivity to attitudes can facilitate the job and community placement process. Understanding the dynamics behind attitudes enables the rehabilitation counselor to effectively deal with attitude change and any resistence that may exist in the environment to participation of clients in employment, housing, transportation, and other areas of functioning. Attitudes toward and by clients may be one of the most overlooked obstacles to rehabilitation success. Attitudes comprise what can be referred to as the social environment.

Accessibility in employment, transportation and housing serve as facilitators to the achievement of rehabilitation goals and objectives. Rehabilitation counselors often deal with these aspects of the environment as secondary factors. However, from the client's perspective, these issues may be of paramount concern. Assisting clients to deal with the concerns can enhance the clients' sense of responsibility and feeling that they can deal successfully with these aspects of the environment. Accessible employment, transportation, and housing facilities are part of what can be called the physical environment.

DEVELOPMENT OF CASELOAD MANAGEMENT SKILLS

Rehabilitation counselors need to be sensitive to the impact the rehabilitation program has on clients. If a client spends a long time waiting for initial diagnostic and evaluative services, the person may lose interest and withdraw his/her application. A client who is ready for job placement may become discouraged if this is not recognized, and he/she spends more time than necessary in a work adjustment program. A client who is sent to a program which does not meet his/her needs may become confused and upset if this is not identified and the client placed in a more appropriate program. Caseload management skills are an essential part of the rehabilitation process. Although they are often administrative functions, it is evident that poor caseload management skills are detrimental to client growth and development. Counselors with excellent counseling and interpersonal skills may lose clients if they are not cognizant of the status of clients in their caseload. The vocational rehabilitation program is a critical part of the overall rehabilitation process. Its impact on clients is closely related to caseload management.

DEVELOPMENT OF SELF-MONITORING
AND EVALUATION SKILLS

As indicated, counseling in rehabilitation is a process through which the client and counselor work together to identify client needs, establish the goals of the rehabilitation process, specify objectives which are intermediary steps toward the attainment of client goals, relate client needs with rehabilitation services, and finally, document what has been achieved—the competencies the client has developed through participation in the rehabilitation process. It is important that rehabilitation counselors develop mechanisms to communicate progress (or lack thereof) to the client. Feedback is necessary for the client to understand how far he/she has come and how much more needs to be done before the rehabilitation goals are achieved. Without feedback, clients may feel they are on a never ending treadmill.

Setting time limits and specifying progress are key ingredients to facilitating client growth. It enables clients to measure improvements and define areas in need of additional work. A key aspect of rehabilitation counseling is for the counselor to be able to monitor the rehabilitation and to be able to document client achievement of objectives. In this way, as the program progresses, the counselor is able to identify and change or modify clients' goals and objectives which may be inappropriate. Rehabilitation counselors will be able to document, for themselves, the client, and external funders, the client outcomes and benefits which have been achieved. As a means of placing the counseling process on a more scientific basis, counselors will then be able to determine changes in client functioning which were anticipated and can be attributed to counseling, and changes in clients which were unanticipated. Documenting client outcomes or competencies is especially important as rehabilitation programs serve more severely disabled clients and provide rehabilitation services for independent living which may not lead directly to a vocational outcome.

IMPLICATIONS FOR REHABILITATION COUNSELING

A consideration that has been neglected in the specification of a core curriculum for rehabilitation counseling programs and the identification of rehabilitation counselor knowledge and skill requirements is the interrelationships that occur between the components in the rehabilitation process as presented in this paper. Rehabilitation counselors in their daily work deal with these interrelationships. By thinking through the issues presented, practitioners can become better able to organize the ways in which they provide rehabilitation services. By understanding the way variables in the rehabilitation process interact, counselors can develop skills which enable them to anticipate potential problems and deal with them before they interfere with the client's rehabilitation program. The consequences of this will be a more efficient and effective service delivery system. With accountability a major concern of administrators and counselors the model suggested can serve as a rationale and a framework for the provision of rehabilitation services.

The model suggested is a way to view the rehabilitation process as a dynamic, ever-changing interaction between the client, the counselor, the rehabilitation environment and the external environment. What is called for is to understand the ways in which the variables in the model interact. In this regard, rehabilitation counselor educators and practitioners can work together to develop a training model that is responsive to clients' needs while maintaining traditional academic standards. From research into this model, it is possible that a unique theory of rehabilitation might emerge and be substantiated.

REFERENCES

American Personnel and Guidance Association. A report of the committee on professional preparation and standards. *Personnel and Guidance Journal*, 1964, *42*, 535-541.

American Rehabilitation Counseling Association. Professional preparation of reha-
    bilitation counselors: A statement of policy. *Rehabilitation Counseling Bulletin,* 1974,
    12, 20-35.
Division of Counseling Psychology, American Psychological Association ad hoc com-
    mittee in the role of psychology in the preparation of rehabilitation counselors,
    1963. In H.A. Moses & C.H. Patterson (Eds.), *Reading in Rehabilitation Counseling.*
    Champaign: Stipes Publishing Company, 1971.
Hall, J.H. & Warren, S.H. *Rehabilitation counselor preparation.* Washington: National
    Rehabilitation Association, National Vocational Guidance Association, 1956.
Harrison, D.K. & Lee, C.C. Rehabilitation counseling competencies. *Journal of Ap-
    plied Rehabilitation Counseling,* 1979, *10,* 135-141.
Joint Liaison Committee of the Council of State Directors of Vocational Rehabilita-
    tion and the Rehabilitation Counselor Educators. Guidelines for supervised
    clinical practice. Washington, D.C.: Vocational Rehabilitation Administration,
    1963.
McGowan, J.F. & Porter, T.L. *An introduction to the vocational rehabilitation process.*
    Washington, D.C.: Department of Health, Education, and Welfare, Vocational
    Rehabilitation Administration, 1967.
Maki, D.R., McCracken, N., Pope, D.A., & Scofield, M.E. The theoretical model
    of vocational rehabilitation. *Journal of Rehabilitation,* 1978, *44,* 26-28.
Muthard, J.E. & Salomone, P.R. The roles and functions of the rehabilitation coun-
    selor. *Rehabilitation Counseling Bulletin,* 1969, *13,* (1-2).
National Rehabilitation Counseling Association. Professional Standards Committee.
    The rehabilitation counselor: What he is and does. *Journal of Rehabilitation,* 1962,
    28, 17.
Scorzelli, J. Reactions to program content of a rehabilitation counseling program.
    Journal of Applied Rehabilitation Counseling. 1975, *6,* 172-177.
Tripp, J.E. *Perceptions of state vocational rehabilitation counselors, supervisors, and administra-
    tors of core competencies for professional vocational rehabilitation counseling.* Unpublished
    doctoral dissertation, University of Northern Colorado, 1975.
Traux, C.B. & Carkhuff, R.R. Concreteness: A neglected variable in research in
    psychotherapy. *Journal of clinical psychotherapy,* 1964, *29,* 119-124.
Traux, C.B. & Carkhuff, R.R. *Introduction to counseling and psychotherapy: Training and
    practice.* Chicago: Aldine, 1966.
Wright, G.N. & Fraser, R.T. *Wisconsin studies in vocational rehabilitation: Task analysis for
    the evaluation, preparation, classification, and utilization of rehabilitation counselor-track per-
    sonnel.* Madison, Wisconsin, Regional Rehabilitation Institute, 1975.

CHAPTER 5

A FUTURISTIC MODEL OF REHABILITATION EDUCATION

WILLIAM G. EMENER AND FRED R. McFARLANE

Abstract

Current and future changes in American society and the field of rehabilitation are highlighted in a demonstrated need for rehabilitation education to develop a more responsive, proactive, futuristic approach to the professional preparation and development of rehabilitation professionals. A proposed futuristic model of rehabilitation education, with foci on identified Learning Modules and Educational Approaches, is offered in a learning continuum from bachelor's degree level through continuing education.

A FUTURISTIC MODEL OF REHABILITATION EDUCATION

When I outgrow my names and facts and theories, or when reality leaves them behind, I become dead if I don't go on to new ways of seeing things.

Prather, 1970

FOR OVER SIX decades, American society has demonstrated its commitment to its disabled citizens. This aspect of the American dream, as most rehabilitationists know, has been well documented (Bitter, 1978; Garrett, 1969; Lassiter, 1972; Rubin & Roessler, 1978; Rusalem, 1976; Wright, 1980). Moreover, the quality and quantity of rehabilitation services have been predicated upon the continued development of unique rehabilitation professionals, such as rehabilitation counselors, vocational evaluators, work adjustment specialists, placement specialists, and rehabilitation administrators and supervisors.

Reprinted by permission from the *Journal of Applied Rehabilitation Counseling* (in press).

Developments such as these, however, have been predominantly reactionary in nature — the field of rehabilitation has changed in response to changes in American society, rehabilitation service delivery has changed in response to changes in the field of rehabilitation, and rehabilitation education has changed in response to changes in rehabilitation service delivery. To a large extent, this observed change-response phenomenon has exemplified Prather's (1970) above-quoted, rather well-known observation. While change to accommodate the present is important, change to accommodate the future is equally, if not more, important.

In discussing critical aspects of the field of rehabilitation almost two decades ago, A.P. Jarrell (1966) wisely cautioned: "The future growth and development of rehabilitation is largely a function of your capacity and my capacity to change" (p. 20). In their recent discussion of rehabilitation counselor education, Scalia and Wolfe (1984) fittingly observed: "Pre-service is viewed as a beginning, not an end, of professional training. It is designed to orient the new counselor to the present condition and prepare the counselor for the future and change" (p. 37). In spite of such cautions and observations, however, the authors of this manuscript suggest that rehabilitation education is currently amid a period of time in which it could be resembling mediocrity and sameness. To hopefully prevent this trend, this article attempts: (a) to articulate ways in which rehabilitation education's ways are quickly being left behind by reality and (b) to offer a blueprint for a futuristic model of rehabilitation education.

Change and the Future

The most prevalent concept associated with the future is the concept of CHANGE. Smits, Emener and Luck (1981), moreover, observed that "In the last half of the twentieth century the most important change has been the rate of change" (p. 1). Rapid change is the benchmark of the eighties, not only in American society but in the world. Professional literature has documented rapid changes in the United States relevant to the field of rehabilitation:

1. *Technological Advances* — "Medical science . . . is capable of keeping people almost indefinitely on the very borderline of life and death. . . . In the past few decades, medical science has produced an ever-increasing population of disabled persons" (Dowd & Emener, 1978, p. 35).
2. *Humanitarian Advancements* — "Handicapped people are . . . in courtrooms throughout the land asserting their rights . . ." (Laski, 1974, p. 15). We are "a post-industrial cybernetic society" (Gross, 1971, p. 260).
3. *Changes in Government* — "The emerging public administration . . . will have to anticipate and deal with changes in a society that is changing

more rapidly than any in human history" (Mosher, 1978, p. 379-380).

4. *Scarce Natural Resources* — "Elected officials are attending to economic concerns rather than programs of service to people" (Smits, Emener & Luck, 1981, p. 5).

5. *Changes in Values, Attitudes and Beliefs* — changes in work patterns (Miller, 1978), interpersonal power within the work place (Salancik & Pfeffer, 1977), and in the attitudes of workers toward their organization and employers (Nord, 1977).

Since 1973, even though the state-federal rehabilitation program has experienced cost-of-living growth in actual dollars available for the delivery of services, the employment market for new professionals from established rehabilitation education programs (especially in rehabilitation counselor education) has shifted from public sector employment to other employment settings (Feinberg & McFarlane, 1979).

Technology is moving to the forefront. Modern technology (e.g., computer-assisted service delivery techniques) is being used to increase the efficiency of service delivery, to expand the range and capacity of services without expanding personnel, and to expand and enrich education and training programs for rehabilitation personnel (see Chan & Questad, 1981; Crimando & Baker, 1984; Nave & Browning, 1983). It is interesting to note the concomitant alterations emerging from changing legislative mandates such as "Order of Selection," "Focus on Severely Disabled," and "Competitive Employment as *the* Outcome" are being used to maximize the purchasing power of the available dollars in a financially stabilized state-federal rehabilitation program. Overall, the increased knowledge base due to research advances in disability, changing employer demands and expectations, and a shift from product-based industries to service and information exchange industries, place increasing needs and demands on the education and training of rehabilitation professionals.

Concomitant to rapid change is the observed resistance to change, especially in public bureaucracy (Bennis, 1966; Downs, 1967; Drucker, 1966, 1980). Relevant to the field of rehabilitation, Spears (1983) recently observed: "The quest for the dimensions of the future are in us all. . . . Since we carry in our heads visions of the future, we tend to act in response to them. For visions that we abhor, we fight their emergence. For the visions we desire, we behave to assure their appearance" (p. 4).[1] Thus, it would appear fitting to assert that the *ability to accommodate rapid change* (within society and specifically within the field of rehabilitation) is sine qua non to any top quality rehabilitation education program. It is important to note, however, that rehabilitation itself is amid higher educational systems and technologies which are also experiencing rapid change.

Rehabilitation education programs, typically housed within public colleges and universities, are experiencing rapid changes in policy issues associated with costs (Morgan, 1982). For example, they are faced with an increased emphasis on maximizing class enrollments for student credit-hour productivity. Since 1954 (Law 565), rehabilitation education programs have heavily relied on federal support. It must be remembered, however, that "Basic public funding for American colleges and universities has developed historically as a state function" (Arnold, 1982, p. 39). Thus, circa 1984, rehabilitation education programs are experiencing funding problems on two fronts: (a) federal support for rehabilitation education is being reduced (Duncan, 1982; Emener, Lauth, Renick & Smits, in press); and (b) increases in future state funds are expected to be reduced. "A survey of the fiscal condition of the fifty states strongly indicates that for them—and for higher education—the recession is not over" (Magarrell, 1983, p. 1). In many ways higher education is in trouble. For example, Bowen (1981) recently observed: "The increasing vocational interests of students combined with the market orientation of institutions has led to the weakening of the liberal arts ideal in higher education and also to a lowering of academic standards" (p. 56).[2]

A review of the history of rehabilitation education (see Emener, in press; Wright, 1980) reveals: (a) continued growth and expansion contingent upon federal support and marketplace orientation trends (e.g. the placement emphasis of the early seventies, the independent living emphasis of the mid-seventies, the psychiatric rehabilitation emphasis of the late seventies, and the private sector emphasis of the eighties); and (b) a national rehabilitation education program model replete with disjointedness, minimal synergy, and shallowness. For example, while one of the original goals for establishing and fostering bachelor's degree programs was to provide educated-in-rehabilitation applicants for master's degree programs (Culberson, Alcorn & Daniels, 1982; Feinberg, Sunblad & Glick, 1974), very few (if any) master's programs require a bachelor's degree in rehabilitation as a prerequisite for admission, not to mention that many state vocational rehabilitation agencies express a preference for hiring bachelor's level graduates anyway (Witten, 1980).[3] Nonetheless, many graduate programs are still trying to augment their graduate curricula without clearly establishing a strong minimum body of knowledge as an a priori prerequisite. Pipes, Buckhalt, and Merrill (1983) recently observed: "This 'psychology of more' seems to be founded on the assumption that the curriculum for counselors may be continually expanded without sacrificing any present curriculum components" (p. 282).[4] The bottom line is that rehabilitation education cannot simply continue doing what it has been doing for the past five years or more (i.e. continue to add here and there—the "psychology of more"; perpetuate mediocrity with uncoordinated accreditation efforts; continue to offer bachelor's, master's and continuing education programs with loosely defined knowledge and competency-based prerequisite linkages; etc.). The time has come for the field of rehabilitation education to explore a conceptualization or model of rehabilitation education that would: (a) operationalize a lifelong continuum of learning; (b) combine a liberal arts and a professional school approach to human resources development; and (c) prepare professionals for a future of change who cannot only accommodate future change but also be a proactive and meaningful part of its shaping forces.

A Proposed Futuristic Model of Rehabilitation Education

The purpose of the following discussion is to provide an overall conceptualization or blueprint of rehabilitation education from a baccalaureate through a continuing education perspective. Existing guidelines and approaches to bachelor's level rehabilitation education (see Culberson et al., 1982; Feinberg, Sunblad & Glick, 1974; Hylbert, 1963), master's level rehabilitation education (Council on Rehabilitation Education, 1978), and continuing education for rehabilitation personnel (Bruyere & Elliot, 1979) are not being individually critiqued.[5] Moreover, a detailed view of alternative models of rehabilitation education[6] and recommendations for specific coursework and specific hours of coursework[7] are not within the scope of this article (e.g., space limitations would not allow just discourse and thoroughness of coverage). Rather, an overall or bigger picture of rehabilitation education is presented with foci on two critical foundations which provide a framework for the establishment of specific coursework and hours of coursework: *Learning Modules* and *Educational Approaches*. These are displayed in Figure 5-1.

Common to each of the areas and approaches is a recommended fiber of commitment to the practice of helping disabled individuals and the declaration of a life-style of competency development. An appreciation of these key commonalities and a "life-style of competency development" was offered by Emener, Luck and Smits (1981): "Too many people have gotten into rehabilitation and are where they are because they care, not because they're competent!" (p. xiii).

The following discussion is designed to enrich the reader's appreciation of the recommended Learning Modules and their respectively recommended Educational Approaches within the three educational levels.

At the baccalaureate level, it is suggested that future rehabilitationists study human difference—from psychological, sociological, gerontological, political, and anthropological perspectives. Moreover, solid grounding in the theory and practice of business (including industrial-organization and marketing components), business trends, computer application and technology, and robotics would appear essential. These areas of study, including a basic philosophy-humanities component, should be offered within an arts and sciences educational approach.[8] It is also suggested that these areas be studied via the tutelage of respective experts—viz., psychology from psychologists, philosophy from philosophers, etc. With appropriate seminar-experiential courses (e.g., a

FIGURE 5–1
Recommended Continuum of Rehabilitation Education with Foci on Level, Learning Modules, and Education Approaches

Educational Level	Learning Modules	Educational Approaches
Bachelors	• individual human difference • cultural/societal difference • business theory and practice • computer application/tech-nology • robotic and business trends	Primarily an Arts and Sciences approach to education
Masters	• experiential self-awareness • philosophy (ies) of living • philosophical and legal tenets of rehabilitation • medical aspects of disability • psychosocial aspects of disability • occupational/vocational develop-ment • business and industry	Combination of Arts and Sci-ences *and* Professional School approaches
Continuing Education	• placement • counseling theory and practice • Specialization Study Emphasis: e.g., rehabilitation coun-seling; administration and supervision; vocational evaluation/work adjustment; placement specialist . . . • curricula specifically designed for real and perceived con-tinuing education needs specific skill building, etc. (e.g. case work practice)	Primary Professional School approach; heavy experiential components Specific coursework, relevant supervised field work (e.g., practical and intern-ship) A model of lifelong learn-ing with a Human Re-sources Development perspective

human relations seminar), the students could personalize and enrich their learnings by exploring themselves, their relationships with others and the world around them, and "what life is all about" from an ideographic and non-menthetic perspective. It is argued that educational components such as these would render a person as having a knowledge base upon which the basic ele-ments of rehabilitation rest.

At the master's level, a combination of an arts and sciences model and a professional school model would facilitate maximum learning in the areas of philosophical and legal aspects of disability (see Emener & Ferrandino, 1983), medical and psychosocial aspects of disability (see Deloach & Greer, 1981), occupational and vocational development (including vocational appraisal), and business and industry (including industrial psychology, high technology development, and the business side of enterprise). An emphasized professional school approach with coordinated and integrated experiential learning components would appear most appropriate for modules in the areas which include skill-based, behavioral competency development: placement (including job analysis, job development, job seeking and job retention skills, job engineering, marketing skills, and industrial personnel relations), counseling theory and practice (including human relations practices), and assorted "non-counseling" variables necessary for successful professional functioning (see Morgan, 1982). Areas of specialization from which students could choose, areas commensurate with their anticipated area of professional practice, would include required relevant coursework with associated relevant practica and an internship. These might include rehabilitation counseling (see Council on Rehabilitation Education, 1978, vocational evaluation and work adjustment (see Coffey & Ellien, 1979), administration and supervision (see Matkin, Sawyer, Lorenz & Rubin, 1982), and placement and job development (see Usdane, 1974). (These specialization areas would require relevant coursework and associated relevant practica and internship.)

The continuing education level should operationalize a lifelong learning model with a human resources development perspective (see Nadler, 1979). It is critical to remain cognizant of Stephens and Kniepp's (1981) suggestion: "While development programs may include activities generally classified as training or education, they are most concerned with moving the organization and employees for organization change, e.g., growth or decline" (p. 93). Tantamount to the success of continuing education programming is the relevance of content to the perceived and real training and development needs of the participants (see McFarlane & Sullivan, 1979).

Concluding Comment

Rimmer (1981) recently offered a systems approach model for counselor education program development and redefinition which provides helpful guidelines to those rehabilitation educators who wish to embellish the coordinated, integrated, synergistic, and futuristic rehabilitation education model proposed herein. Fittingly, an investigation of Scofield, Berven and Harrison's (1981) assumptions underlying current rehabilitation education practices would also be exceptionally helpful. Expertise in rehabilitation education development exists. Nonetheless, it is suggested that current rehabilitation education practices in the United States simply are not attending to futuristic indices in the field of rehabilitation. Compounding the current scene is the simultaneous cutback in federal and state support of rehabilitation education programs. Rehabilitation education programs must abandon current crisis management and bandaid-expansion trends and design a lifelong model of rehabilitation education for the rehabilitation careerists of tomorrow. As Emener (in press) recently suggested, rehabilitation education has to become "(a) less re-active—more pro-active; (b) less defensive—more open to inspection and forward moving, and (c) less threatened—more confident in its strengths and future" (p. 27).

While the field of rehabilitation is proactively exploring new, future directions (vis-à-vis "famine or extinction in the 1980s," McFarlane & Frost, 1981), rehabilitation education needs to develop a futuristic, developmental change of direction. The approach suggested in this paper is not one which is dramatically revolutionary but one which attempts to integrate within the rehabilitation education curriculum a variety of learning modules beyond the traditional scope of rehabilitation education. The rehabilitationist in the present and in the future is and should be required to utilize a multiplicity of skills, knowledges, and attitudes which historically were nonexistent. The current rehabilitation education curriculum ultimately needs to develop a future-responsive model by modifying courses, changing curriculum, and offering an integrated approach which provides students in rehabilitation a continuum of learning in an effective, efficient, and stimulating manner.

NOTES

1. Interested readers are urged to consult Spears (1983, pp. 4-7). He offers relevant, specific discussion of (a) the changing nature of disablement, (b) the changing nature of work, and (c) the changing nature of society.
2. Bowen's (1981) discussion of higher education in general is extremely relevant to rehabilitation education. For example, the "market orientation" of rehabilitation education toward the mushrooming private sector rehabilitation has been clearly evident in the past five years (see Matkin, 1980; McMahon, 1979; McMahon & Matkin, 1983; Sales, 1979).
3. For further information on graduates of undergraduate programs and agencies' perceptions of their graduates, see Culberson (1979) and Gandy (1983).
4. An excellent critique of specialization trends in rehabilitation counselor education is offered by Thomas (1982). Examples of such trends can be seen in the areas of independent living (Roessler, 1981) and psychiatric rehabilitation (Weinberger & Greenwald, 1982), among others.
5. For examples of assessments, evaluations, and critiques of rehabilitation education curricula and programs, consult Emener and Rasch (1984), Janes and Emener (1983), and Scorzelli (1975, 1979).
6. Rehabilitation literature contains many discussions on alternative models of rehabilitation education, for example: the traditional versus the experiential model (Holbert & Miller, 1970), the reality model (Thomason & Saxon, 1973), the training model (Anthony, Dell Orto, Lasky, Marinelli, Power & Spaniol, 1977), the competency-based model (Diamonti & Murphy, 1977), and the integrative model (Crystal, 1981).

7. For examples of specific coursework recommendations, see the Council on Rehabilitation Education (1978) and the (private sector) recommendations of Lynch and Martin (1982).

8. Among other constructs, the arts and sciences approach encourages coursework in the traditional, basic disciplines (e.g., sociology, psychology, humanities). The professional school approach, addressed in the next paragraph, encourages coursework in applied, within-the-specific-professional-discipline area (e.g., social work, rehabilitation counseling), and also emphasizes supervised clinical practice (practica and internship). The arts and sciences model is more basic and generic in nature; the professional school model is more focused and applied in nature and has a strong "practice" component.

REFERENCES

Anthony, W.A., Dell Orto, A.E., Lasky, R.G., Marinelli, R.P., Power, P.W., & Spaniol, L.J. (1977). A training model for rehabilitation counseling education. *Rehabilitation Counseling Bulletin, 20*(3), 218-235.

Arnold, C.K. (Spring, 1982). The federal role in funding education. *Change,* 39-34, 54.

Bennis, W.G. (1966). *Changing organizations: Essays on the development and evolution of human organization.* New York: McGraw-Hill.

Bitter, J.A. (1978). Continuing education for new rehabilitation counselors. *Rehabilitation Counseling Bulletin, 22*(1), 74-77.

Bowen, H.R. (1981). Observations on the costs of higher education. *Quarterly Review of Economics and Business, 21*(1), 47-57.

Bruyere, S.M., & Elliot, J.K. (1979). RRCEPs and Continuing education for rehabilitation personnel. *Rehabilitation Counseling Bulletin, 23*(2), 131-135.

Chan, F., & Questad, K. (1981). Microcomputers in vocational evaluation: An application for staff training. *Vocational Evaluation and Work Adjustment Bulletin, 14*(4), 153-158.

Coffey, D., & Ellien, V. (1979). *Work adjustment curriculum development project: A summary.* Menomonie, WI: University of Wisconsin — Vocational Rehabilitation Institute, Research and Training Center.

Council on Rehabilitation Education (1978). *Accreditation Manual for Rehabilitation Counselor Education Programs.* Chicago, IL: Author.

Crimando, W., & Baker, R. (1984). Computer-assisted instruction in rehabilitation education. *Rehabilitation Counseling Bulletin, 28*(1), 50-54.

Crystal, R.M. (1981). An integrative model for rehabilitation training and practice. *Journal of Applied Rehabilitation Counseling, 12*(4), 191-194.

Culberson, J.O. (1979). Undergraduate education for rehabilitation: Agency perceptions of training and characteristics preferred of job applicants. *Journal of Rehabilitation, 45*(2), 39-43, 88.

Culberson, J.O., Alcorn, J.D., & Daniels, J.L. (1982). Making undergraduate rehabilitation education relevant: A cooperative project. *Rehabilitation Counseling Bulletin, 25*(4), 228-230.

Deloach, C., & Greer, B.G. (1981). *Adjustment to severe physical disability: A metamorphosis.* New York: McGraw-Hill.

Diamonti, M.C., & Murphy, S.T. (1977). The realities of competency-based rehabilitation counselor education: A reply. *Rehabilitation Counseling Bulletin, 21*(1), 63-66.

Dowd, E.T., & Emener, W.G. (1978). Lifeboat counseling: The issue of survival decisions. *Journal of Rehabilitation, 44*(3), 34-36.

Downs, A. (1967). *Inside Bureaucracy*. Boston: Little, Brown. (Chapter II. The life cycle
of bureaus.)

Drucker, P.F. (1966). *The effective executive*. New York: Harper & Row.

Drucker, P.F. (1980). The deadly sins in public administration. *Public Administration Review, 40,* 103-106.

Duncan, J.G. (Spring, 1982). Highlights on the Washington scene. *NCRE Report*
(Newsletter), National Council on Rehabilitation Education, Washington, D.C.,
pp. 1, 3.

Emener, W.G. (in press). Rehabilitation counselor education: A state of the art perspective. In E. Pan, T.E. Backer, & C.L. Vash: *1984 Annual Review of Rehabilitation*.
New York: Springer.

Emener, W.G., & Ferrandino, J.A. (1983). A philosophical framework for rehabilitation: Implications for clients, counselors, agencies. *Journal of Applied Rehabilitation
Counseling, 14*(1), 62-67.

Emener, W.G., & Rasch, J.D. (1984). Actual and preferred instructional areas in
rehabilitation education programs. *Rehabilitation Counseling Bulletin, 27*(5), 269-
280.

Emener, W.G., Lauth, T.P., Renick, J.C., & Smits, S.J. (in press). Impact of government retrenchment on professionalism: The cases of rehabilitation counseling and
social work. *Journal of Rehabilitation Administration*.

Feinberg, L.B., & McFarlane, F.R. (1979). Setting-based factors in rehabilitation
counselor role variability. *Journal of Applied Rehabilitation Counseling, 10,* 95-106.

Feinberg, L.B., Sunblad, L.M., & Glick, L.J. (1974). *Education for the rehabilitation services: Planning undergraduate curricula*. Syracuse, NY: Syracuse University, School of
Education.

Gandy, G.L. (1983). Graduates of an undergraduate rehabilitation curriculum. *Rehabilitation Counseling Bulletin, 26*(5), 357-359.

Garrett, J.F. (1969). Historical background. In D. Malikin and H. Rusalem (Eds.),
Vocational rehabilitation of the disabled. New York: New York University Press.

Gross, B.M. (1971). Planning in an era of social revolution. *Public Administration Review, 31,* 259-297.

Holbert, W.M., & Miller, J.H. (1970). Traditional versus experiential model for counselor education. *Journal of Applied Rehabilitation Counseling, 1*(3), 21-30.

Hylbert, K.W. (1963). Experiment at Penn State: Bachelor of rehabilitation. *Journal of
Rehabilitation, 29*(2), 23-24.

Janes, M.W., & Emener, W.G. (1983). Graduates' views of instructional/competency
areas in rehabilitation counselor education programs: A hypotheses generating
study. *Journal of Applied Rehabilitation Counseling, 15*(2), 38-43.

Jarrell, A.P. (1966). The courage to change. *Journal of Rehabilitation, 32*(1), 20.

Laski, F. (1974). Civil rights victories for the handicapped. I. *Social and Rehabilitation
Record, 1*(5), 15-20.

Lassiter, R.A. (1972). History of the rehabilitation movement in America. In J.G.

Cull, & R.E. Hardy (Eds.), *Vocational rehabilitation: Profession and process.* Springfield, IL: Charles C Thomas.

Lynch, R.K. & Martin, T. (1982). Rehabilitation counseling in the private sector: A training needs survey. *Journal of Rehabilitation, 48*(3), 51-53, 73.

Magarrell, J. (1983). Growth in state funds for colleges expected to slow further in 1984. *Chronicle of Higher Education,* Spring, 1, 6.

Matkin, R.E. (1980). The rehabilitation counselor in private practice: Perspectives for education and preparation. *Journal of Rehabilitation, 46*(2), 60-62.

Matkin, R.E., Sawyer, H.W., Lorenze, J.R., & Rubin, S.E. (1982). Rehabilitation administrators and supervisors: Their work assignments, training needs, and suggestions for preparation. *Journal of Rehabilitation Administration, 6,* 170-183.

McFarlane, F.R., & Frost, D.E. (1981). Rehabilitation directions: Feast, famine, or extinction in the 1980's. *Journal of Rehabilitation,* 1981, *47*(3), 20-23.

McFarlane, F.R., & Sullivan, M. (1979). Educational and training needs of rehabilitation counselors: Implications for training. *Journal of Applied Rehabilitation Counseling, 10*(1), 41-43.

McMahon, G.T. (1979). Private sector rehabilitation: Benefits, dangers, and implications for education. *Journal of Rehabilitation, 45*(3), 56-58.

McMahon, B.T., & Matkin, R.E. (1983). Preservice graduate education for private sector rehabilitation counselors. *Rehabilitation Counseling Bulletin, 27*(1), 54-60.

Miller, A.R. (1978). Changing work life patterns: A twenty-five year review. *The Annals of the American Academy, 435,* 83-101.

Morgan, C.A. (1982). An evolving practicum for the World of IS—one approach. Counselor survival and noncounseling skills. Preservice conditioning for "The World of IS." *Journal of Rehabilitation, 48*(2), 29-32, 72.

Mosher, F.C. (1978). The public service in a temporary society. In J.M. Shafritz & A.C. Hyde (Eds.), *Classics in Public Administration.* Oak Park, IL: Moore.

Nadler, L. (1979). *Developing human resources.* 2nd ed. Austin: Learning Concepts.

Nave, G., & Browning, P. (1983). Preparing rehabilitation leaders for the computer age. *Rehabilitation Counseling Bulletin, 26*(5), 364-367.

Nord, W.R. (1977). Job satisfaction reconsidered. *American Psychologist, 32,* 1026-1035.

Patterson, C.H. (1969). *Rehabilitation counseling: Collected papers.* Champaign, IL: Stipes Publishing Co.

Pipes, R.B., Buckhalt, J.A., & Merrill, H.D. (1983). Counselor education and the psychology of more. *Counselor Education and Supervision, 22*(4), 282-286.

Prather, H. (1970). *Notes to myself.* Moab, Utah: Real People Press.

Rimmer, S.M. (1981). A systems approach model for counselor education program development and redefinition. *Counselor Education and Supervision, 21*(1), 7-15.

Roessler, R.T. (1981). Training independent living rehabilitation specialists. *Journal of Rehabilitation, 47*(2), 36-39.

Rubin, S.E., & Roessler, R.T. (1978). *Foundations of vocational rehabilitation process.* Baltimore: University Park Press.

Rusalem, H. (1976). A personalized recent history of vocational rehabilitation in America. In H. Rusalem & D. Malikin (Eds.), *Contemporary Vocational Rehabilitation.* New York: New York University Press.

Salancik, G.R., & Pfeffer, J. (Winter, 1977). Who gets power — and how they hold on to it: A strategic-contingency model of power. *Organizational Dynamics,* 3-21.

Sales, A. (1979). Rehabilitation counseling in the private sector: Implications for graduate education. *Journal of Rehabilitation, 45*(3), 59-61, 72.

Scalia, V.A., & Wolfe, R.R. (1984). Rehabilitation counselor education. *Journal of Applied Rehabilitation Counseling, 15*(3), 34-38.

Scofield, M.E., Berven, N.L., & Harrison, R.P. (1981). Competence, credentialing, and the future of rehabilitation. *Journal of Rehabilitation, 47*(1), 31-35.

Scorzelli, J.F. (1975). Reactions to program content of a rehabilitation counseling program. *Journal of Applied Rehabilitation Counseling, 6*(3), 172-177.

Scorzelli, J.F. (1979). Assessing the content of a rehabilitation counseling program. *Journal of Applied Rehabilitation Counseling, 9*(4), 184-186.

Smits, S.J., Emener, W.G., & Luck, R.S. (1981). Prologue to the present. In Emener, W.G., Luck, R.S., & Smits, S.J. (Eds.), *Rehabilitation Administration and Supervision,* Baltimore: University Park Press.

Spears, M. (1983). Rehabilitation in the third wave. *Journal of Rehabilitation, 49*(3), 4-7.

Stephens, J.E., & Kniepp, S. (1981). Managing human resource development in rehabilitation. In W.G. Emener, R.S. Luck & S.J. Smits. *Rehabilitation administration and supervisor.* Baltimore: University Park Press.

Thomas, K.R. (1982). A critique of trends in rehabilitation counselor education toward specialization. *Journal of Rehabilitation, 48*(1), 49-51.

Thomason, B., & Saxon, J.P. (1973). A reality model for rehabilitation counselor education. *Journal of Applied Rehabilitation Counseling, 4*(1), 23-31.

Usdane, W. (1974). Placement personnel: A graduate program concept. *Journal of Rehabilitation, 40*(2), 12-13.

Weinberger, J., & Greenwald, M. (1982). Training and curricula in psychiatric rehabilitation: A survey of core accredited programs. *Rehabilitation Counseling Bulletin, 25*(5), 287-290.

Witten, B.J. (1980). Preparation and utilization of undergraduate workers in rehabilitation: Comparative perceptions of respondents. Unpublished doctoral dissertation, Syracuse University.

Wright, G.N. (1980). *Total rehabilitation.* Boston: Little, Brown, and Company.

CHAPTER 6

KNOWLEDGE ADEQUACIES AND TRAINING NEEDS OF REHABILITATION EDUCATORS

WILLIAM G. EMENER, JOHN D. RASCH, AND PAUL E. SPECTOR

Abstract

This article describes results of a national survey of rehabilitation educators concerning their perceptions of their knowledge adequacies and training needs. Twelve vital instructional areas were identified and respondents were asked to rate each area for their adequacy of knowledge, need for inservice training, and willingness to attend inservice training. Findings showed that educators rated their knowledge adequacy high and their need for inservice training low. Although there was a significant inverse relationship between knowledge adequacy and need for inservice training, there was no significant relationship between willingness to attend inservice training and knowledge adequacy, or between willingness to attend inservice training and need for inservice training.

WITHIN THE FIELD of rehabilitation counseling, practitioner competencies have been discussed by a number of authors (e.g., Berven & Scofield, 1980; Harrison & Lee, 1979; Porter, Rubin, & Sink, 1979; Rubin & Emener, 1979; Sink & Porter, 1978). At least three lists of instructional areas typically taught in rehabilitation counseling programs have been outlined (Council on Rehabilitation Education (CORE), 1978; Harrison & Lee, 1979; Sink & Porter, 1978). The ability of a faculty to prepare students in these instructional areas, however, is predicated upon their own level of knowledge and mastery of those areas. The changing roles and functions of rehabilitation counselors (see Emener & Rubin, 1980) and the continuing expansion of rehabilitation literature and technology place many rehabilitation educators in a position where they are hardpressed to remain abreast of the field.

This study synthesized the instructional areas of Sink and Porter (1978).

Reprinted by permission from Volume 22 (1983), *Counselor Education and Supervision*, pp. 242-249.

Harrison and Lee (1979), and CORE (1978) into twelve distinct instructional areas. The purpose of this study was to determine, for each instructional area, educators' perceptions of their: (a) knowledge adequacies for effective teaching: (b) need for inservice training; and (c) willingness to attend inservice training.

METHOD

Sample

This study was conducted as a component of *The 1981 Rehabilitation Education Survey*. (The survey consisted of 23 items, 14 of which focused on respondent demographics. Other areas investigated by the survey were: (a) actual and preferred instructional area emphases in bachelor's, master's, doctoral, and continuing education training programs; and (b) sources and availability of rehabilitation education and training resource materials). The survey population consisted of all 459 members of the National Council of Rehabilitation Education (NCRE). NCRE is a professional organization of rehabilitation educators dedicated to quality services for persons with disabilities through education and research. Participants for this survey were identified through the 1980 *NCRE Directory*. Usable surveys were returned by 235 respondents (51.2% response rate).

Analyses of the respondents' demographic data revealed that: (a) the majority were male (84%); (b) their average age was 42.2 ($SD=9.0$); (c) they primarily had master's (M) and doctoral (D) degrees in rehabilitation (M=55%; D=42%), counseling (M=17%; D=33%), and psychology (M=12%; D=11%); (d) they were predominantly assistant professors (31%), associate professors (24%), and professors (29%); (e) they had a geographic representation commensurate with the NCRE population; (f) they had been employed in the field of rehabilitation an average of 13.3 years ($SD=6.9$) and as rehabilitation educators an average of 8.6 years ($SD=5.2$); (g) they worked with bachelor's (54%), master's (84%), and doctoral (46%) students and with continuing education professionals (54%) and paraprofessionals (18%); (h) for most (82%), rehabilitation education was the primary nature of their work; and (i) almost half (45%) had rehabilitation training program administrative responsibilities.

Instruments

As previously indicated, instructional areas were delineated through a synthesis of findings from earlier studies and the training content recommendations of CORE's Commission on Standards and Accreditation for Rehabilitation Counselor Education (1978). The twelve rehabilitation education

FIGURE 6-1
Operational Definitions of 12 RC Competency Areas

1. *Basic Principles:* Knowledge of principles and concepts underlying rehabilitation, including history, philosophy, structure, and legislation.

2. *Counseling Theories and Techniques:* Knowledge and historical and current approaches to individual and group counseling with application to the field of rehabilitation. Training in basic counseling skills used in relationship building, problem/need identification, and action on rehabilitation problems.

3. *Medical Aspects:* Knowledge of the structure of medicine in the United States, medical specialties, medical terminology, and the medical examination. Knowledge of body systems, basic functions, common malfunctions, therapeutic services, restorative techniques, and disability evaluation. Knowledge of the unique characteristics of various disability groups, especially the severely disabled.

4. *Psychosocial Aspects:* Knowledge of behavioral and psychodynamic principles underlying personal adjustment to disability. Knowledge of adjustment issues in the family and community at large.

5. *Occupational Information and Job Analysis:* Knowledge of the vocational structure of society, including skill requirements of occupations, entry level requirements, and physical and emotional demands. Ability to effectively use occupational information and to analyze jobs.

6. *Evaluation:* Ability to determine diagnostic and assessment procedures needed, analyze and synthesize information, interpret data to client, and determine eligibility. Includes knowledge of psychometric tests, work samples, on-the-job evaluation, and situational assessment procedures.

7. *Case Management:* Ability to move and monitor clients through the rehabilitation process. Includes knowledge of case finding, rehabilitation plan development, service delivery/coordination, and follow-up.

8. *Community Organization and Resources:* Knowledge of community (local) organization and resources. Knowledge of service delivery systems, issues in linking and coordinating services with other agencies, and inter-agency cooperation.

9. *Job Development and Placement:* Knowledge of job development and placement procedures, including methods for contacting and interfacing with employers, and job modification.

10. *Fieldwork:* Ability to arrange practicum and internship placements in suitable agencies, monitor field work, maintain a working relationship with field supervisors, and supervise students on an individual and/or group seminar basis.

11. *Research:* Knowledge of research methodology, including design, sampling data analysis and interpretation, and familiarity with rehabilitation research literature.

12. *Professional Issues:* Knowledge of professional issues and current developments in rehabilitation, including ethics, legal issues, certification, program accreditation, and professional associations.

instructional areas are defined in Figure 6-1. It was believed that these twelve areas adequately represent essential competency needs of rehabilitation practitioners as well as the typical instructional areas in rehabilitation education programs.

Respondents were asked to rate each instructional area in reference to their own: (a) adequacy of knowledge for teaching, (b) professional need for inservice training, and (c) willingness to attend formal inservice training programs for rehabilitation educators (if stipends were available). Ratings were made on a seven-point scale ranging from Very Low to Very High for adequacy of knowledge and need for training, and Definitely No to Definitely Yes for willingness to attend inservice training programs.

Procedure

All NCRE members were sent introductory letters informing them that the Rehabilitation Education Survey would soon arrive in the mail. It was requested that they promptly complete and return the survey after receiving it. The Survey was mailed with a cover letter and prepaid return envelope one week after the introductory letter was mailed. Respondents and nonrespondents were assured of complete anonymity. Accordingly, no questionnaire numbering system was employed (which would have allowed for additional mailings to nonrespondents). A follow-up letter was mailed to all NCRE members two weeks after the survey encouraging them to complete and return it if they had not already done so.

RESULTS

Means and standard deviations were calculated for all three questions and all twelve instructional areas (see Table 6-1). Also included are the rank orders of the twelve areas for each of the three questions. Spearman Rank Order Correlations were computed to compare each pair of the three ranks.

No instructional area received a Very High average knowledge rating ($\overline{X}=6.0-7.0$). Seven instructional areas (Fieldwork, Professional Issues, Basic Principles, Counseling Theories and Techniques, Psychosocial Aspects, Community Organization and Resources, and Evaluation) received High knowledge ratings ($\overline{X}=5.0-5.9$). The lowest knowledge rating was for Medical Aspects.

Three of the twelve instructional areas (Basic Principles, Counseling Theories and Techniques, and Fieldwork) were rated Low ($\overline{X}=2.0-2.9$) on need for inservice training. Nine of the twelve instructional areas were rated Slightly Low ($\overline{X}=3.0-3.9$) in terms of need for inservice training, and the greatest expressed need for inservice training was in Research and Medical Aspects.

No instructional area was rated Very High ($\overline{X}=6.0-6.7$) in terms of willingness to attend inservice training, and only three (Professional Issues, Research, and Psychosocial Aspects) were rated High ($\overline{X}=5.0-5.9$). Two of the twelve instructional areas (Basic Principles and Fieldwork) were rated Slightly Low ($\overline{X}=3.0-3.9$) in terms of willingness to attend inservice training.

Spearman Rank Correlation Coefficients were calculated for the three sets of ratings. There was a significant inverse relationship between educators'

Table 6-1

Means and Mean Rankings of Rehabilitation Educators' Ratings:
Teaching Knowledge Adequacy and Need/Willingness to Attend Inservice Training Across 12 RC Competency Areas

RC Competency Areas		Mean Ratings on Adequacy of Knowledge for Teaching	Mean Rankings	Teaching Adequacy, Need/Will to Attend Inservice Training			
				Mean Ratings on Perceived Need for Inservice Training	Mean Rankings	Mean Ratings on Willingness to Attend Inservice Training	Mean Rankings
1. Basic Principles:	x̄	5.7	2.5	2.3	12	3.4	12
	sd	1.4		1.4		1.8	
	n	226		216		182	
2. Counseling Theory and Techniques:	x̄	5.5	4	2.8	10.5	4.3	8
	sd	1.4		1.5		1.8	
	n	225		213		183	
3. Medical Aspects:	x̄	4.4	12	3.7	2	4.9	4
	sd	1.7		1.7		1.7	
	n	226		216		184	
4. Psychosocial Aspects:	x̄	5.4	5	3.2	9	5.0	2.5
	sd	1.3		1.6		1.6	
	n	225		217		182	
5. Occupational Information and Job Analysis:	x̄	4.9	9.5	3.5	4	4.5	7
	sd	1.6		1.7		1.7	
	n	225		213		183	
6. Evaluation:	x̄	5.1	7	3.4	6.5	4.8	5
	sd	1.6		1.6		1.5	
	n	224		214		183	
7. Case Management:	x̄	4.9	9.5	3.4	6.5	4.1	9
	sd	1.5		1.6		1.7	
	n	224		214		184	

Table 6-1 *(Continued)*

Competency							
8. Community Organization and Resources	x̄	5.2	6	3.4	6.5	4.0	10
	sd	1.4		1.5		1.7	
	n	225		215		183	
9. Placement:	x̄	4.9	9.5	3.6	3	4.6	6
	sd	1.5		1.8		1.8	
	n	225		216		184	
10. Fieldwork:	x̄	5.9	1	2.8	10.5	3.8	11
	sd	1.3		1.5		1.9	
	n	224		215		183	
11. Research:	x̄	4.9	9.5	3.8	1	5.0	2.5
	sd	1.5		1.9		1.7	
	n	224		218		184	
12. Professional Issues:	x̄	5.7	2.5	3.4	6.5	5.2	1
	sd	1.2		1.7		1.7	
	n	225		218		182	
Averages:		5.21		3.27		4.47	

Notes. Questionnaire Item #15: Using the following scale, rate the present adequacy of your knowledge for teaching in each of the following competency areas:

Questionnaire Item #19: Rate your professional need for inservice training in each of the following competency areas:

Scale Used for Items 15 and 19: 1 = Very Low; 2 = Low; 3 = Slightly Low; 4 = Adequate; 5 =Slightly High; 6 = High; 7 = Very High.

Questionnaire Item #22: Rate your willingness to attend formal inservice training program for rehabilitation educators (if stipends were available) in each of the following competency areas:

Scale for Item 22: 1 = Definitely No; 2 = No; 3 = Probably No; 4 = Maybe; 5 = Probably Yes; 6 = Yes; 7 = Definitely Yes.

Spearman Rank Correlation Coefficients between the mean rankings:

1. (a) Adequacy of Knowledge for Teaching vs (d) Perceived Need for Inservice Training: rho = −.8532; t = 2.68; df = 10; p .05 (two-tailed).
2. (a) Adequacy of Knowledge for Teaching vs (e) Willingness to Attend Inservice Training: rho = −.3105; t = 1.19; df = 10; p − NS.
3. (b) Perceived Need for Inservice Training vs (e) Willingness to Attend Inservice Training: rho = .5126; t = 1.58; df = 10; p − NS.

reported adequacy of knowledge for teaching and their perceived need for inservice training (rho $= -.85$, $p < .05$). There were nonsignificant correlations between the educator's: (a) knowledge adequacy for teaching and personal willingness to attend inservice training, and (b) perceived need for inservice training and willingness to attend inservice training.

DISCUSSION

The results of this survey of rehabilitation educators presented several interesting findings. The educators tended to rate their knowledge adequacy high and their need for inservice training low. Although there was the expected negative relationship between adequacy of knowledge and need for training, the nonsignificant relationship between willingness to attend inservice training and training need or knowledge adequacy were not anticipated.

The results for knowledge adequacy indicated that Fieldwork was rated highest. Fieldwork is probably one of the less intellectually demanding of the twelve instructional areas in that formal presentations in Fieldwork courses are less common than site visits and group and individual clinical supervision. The lowest knowledge rating was reported for Medical Aspects, and this is perhaps the most information-specific of the twelve instructional areas. This perceived inadequacy is possibly reflected in the common instructional practice of bringing in medical specialists for guest lectures in Medical Aspect courses.

It is interesting to note that the two instructional areas related most strongly to vocational service delivery (i.e., Occupational Information and Job Analysis, Job Development and Placement) were not included among the highest educator knowledge ratings. In the work of vocational rehabilitation counselors, competency in these areas is critical to successful service delivery. Because these areas apply to working with handicapped individuals, they are instrumental in differentiating rehabilitation counseling from other counseling professions.

The ratings on need for inservice training indicated that educators generally believe they do not need inservice training. They reported very little for inservice training in Basic Principles, Counseling Theories and Techniques, and Fieldwork. Educators seem to believe they could benefit most from inservice training in Research and Medical Aspects. Medical Aspects was also the area of their lowest teaching knowledge adequacy. Other areas where inservice training was perceived as potentially being most helpful were Job Development and Placement and Occupational Information and Job Analysis.

The ratings on willingness to attend inservice training suggest that educators might participate in inservice training programs in the areas of Professional Issues, Research, and Psychosocial Aspects. It is interesting that the willingness to attend inservice training was not necessarily consistent with their reported knowledge adequacy or need for inservice training. The Professional Issues area reflects continually changing content of importance to the field of rehabilitation. The issues addressed in this area are broad and may affect rehabilitation education directly, as in the cases of legislation and appropriation. Because professional issues may change markedly with time, a greater willingness to attend inservice training programs in this area is understandable. In relation to the Research area, rehabilitation counseling has an empirically based literature, and many rehabilitation educators may believe they need to improve their skills in statistics and research methodology. Research is also a skill area necessary for promotion and tenure in university settings. The Psychosocial Aspects area overlaps many disciplines (e.g., psychology, sociology, economics), and, as in the case of Professional Issues, the social implications of disability (which educators must remain aware of) are constantly changing.

The obvious limitations of this study notwithstanding (e.g., low response rate), the need for similar research investigations across the variety of counselor education specializations seems evident and warranted. Such research would enrich the field of counselor education and would ultimately enhance the practice of counseling across all specializations.

REFERENCES

Berven, N.L., & Scofield, M.E. Evaluation of professional competence through standardized simulation: A review. *Rehabilitation Counseling Bulletin*, 1980, *24*, 178-202.

Council on Rehabilitation Education. *Accreditation manual for rehabilitation counselor education programs*. Chicago: Author, 1978.

Emener, W.G., & Rubin, S.E. Rehabilitation counselor roles and functions and sources of role strain. *Journal of Applied Rehabilitation Counseling*, 1980, *11*, 57-69.

Harrison, D.K., & Lee, C.C. Rehabilitation counseling competencies. *Journal of Applied Rehabilitation Counseling*, 1979, *10*, 135-141.

Jones, L.K. *U.S. counselor education programs: Nature, numbers, CBE, traditional and nontraditional*. Paper presented at the annual meeting of the American Personnel and Guidance Association, New York City, 1975.

Porter, T.L.; Rubin, S.E.; & Sink, J.M. Essential rehabilitation counselor diagnostic, counseling, and placement competencies. *Journal of Applied Rehabilitation Counseling*, 1979, *10*, 158-162.

Rubin, S.E., & Emener, W.G. Recent rehabilitation counselor role changes and role strain—a pilot investigation. *Journal of Applied Rehabilitation Counseling*, 1979, *10*, 158-162.

Sink, J., & Porter, T. Convergence and divergence in rehabilitation counseling. *Journal of Applied Rehabilitation Counseling*, 1978, *9*, 5-20.

CHAPTER 7

CONTEMPORARY REHABILITATION
COUNSELOR EDUCATION

GEORGE N. WRIGHT

Abstract

Rehabilitation counselors must have knowledge and skills in not only counseling but also many other professional functions (e.g., selective job placement). Consequently, graduate study is even more important for counselors in rehabilitation than for school guidance workers. In addition to the required two-year master's degree, the rehabilitationist needs continuing (outservice) education to keep up with expanding technology and to prepare for specialization.

ONLY FUNDAMENTAL errors of fact and reasoning can lead to the invalid conclusion that a bachelor's degree (approximately 120 weeks of college education) is sufficient preparation in rehabilitation counseling (RC). Unfortunately, such misinformation and misconceptions about this profession can be misused in our nation's current political climate. For many years, persons without vocational rehabilitation (VR) experience have failed to appreciate the nature and value of preprofessional RC preparation at the master's degree level. Most Americans associated with VR service, however, realize that its effectiveness depends on a well-qualified rehabilitation counselor. Moreover, the consensus within all facets of rehabilitation education and practice is that RC qualification is based on one or two years of graduate (master's degree) education.

The technological basis of our profession has advanced greatly since the mid-1950s with federal support for rehabilitation counselor education (RCE) and research. Most of the early RCE programs, however, were in school guidance departments and therefore shaped by a narrow view of psychology that

Reprinted by permission from Volume 25(4), *Rehabilitation Counseling Bulletin*, pp. 254-256.

equates it with psychotherapy. Many early RCE professors had never worked as vocational rehabilitation counselors; consequently, they tried to redefine the RC role to exclude other professional functions (e.g., client assessment and selective placement) in order to teach their kind of "counseling," which was held to be synonymous with "psychotherapy."

Today's RCE curriculum and professors generally recognize that the effective rehabilitation counselor must be qualified for a variety of professional functions including, but not limited to, vocational and personal-social adjustment counseling. Moreover, the complexity of these RC functions and the required psychological knowledge and skills require a specific program of classroom and clinical instruction at the graduate level. Fortunately, however, many doctoral graduates of RCE programs—the new breed of rehabilitation professors—are identified with rehabilitation and have learned through their own experience in VR agencies that RC practitioners have a variety of high level and critical responsibilities. Job placement, for example, is viewed now as an RC professional function involving a detailed knowledge of both the client and the world of work.

Guidance professors once said that the only professional function of the rehabilitation counselor was counseling (therapy), and that placement and the like should be assigned to a "subprofessional," a salesperson or aide of something less than master's level preparation. Some of these early professors who wrote and taught about their notions of the roles and functions of rehabilitation counselors were enamored of a simplistic Rogerian approach and so rejected psychological measurement and client assessment as components of rehabilitation counseling; such views reflect a very narrow conception of counseling and other fields of psychology.

To say that agency employers have made RC work routine with such unchallenging tasks as report-writing and job placement reflects the older RCE notion that counseling is psychotherapy and that only this counselor function and goal is professionally appropriate and challenging in rehabilitation. Contemporary educators see counseling as a basic responsibility that facilitates other critically important RC functions, most of which are scientifically based in one or another branch of psychology. While there is a pecking order in psychology, psychotherapy should not be regarded as more important, more challenging, or more professional than areas of other psychology.

Undergraduate rehabilitation education serves as a feeder to RCE master's degree programs. Although many occupational options can be built into a flexible undergraduate rehabilitation curriculum, professional counseling courses are reserved for graduate level instruction. Many of the traditional RCE courses, however, are appropriate for upper class undergraduate students (e.g., courses on the medical, psychosocial, and occupational aspects of disability). A master's RCE student who has completed such courses as an undergraduate in rehabilitation services should be able to shorten the usual two-year graduation requirement.

The master's degree in RCE should not be changed from one of professional preparation for clinical practice with disabled clients to providing preparation for research. Most educators, even in the professional areas, generally regard the Ph.D. as necessary for a research career. All levels of graduate preparation in rehabilitation would be lessened by downgrading present requirements. It is not true that most rehabilitation counselors entering doctoral programs end up by changing their professional identity. Doctoral graduates of many RCE programs are prepared for and often placed in rehabilitation research and education. Most RCE graduates (both master's and Ph.D. degree level) at the University of Wisconsin-Madison are in rehabilitation. Our experience does not suggest that employers reject the present master's level RCE graduate; demand for Wisconsin's RCE graduates for rehabilitation jobs is greater than ever and at the highest salary level. Exception must be taken regarding the implication that federal training grant officials exerted influence on university RCE faculty by forming guidelines for developing curriculum. The fact is that many of the earlier RCE programs were funded despite inappropriate instruction and inadequate contribution to the rehabilitation community.

Finally, there is the criticism of "the small army" of professionally trained rehabilitation counselors in the United States and their effectiveness compared to unspecialized rehabilitation workers in West European countries. Such data are misleading because of the great differences in rehabilitation programming abroad. The fact is that there is a worldwide interest in both the American technology of vocational rehabilitation and in the professional preparation of its rehabilitation counselors.

The explosion of knowledge in RC, as in many other professions, calls for more learning, not less. The RCE master's degree graduate can practice adequately as a generalist (c.f., general practitioner in medicine). But the growth of our profession calls for RC specialization (according to type of client handicap or service emphasis). University RCE programs consequently should accommodate the graduates' need for continuing education, keeping up with the expanding technology and advancing in a specialized area of rehabilitation counseling practice. Professional counseling, particularly in rehabilitation, cannot be mastered at the baccalaureate level.

CHAPTER 8

THE CHANGING ROLE AND FUNCTION OF
THE REHABILITATION COUNSELOR

Stanford E. Rubin and Frank D. Puckett

Abstract

Historically, it has been difficult to trace changes in the role and function of the
rehabilitation counselor (RC) because of differences in instrumentation among
existing studies. In an attempt to address the question of the changing role of the
rehabilitation counselor in the most valid manner possible, the authors analyzed
data from three existing studies in which the Muthard and Salomone (1969) Abbreviated Task Inventory was administered to RC's. The results of the analyses
suggest that changes in the RC's job have occurred, but not to the degree that
would support the conclusion of a major modification in the basic dimensionality
of that job role.

THE ROLE and function of the rehabilitation counselor (RC) has been
addressed frequently in the rehabilitation counseling literature during the
last three decades (Roessler & Rubin, 1982). Empirical research reported in
that literature (Emener & Rubin, 1980; Rubin & Emener, 1979) suggests a
shift in RC time allocation across job tasks since the mid-1960s. Examples of
such suggested changes include a reduction in the amount of RC time devoted
to counseling and guidance and an increase in RC time spent on paperwork
and arranging for services (Rubin & Emener, 1979).

Historically, it has been difficult to trace changes across time in the role and
function of the RC due to methodological variability among studies. For example, Rubin and Emener (1979) identified high variability across five RC role
and function studies "in regard to the number of role categories used as well as
the labels of those categories" (p. 145). Three studies (Emener & Rubin, 1980;
Muthard & Salomone, 1969; Rubin, Matkin, Ashley, Beardsley, May, Onstott,

Reprinted by permission from Volume 27 (1984), *Rehabilitation Counseling Bulletin*, pp. 225-231.

& Puckett, 1984) stand out as allowing for the most valid comparison to date, as they all used the 40-item Abbreviated Task Inventory (ATI) to study RC role and function. The current study attends to the issue of the changing role of the rehabilitation counselor by drawing on available data from those three studies.

The following specific research question was addressed: To what extent are the roles and functions of certified rehabilitation counselors today similar to those reported by rehabilitation counselors in previous research? Further attention to this question could be justified as being relevent to the RC's professional identity, education curriculum, and certification and licensure process.

METHOD

Source of Data

Data for this study were drawn from three RC role and function studies (Emener & Rubin, 1980; Muthard & Salomone, 1969; Rubin et al., 1984). In all three studies a sample of rehabilitation counselors rated each of the 40 items on the ATI (see Appendix C for actual items) on the Muthard and Salomone (1969) 8-point rating scale (see Appendix A). A few of the 40 items were very slightly modified by Rubin et al. (1984) to remove sexist language (e.g., his was changed to his/her). The wording of three items of the ATI (5, 15, and 21) was also modified by Rubin et al. during the process of developing their Job Task Inventory (JTI).

The Muthard and Salomone data were collected in 1966 and the Emener and Rubin data in 1979. The data for the Rubin et al. (1984) study were collected in early 1982. In the remainder of this article, these data will be referred to as 1966, 1979, and 1982 data. Means and standard deviations were available for the 1979 and 1982 data. Only means were available for the 1966 data. Two groups of practicing RCs are found in all three studies. They are:

1. State rehabilitation agency rehabilitation counselors (DVR RCs) (for the 1966 data, $N=218$; for 1979, $N=104$; for 1982, $N=317$); and
2. Private nonprofit rehabilitation facility rehabilitation counselors (PRF RCs) (for the 1966 data, $N=115$; for 1979, $N=29$; for 1982, $N=98$).

Certain differences between the 1966, 1979, and 1982 data with respect to sampling and data collection procedures should be noted. In the Muthard and Salomone (1969) study RCs were gathered together in 15 large cities and administered the 119-team Rehabilitation Counselor Task Inventory (in which was embedded the 40-item ATI). In the Emener and Rubin (1980) study the 40-item ATI was mailed to a random sample of persons on the National Rehabilitation Counseling Association mailing list. For the Rubin et al. (1984)

study, the 130-item JTI was mailed to approximately 7,000 certified rehabilitation counselors. The reader is referred to each of the original articles for a more complete description of the sample selected and data collected.

Data Analysis Procedures

To determine if a trend exists in the direction of change in the mean ratings of the 40 ATI items from 1966 to 1979 and 1979 to 1982, the sign test (Conover, 1971, pp. 121-122) was used. Independent samples t tests (Glass & Stanley, 1970, p. 195) using the means, standard deviations and Ns given for the 1979 and 1982 data sets were performed to test for the significance of change for each individual item. The Bonferroni procedure was used to control for inflating the alpha level when conducting 40 t tests. To obtain a family-wise probability of Type I errors of .05, the alpha level for each t test was set at .001 (Schafer & Dayton, 1981).

RESULTS AND DISCUSSION

Comparison of the 1966, 1979, and 1982 ATI item means showed that: (a) 77.5% of the DVR RCs' item means increased from 1966 to 1979; (b) 87.5% of the DVR RCs' item means increased from 1979 to 1982; (c) 85% of the PRF RCs' item means increased from 1966 to 1979; and (d) 85% of the PRF RCs' item means increased from 1979 to 1982. Sign tests (Hull & Nie, 1981, p. 327) of the significance of the directionality of change in the 40 matched pairs of means for each of the above four comparisons (DVR RCs 1966 vs. 1979 and 1979 vs. 1982; PRF RCs 1966 vs. 1979 and 1979 vs. 1982) were statistically significant at the .001 level. These results indicate that as one moves across the years 1966, 1979, and 1982, the ratings of RCs for the majority of ATI items increased.

Although the sign test results showed a statistically significant trend in direction of change, they did not address the significance of size of change for individual job task items. Independent samples t tests were used to address this latter area where possible (i.e., both means and standard deviations available). Independent samples t test comparisons of PRF RCs ratings for each of the 40 ATI items between 1979 and 1982 yielded no significant differences ($p < .001$). Independent samples t test comparison of DVR RCs' ratings for each of the 40 items between 1979 and 1982 yielded significant differences for only three of the ATI items. They were: (a) item 9, $t(419) = 3.58$, $p < .001$; (b) item 12, $t(419) = 4.08$, $p < .001$; and (c) item 32, $t(419) = 3.59$, $p < .001$. These items read as follows:

9. Discusses factors related to good work adjustment with the client to help him/her improve his/her employability.

12. Evaluates the client's past work adjustment by securing employer recommendations and evaluations.

32. Discusses the client's work skills with an employer and enumerates the client's work skills with an employer and specific tasks the client can do.

Two themes covered by these three job task items are work adjustment and dealing with employers. These findings suggest a recent increase in DVR RCs' focus on client job readiness and employer contacts. Possibly these increased emphases have been stimulated by the depressed economic conditions and increased unemployment rate during the last few years.

Although the absence of standard deviations for the 1966 data precluded comparison of individual item ratings via Independent samples *t* tests, observation of 1966 and 1979 DVR RCs' item means suggests that the following ATI items might have shown significant 1966 versus 1979 *t* test results if standard deviations (assuming that they were similar to 1979 *SD*s) were available:

16. Assess the consistency of the client's vocational choice with his/her personality.

19. Interprets results (may use test forms and protocols) and answers any questions the client has about group intelligence and special aptitude tests (e.g., GATB, Bennett Mechanical, Minnesota Clerical, Purdue Pegboard).

21. Recommends and makes available occupational files (briefs, abstracts, etc.) to explain job titles, duties, and requirements relevant to the client's general vocational goals.

22. Uses the Occupational Outlook Handbook and occupational files (brief, abstracts, etc.) to explain job titles, duties, and requirements that are relevant to the client's vocational goals.

23. Incorporates information covering broad occupational areas and specific jobs into the counseling interview.

25. Determines which special medical examinations the client requires.

29. Decides if medical or psychological services will reduce the vocational handicap.

36. Writes case notes and summaries (including analysis, reasoning, and comments) so that others can understand the client's progress.

38. Establishes working relationships with community organizations and leaders to secure referrals.

Each of the nine items listed above contains a difference between 1966 and 1979 means that exceeds the largest 1979 to 1982 difference (.82) between means found among the items that yielded significant ($p < .001$) *t* test results. Observation of the above list suggests that the diagnostic aspect of the RC's job (items 16, 19, 25, 29) expanded between 1966 and 1979. Similar 1966 versus 1979 findings can be observed for the expanded use by DVR RCs of formal sources of occupational information (items 21, 22, 23). Case recording (item 36) and case finding (item 38) also seem to have become a more substantial part of the RC's job.

Clearly absent on the above list are any items from the Beardsley and Matkin (1984) Vocational Counseling and Affective Counseling factors. This absence of potentially significant change in the extent to which vocational and affective counseling activities are a substantial part of the DVR RC's job role brings into question the results of research in the late 1970s (Fraser & Clowers, 1978; Rubin & Emener, 1979; Zadny & James, 1977) suggesting a decline in that aspect of the RC's job. Those studies all asked RCs to estimate the percentage of time they spent on each of several job activities. Possibly such research instrumentation (e.g., estimate percentages — all must add to 100%) is too "crude" to provide a valid picture of the RC's work role.

Observation of 1966 and 1979 PRF RCs' item means suggests that the following ATI items might have shown significant 1966 versus 1979 *t* test results if standard deviations (again assuming that they were similar to 1979 *SD*s) were available:

11. Helps clients, through group procedures, to learn and use new ways to deal with their problems.
24. Refers clients for psychiatric treatment.
29. Decides if medical or psychological services will reduce the vocational handicap.
36. Writes case notes and summaries (including analysis, reasoning, and comments) so that others can understand the client's progress.
37. Reports verbally on the client's progress to a rehabilitation team or other collaborators.
39. Collaborates with cooperating rehabilitation workers in planning and executing the client's rehabilitation plan.
40. Prepares a summary report or letter to describe the client to cooperating individuals or agencies.

Each of these seven items also contains a difference between their 1966 and 1979 means that exceeds .82. Examination of the content of the seven items suggests that compared to 1966, PRF RCs in 1979 were doing more group work (item 11), more services arrangement (items 24, 29, 39, 40), and more recording and reporting (items 36, 37).

SUMMARY AND CONCLUSIONS

The rehabilitation counselor role and function literature contains numerous studies that build the case for substantial change in the role and function of rehabilitation counselors (Emener & Rubin, 1980; Fraser & Clowers, 1978;

Rubin & Emener, 1979). The literature also contains the contradictory argument that the basic dimensionality of the RC's job has remained the same over time (Cobb, 1972; Livneh, 1980). The results of this study tend to suggest that changes in the RC's job have occurred, but not to the degree that would support the conclusion of a major modification in the basic dimensionality of that job role. As in the past, current RCs still do case management, counseling, service arrangement, placement and so forth.

It may very well be that any observable changes in rehabilitation education curriculums during the 1970s demonstrate more of an attempt to become consistent with an already established RC job role than to be responsive to changes in that role. In regard to certification and licensure exams, it is likely that the content focus that would be appropriate today would also have been appropriate in the early 1970s. Future major modification in the content emphasis of such exams would seem to be unwarranted unless distinct changes in the dimensionality of the RC's role occur.

ACKNOWLEDGMENTS

This research emanated from the responsibilities assigned to the Examinations Committee of the Commission on Rehabilitation Counselor Certification. The CRCC Examinations Committee is chaired by Stanford E. Rubin. Sincerest appreciation is extended to Eda Holt, Executive Director of CRCC, and to Art Bowers for their invaluable technical assistance with this project. Sincerest appreciation is extended also to W. Russell Wright for his contributory expertise during the analysis phase of the project. Finally, sincerest appreciation is offered to Joseph Ashley, Mark Beardsley, William Garner, Suzanne Johnson, Ralph Matkin, Virgil R. May, Karan Onstott, and Rene Prentki for their critical reading of and valuable suggestions for the early drafts of this paper.

REFERENCES

Beardsley, M.M., & Matkin, R.E. (1984). The abbreviated task inventory: Implications for future role and function research. *Rehabilitation Counseling Bulletin, 27,* 232-237.

Cobb, B. (1972). The challenge of new dimensions in rehabilitation counselor education. In J.G. Cull & R.E. Hardy (Eds.). *Vocational rehabilitation: Profession and process.* Springfield, IL: Charles C Thomas.

Conover, W.J. (1971). *Practical nonparametric statistics.* New York: John Wiley.

Emener, W.G., & Rubin, S.E. (1980). Rehabilitation counselor roles and functions and sources of role strain. *Journal of Applied Rehabilitation Counseling, 11,* 57-69.

Fraser, R.T., & Clowers, M.R. (1978). Rehabilitation counselor functions: Perceptions of time spent and complexity. *Journal of Applied Rehabilitation Counseling, 9,* 31-35.

Glass, G.V., & Stanley, J.C. (1970). *Statistical methods in education and psychology.* Englewood Cliffs, NJ: Prentice-Hall.

Hull, C.H., & Nie, N.H. (1981). *SPSS update 7-9.* New York: McGraw-Hill.

Livneh, H. (1981). Rehabilitation counselor functions and tasks in Rhode Island. *Rehabilitation Counseling Bulletin, 25,* 101-104.

Muthard, J.E., & Salomone, P.R. (1969). The roles and functions of the rehabilitation counselor. *Rehabilitation Counseling Bulletin, 13,* 81-168.

Roessler, R.T., & Rubin, S.E. (1982). *Case management and rehabilitation counseling.* Baltimore: University Park Press.

Rubin, S.E., & Emener, W.G. (1979). Recent rehabilitation counselor role changes and role strain—A pilot investigation. *Journal of Applied Rehabilitation Counseling, 10,* 142-147.

Rubin, S.E., Matkin, R.E., Ashley, J.M., Beardsley, M.M., May, V.R., Onstott, K.L., & Puckett, F. (1984). Roles and functions of the certified rehabilitation counselor. *Rehabilitation Counseling Bulletin, 27,* 199-224.

Schafer, W.D., & Dayton, C.M. (1981). Techniques for simultaneous inference. *Personnel and Guidance Journal, 59,* 631-636.

Zadny, J.J., & James, L.F. (1977). Time spent on placement. *Rehabilitation Counseling Bulletin, 21,* 31-35.

CHAPTER 9

A CRITIQUE OF TRENDS IN REHABILITATION COUNSELOR EDUCATION TOWARD SPECIALIZATION

Kenneth R. Thomas

Abstract

In this article current trends and practices in rehabilitation counselor education with respect to specialization are critiqued in terms of their implications for students, clients, and the profession itself. Four broad categories of specialization are identified and discussed: preparation of students to work with specific disability groups, preparation for employment in particular settings, preparation for counseling in specific life areas, and the development of skills in applying particular treatment methods. Recommendations are offered for restructuring current approaches.

THROUGHOUT the relatively brief history of rehabilitation counseling it has been debated whether counselors should be generalists, specialists, or both. An excellent summary of this debate is presented by Wright (1980), who thoroughly researched both early and current thinking on this issue and then offered recommendations for implementing the specialization concept within the existing state-federal vocational rehabilitation program.

Insofar as rehabilitation counselor education (RCE) is concerned, probably the most visible critic of the specialization concept has been C.H. Patterson (1965, 1967). While Patterson felt that specialization in rehabilitation counseling was both inevitable and desirable, he warned that specialization risks breaking the individual into parts and also pointed out several logistical problems in terms of counselor training and counselor role which he felt would have

Reprinted by permission from Volume 48, 1982, *Journal of Rehabilitation*, pp. 49-51.

This article is based in part on a paper of the same title presented at the annual convention of the American Personnel and Guidance Association, Washington, D.C., March, 1978.

to be dealt with very carefully as the practice of specialization became more universal.

Although Patterson alluded to a post-master's program at the University of Illinois which prepared counselors to work with deaf persons, specialization in RCE was almost nonexistent when he authored his 1967 article on specialization in rehabilitation counseling. Since that time, however, several graduate training programs offering different types of specialization in rehabilitation counseling have emerged.

The purpose of the present article is to provide a critique of current trends and practices in RCE with respect to specialization. While the term *specialization* will be used throughout the article to refer to the preparation of rehabilitation counselors who are to assume special responsibilities, it should be noted from the outset that a better term might be *subspecialization* or *emphasis* since in the author's opinion rehabilitation counseling itself is really a specialization within the generic field of counseling. To draw an analogy from the field of medicine: A physician who specializes in pediatrics with a subspecialty in hematology (i.e., a pediatrician, who, for example, is an expert on child leukemia) is a physician none the less. Similarly, a counselor who specializes in rehabilitation (a rehabilitation counselor) and who has developed a subspecialty in some aspect of rehabilitation (e.g., Workers' Compensation) is still a counselor. Therefore, the major concern of this article is not really the pros and cons of specialization, but rather the pros and cons of subspecializations or emphases.

The above-expressed semantic considerations notwithstanding, let it be stated immediately, lest the author be forever cursed as the Don Quixote of rehabilitation counseling, that further "specialization" in RCE is virtually inevitable. Among the reasons for this probable eventuality are the following:

1. Rehabilitation students, counselors, and counselor educators differ in their interests and abilities;
2. University training programs differ in their capacity to offer varying types of didactic and clinical instruction;
3. The variety of roles and functions expected of the rehabilitation counselor is really quite extensive;
4. Clients bring an enormous variety of disabilities and handicapping problems to the rehabilitation process;
5. Rehabilitation counselors work in a wide range of employment settings which may have different requisites for success;
6. The additional knowledge gained about various client groups and about different aspects of the rehabilitation process will ultimately limit the effectiveness of the generalist;
7. The field is constantly being bombarded with new priorities such as vocational evaluation culturally disabled persons, program evaluation,

severely disabled persons, job placement, and independent living; and

8. The federal government has deemed it appropriate to separately subsidize graduate programs which do not conform to the traditional generic RCE training model.

As a result of these factors, several types of master's level training programs have been developed which either purport to train students to work with a specific disability group or to become especially proficient in performing a particular aspect of the rehabilitation process. For the purposes of this article, four broad categories of specialization in rehabilitation counselor education have been identified which will be critiqued in terms of their implications for students, clients, and the profession itself.

PREPARATION TO WORK WITH SPECIFIC DISABILITY GROUPS

Probably the most obvious form of specialization in RCE is the preparation of students to work with a specific disability group such as blind, deaf, or mentally retarded persons. These programs are usually offered by the universities involved either because special monies have been provided for this purpose by the federal government or because the strengths of the faculty and community resources naturally facilitate the development of expertise with a particular disability group.

Justification for this type of specialization should be based on the meeting of at least three assumptions. First, it must be assumed that members of the particular client group involved differ significantly from other clients in terms of their overall personality and behavioral characteristics. Secondly, it must be assumed that special counselor competencies and knowledges are necessary to be effective with this particular client group. And finally, it must be assumed that a large enough body of knowledge exists about this particular client group to warrant or require intensive study. The first two of these assumptions have yet to be demonstrated in the research literature, and the third is at least debatable.

Although it is likely that certain patterns of functional limitations could be universally associated with persons possessing the same type of disability, existing research data tend to contraindicate the idea that persons with different disabilities have different personality characteristics (Shontz, 1975). There is also little research evidence to suggest that different client groups require different counselor competencies or rehabilitation methods. Obviously, rehabilitation counselors working with deaf persons should be able to sign, and those working with Spanish-speaking clients should be able to speak Spanish. However, whether the development of such competencies should constitute the bulk of a graduate program in rehabilitation counseling is highly debatable. It is also debatable, unless clients are broadly classified into groups such as the physically disabled, the emotionally disturbed or the mentally retarded, whether a large enough body of rehabilitation-related knowledge exists about any particular disability group to require more than one or two additional courses of study.

Unfortunately, by calling attention to the *categorical* differences between persons with different types of disabilities, either through specialization or by earmarking such persons for special study or services. legislators and educators reinforce the act of labeling and the potentially negative consequences thereof. Through the offering of specialization options at the master's level, educators may also be unnecessarily limiting the employment opportunities of students by encouraging them to focus on a client group which may have little legislative or administrative priority in the future.

PREPARATION FOR EMPLOYMENT IN PARTICULAR SETTINGS

A second type of specialization in master's level RCE programs involves the preparation of students for employment in particular work settings. This type of specialization is usually not advertised or even explicitly stated; it results primarily from the orientation of the faculty and the types of university and community resources available.

Probably the most obvious example of this kind of specialization is the inordinate amount of emphasis placed by some RCE programs on preparing graduates for employment with state vocational rehabilitation agencies. (In fact, it is rumored that several years ago at least one RCE program went so far as to require students in "Foundations" to memorize the state agency operations manual). While some might argue that such an emphasis is justifiable because many RCE programs and students are at least partially funded under the auspices of the state-federal vocational rehabilitation program, limiting graduate instruction to the preparation of students for employment in state rehabilitation agencies raises serious questions about the vitality and status of rehabilitation counseling as a field and academic discipline. Not to be outdone, other programs may place almost exclusive emphasis on the preparation of students for employment in medical settings, sheltered workshops, mental health centers, or *any place but a state vocational rehabilitation agency.*

Considered collectively, specializations which prepare students for employment in a particular work setting can be justified to the extent that they clearly reflect student interest and the strengths of the faculty and the community resources available. However, such specializations invariably result in giving students a narrow, unrealistic perspective on the profession and many also limit the range of employment opportunities available after graduation.

PREPARATION FOR COUNSELING IN SPECIFIC LIFE AREAS

Another type of specialization in RCE involves what may be called the emphasis given to remediating particular aspects of the client's adjustment problems. It refers to the relative importance placed by RCE programs on preparing students to be able to deal with clients' vocational, personal, or social adjustment problems. This type of specialization typically results from a bias (sometimes unconscious) on the part of the faculty. Specializations resulting from this kind of bias are so prevalent that one easily gets the impression that many rehabilitation counselor educators feel some moral obligation to commit either for or against the relative importance of personal versus vocational adjustment.

It almost goes without saying that an approach to counseling which treats vocational and personal adjustment as autonomous entities is likely to be ineffective. Similarly, it is inappropriate to practice RCE as though personal and vocational counseling were separate entities. Not only does overemphasis (or deemphasis) of the importance of vocational versus personal adjustment counseling handicap students in terms of their clinical effectiveness, it may also confuse them about their future roles as counselors. For example, overemphasis on the personal adjustment aspects of counseling is quite unrealistic in terms of the primary mission of most rehabilitation agencies and facilities and may also ignore the considerable impact of one's vocational competencies on personal adjustment. Overemphasis on vocational counseling, on the other hand, often negates the importance that personal adjustment can play in employability. Overemphasis on the vocational aspects also tends to overlook the long-standing trend in the field of rehabilitation toward a broader definition of program objectives.

The practice of viewing clients holistically is deeply rooted in rehabilitation tradition and philosophy. For rehabilitation counselors or educators to disregard either the vocational or personal aspects of adjustment risks, as pointed out by Patterson (1965, 1967), breaking the individual into parts is neither good rehabilitation practice or philosophy.

PREPARATION FOR EXPERTISE IN APPLYING PARTICULAR TREATMENT METHODS

The fourth and final type of specialization in RCE is the emphasis placed by some programs on helping students to develop expertise in applying particular treatment techniques or in performing specific aspects of the rehabilitation process. Included in this category are emphases on specific treatment techniques such as behavior modification and affective counseling and emphases on particular aspects of the rehabilitation process such as vocational evaluation, work adjustment, and job placement.

Specialization in applying particular treatment techniques offers both advantages and disadvantages. One advantage is that students receive a consistent theoretical frame of reference from which to view client behavior and development. Moreover, the students probably become especially adept and effective in applying at least one treatment strategy. A disadvantage, however, is that the students may receive little exposure to other treatment strategies which would be just as effective. Also, of course, the assumption that *all* clients will respond to the same treatment strategy is a tenuous one at best — not to mention the problem of assuming that *all* students can be trained to effectively use a particular treatment strategy.

Specializations in vocational evaluation and job placement are really in their own league since both are represented by some educators as being "professions" distinct from rehabilitation counseling. The question is whether the development of separate training programs at the master's level in either of these areas was very appropriate. Studies have consistently shown that vocational evaluation (assessment) and job placement are included in the roles and functions of the rehabilitation counselor (Emener & Rubin, 1980; Muthard & Salomone, 1969; Wright, Smits, Butler, & Thoreson, 1968). Moreover, it is dubious that anyone who exclusively practices vocational evaluation or job placement could be particularly effective without possessing considerable knowledge about disability and skills in counseling and communication. As such, one wonders whether these specializations might have been better offered at the post-master's level rather than as a substitute for a master's degree in rehabilitation counseling. Unfortunately, the way these training programs are presently structured they are preparing students for entrance into "professions" which are not even listed in the *Dictionary of Occupational Titles* or the *Occupational Outlook Handbook*.

RECOMMENDATIONS

While recognizing the inevitability and inherent advantages of some amount of specialization in RCE, at least two considerations are recommended before establishing such programs:

1. Make certain that graduates are not locked into something which affords limited employment opportunities or exclusive identification with a "profession" only a few recognize; and

2. Make certain that other disability groups, work settings, life adjustment areas, counseling theories and techniques, and other areas of the rehabilitation process are not ignored at the expense of the specialization.

In other words, consider providing a comprehensive, generic orientation to rehabilitation counseling before worrying about the specialization.

This orientation would include clinical practice experience in a variety of employment settings and the opportunity to work with a variety of client groups. In fact, it probably makes the most sense to encourage specialization at the post-master's level only. At least by that time students will have obtained a thorough orientation to the theory and practice of rehabilitation counseling and will have had the opportunity to sample many aspects of the profession before opting to specialize in one.

REFERENCES

Emener, W.G. & Rubin, S.E. Rehabilitation counselor roles and functions and sources of role strain. *The Journal of Applied Rehabilitation Counseling,* 1980, *11*(2), 57-69.

Muthard, J.E. & Salomone, P.R. The roles and functions of the rehabilitation counselor. *Rehabilitation Counseling Bulletin,* 1969, *13*(1-SP), 81-168.

Patterson, C.H. Specialization in rehabilitation counseling. In W. Holbert (Ed.), *Proceedings of a conference on vocational rehabilitation counselor specialization: Cause and effects.* Atlanta, GA: April 29-30, 1965, pp. 11-20.

Patterson, C.H. Specialization in rehabilitation counseling. *Rehabilitation Counseling Bulletin,* 1967, *10*(4), 147-154.

Shontz, F.C. *The psychological aspects of physical illness and disability.* New York, NY: MacMillan, 1975.

Wright, G.N. *Total rehabilitation.* Boston, MA: Little, Brown and Company, 1980.

Wright, G.N.; Smits, S.J.; Butler, A.J.; & Thoreson, R.W. *A survey of counselor perceptions.* Madison, WI: University of Wisconsin, Regional Rehabilitation Research Institute, 1968.

CHAPTER 10

TRAINING INDEPENDENT LIVING REHABILITATION SPECIALISTS

Richard T. Roessler

Abstract

The growth of independent living rehabilitation has created the need for graduate training in independent living rehabilitation. Independent living training programs should be multidisciplinary in nature and focus on the needs which must be met if individuals with disabilities are to participate more fully in life of the home, community, and work place. The article to follow discusses the efforts underway at the University of Arkansas to develop an independent living rehabilitation specialists program at the master's level.

INTRODUCTION

LEGISLATIVE efforts to establish independent living rehabilitation services began 20 to 30 years ago. However, concrete outcomes of those activities have only recently come in the Comprehensive Needs Study of the 1973 Rehabilitation Act and the provisions for independent living services in Title VII, Parts A-C in the 1978 Amendments.

Recognizing the need for independent living services and graduate training in independent living rehabilitation, the Rehabilitation Services Administration awarded an Experimental and Innovative Training grant in independent living to the University of Arkansas Rehabilitation Education program and the Arkansas Rehabilitation Research and Training Center. Independent living rehabilitation students at the University of Arkansas complete a 54 hour master's degree. The program stresses recruitment of handicapped and minority students for placement in independent living programs serving rural areas. In

Reprinted by permission from Volume 47, 1981, *Journal of Rehabilitation*, pp. 36-39.

fact, study of the implications of serving rural areas in independent living rehabilitation is a primary focus of the program. Other major objectives of the
training program include:

1. Integrating more knowledge regarding independent living rehabilitation into existing courses in rehabilitation, special education and related areas.
2. Seeking the advice and support of handicapped consumers, rehabilitation service providers, and others in the design and conduct of the program.
3. Developing and maintaining relations with a wide variety of independent living rehabilitation projects in HHS Region VI.

With input from an Advisory Committee of consumers and rehabilitation
professionals, Rehabilitation Education is broadening its curriculum to include
issues pertinent both to independent living and vocational rehabilitation. In
addition, students specializing in independent living rehabilitation will complete an independent living and community adjustment block of courses. Upon
completion of their course work, these students will enroll in internship experiences which will involve them in supervised service delivery in an independent living rehabilitation setting.

The independent living effort in Rehabilitation Education is also coupled
with similar developments in Special Education. Students in Special Education
preparing for work in school settings will complete core courses in Special Education and then enter the independent living course block with Rehabilitation
Education students. Students in Special Education will also complete an internship in which they will receive supervised practice in the delivery of independent living services.

Independent Living Curriculum

With basic training in Rehabilitation Education as a foundation, students
specializing in independent living complete an independent living and community adjustment block of courses including;

Community Organization

This course is offered by Rural Sociology and focuses on the community in
terms of communication networks, value systems, stratification of social
groups, social control, structure and function of major community systems and
community action and development. Special emphasis is placed on community
attitude formation and change and the role of consumer involvement in affecting social policy.

Recreation for Special Populations

Offered by the Health, Physical Education, and Recreation Department, this course enables students to develop the skills, knowledge, and concepts within recreation which are appropriate for planning and implementing recreation programs and services for the handicapped.

Educational Methods in Adaptive Physical Education

This course provides instruction in the assessment, prescription, adaptation, and use of instructional methods, materials, and equipment relevant to specific handicapping conditions in the physical education setting.

Seminar in Home Management and Family Living for Disabled Individuals

In this seminar, students are introduced to problems, adaptations, and rehabilitation techniques for home management and family relations for various handicapping conditions.

Group Home Living and Administration

The Special Education Department involves students in a study of alternative living arrangements for individuals with disabilities. Techniques of administration, finance, supervision, and programming for group living situations are also discussed.

Independent Living and Community Adjustment

Offered by the Rehabilitation Education program, this course focuses on an intensive study of the problems and practices involved in developing and maintaining independent living and community adjustment by individuals who have severe disabilities of a physical, emotional or intellectual nature. Specific problems focused on in the course include housing, employment, transportation, recreation, health maintenance, home management, family relations, peer counseling, and client advocacy.

Because it addresses independent living in depth, the course on independent living and community adjustment merits further discussion (a course syllabus is available on request). The objective of the course is to provide students with knowledge of the history, philosophy and services of independent living. Special topics to be covered include history and philosophy of independent living rehabilitation, barriers to independent living, evaluation of needs in independent living, methods and models of service delivery in independent living rehabilitation, consumer involvement and advocacy, models of peer counseling, overcoming architectural and transportation barriers, legal rights of individuals with disabilities, financial resources for independent living needs, and service approaches in independent living rehabilitation.

In addition to reading an extensive list of articles and books for the course, students will complete a research paper on a selected topic in independent living rehabilitation. They will also participate in independent living seminars;

e.g., needs in independent living rehabilitation identified by a panel of individuals who have severe disabilities, environmental and community attitude barriers to independent living discussed by the staff of the Disabled Students Office at the University of Arkansas, designing buildings and homes for barrier-free living presented by a member of the School of Architecture faculty, and legal rights of individuals with disabilities presented by a member of the Northwest Arkansas Legal Aid Staff.

Other special assignments in the course include a home visit to assess independent living needs of an individual with a disability and study and classroom demonstration of a service approach responsive to an independent living need. The home visit should be coordinated with a local rehabilitation counselor or facility counselor, the individual being visited, and the instructor. The purpose of the student's visit is to assess the individual's self-care, housing, transportation, daily living needs, etc., to determine whether additional services of an independent living nature are required. The counselor working with the client should then be informed of the individual's need for additional assistance.

Selection of an independent living service to demonstrate in the course could be made from the New Options training materials (Cole, Sperry, Board, & Frieden, 1979), career education literature (Brolin, 1978), and personal adjustment training packages (Means & Roessler, 1976; Roessler & Means, 1977). Other potential service areas in which students might develop presentations include housing referral and adaptation, avocational counseling, client advocacy, job seeking skills, job modification, peer counseling, etc.

Students will also have the opportunity to take field trips to independent living programs in Arkansas and nearby states. These visits will include independent living centers serving both rural and metropolitan areas. During the visit, students will be introduced to the services provided by the agency. Students will also have an opportunity to visit with clients of the program and discuss issues relevant to independent living.

Since the independent living and community adjustment course will be taught for the first time in the spring of 1981, it is not possible to provide feedback on the course readings or experience. However, the course readings which are listed in the syllabus introduce students to the writings of many individuals who have done significant work in the field of independent living (Bowe, 1978 & 1980, Bowe & Williams, 1979; DeJong, 1979; Frieden, 1975; Hull, 1979; Institute on Rehabilitation Issues, 1978 & 1980; Pflueger, 1977; Varella, 1980; Walton, Schwab, Cassatt-Dunn, Wright, 1980).

It is anticipated that students will apply the skills they have learned in the independent living course in their practica and internship placements. These placements will be in independent living rehabilitation centers, group homes, rehabilitation facilities, and rehabilitation agency settings which are offering independent living services. In their practica and internships, students will gain supervised experience in providing the many independent living services listed in the Rehabilitation amendments of 1978, e.g., intake counseling, selection and training of attendants, legal and economic rights of individuals with disabilities, independent living skills training, housing and transportation referral and assistance, housing and transportation surveys and directories, health maintenance, peer counseling, activities of daily living training, recreational counseling, and financial counseling.

SPECIAL CONSIDERATIONS IN INDEPENDENT LIVING TRAINING

In a recent meeting, the Advisory Committee for the Arkansas program made many valuable suggestions about independent living training. For example, independent living rehabilitation training should be responsive to the needs of many individuals. Too often one thinks of independent living as basically a program for the physically disabled. Independent living rehabilitation should also focus on the special needs of individuals with intellectual impairments and individuals with emotional disorders so that issues of accessibility, life competencies, and personal adjustment are considered in as broad a sense as possible.

Students in an independent living rehabilitation program should have close contact with individuals with disabilities. Since many students in independent living training will themselves have disabilities, part of that principle is automatically followed. But, it is important for these students also to learn from individuals who are coping with different sets of problems as a result of different types of disabilities. Experiences such as home visits, joint recreation and travel, seminars, and supervised practice in independent living programs will bring students in the program together with individuals with a wide range of disabilities.

Another resource that would be a great help in developing an independent living rehabilitation program would be a demonstration site. This model independent living laboratory could serve both as a training site for students and as a site for evaluating new service programs in independent living rehabilitation.

Rehabilitation programs moving into independent living should also encouage other departments to develop new courses or modify existing courses to include more information on disability and its effects. Though this interdisciplinary approach is desirable, rehabilitation education departments may have some difficulty stimulating it due to limited resources. One way to encourage such interest is with the promise of new students coming into the course and related department.

Another aspect of curriculum development was pointed out by members of the Advisory Committee. For several reasons, graduates at the master's level in independent living rehabilitation should have management skills. First, many independent living centers will seek such people as directors of their programs. Individuals with master's degree training in independent living may also supervise teams of individuals. This need for management expertise also suggests the development of new specializations focusing on independent living rehabilitation programs within rehabilitation administration programs.

Another important consideration in providing a program in independent living rehabilitation is the accessibility of the campus. Due to the enrollment of many disabled individuals in independent living, the program and campus must be accessible and have adequate educational support and transportation services.

Finally, the traditional, clear-cut outcome in vocational rehabilitation, status "26" or employment, is not inclusive enough for independent living rehabilitation. Therefore, trainees in independent living rehabilitation should have (a) knowledge of the many areas in which environmental change and individual gain is possible, (b) a concrete understanding of service approaches to effect these changes, and (c) a methodology for assessing change as a result of independent living services.

IMPLICATIONS

Implications for the development of independent living training in rehabilitation counselor education include:

1. Independent living students must develop capabilities to assist individuals with disabilities in a broad range of life planning activities. Hence, new courses in home modification, community relations, recreation, adaptive physical activities, independent living rehabilitation, management and administration, and community organization must be added to the curriculum.
2. Practica and internship placements should be developed for students in independent living centers, transitional and group home settings, and comprehensive rehabilitation centers emphasizing independent living training.
3. Independent living rehabilitation should not be limited to serving those with physical disabilities. It has a vital role to play in increasing the autonomy of individuals with intellectual and emotional impairments as well.
4. Throughout their programs, students in independent living should have close contact with individuals who are coping on a daily basis with disability-related problems. Activities such as home visits, joint recreation and travel, seminars, work in an independent living

demonstration site, and supervised internships in independent living programs contribute to this objective.

5. Finally, because the scope of independent living rehabilitation services is extremely broad, students should be encouraged to use their creativity to develop services and resources which enhance individual autonomy and life satisfaction. However, certain services are particularly germane to independent living rehabilitation; e.g., identification, selection, and training of attendants; personal health care; transportation; housing and home modification; financial counseling; and life planning.

CONCLUSION

The need for independent living rehabilitation services was clearly demonstrated by the Comprehensive Needs Study commissioned by the Rehabilitation Act of 1973. Based on this documented need, the 1978 Amendments called for the provision of such services by state agencies (Title VII, Section A) and by centers for independent living (Title VII, Section B). The only missing ingredient at this point is adequate funding to implement the program. With the advent of sufficient state/federal appropriations for comprehensive services, rehabilitation counseling education programs will find many new employment opportunities for program graduates who have a specialization in independent living rehabilitation.

REFERENCES

Bowe, F. *Handicapping America*. New York: Harper & Row, 1978.

Bowe, F. *Handicapping America*. New York: Harper & Row, 1980.

Bowe, F. & Williams, J. *Planning effective advocacy programs*. American Coalition of Citizens with Disabilities, Washington, D.C., 1979.

Brolin, D. *Life centered career education: A competency based approach*. Reston, Va.: Council for Exceptional Children, 1978.

Cole, J., Sperry, J., Board, M. & Frieden, L. *New Options*. Texas Institute for Rehabilitation and Research, Houston, Tex., 1979.

DeJong, G. *The movement for independent living: Origins, ideology, and implications for disability research*. University Centers for International Rehabilitation, Michigan State University, East Lansing, Michigan, 1979.

Frieden, L. Independent living arrangements for the severely disabled. Report of the state-of-the-art conference. Center for Independent Living. RSA grant 45-P-45484/9-01, 1975.

Hull, K. *The rights of physically handicapped people*. New York: Avon Books, 1979.

Institute on Rehabilitation Issues. The role of vocational rehabilitation in independent living. Arkansas Rehabilitation Research and Training Center, Hot Springs, Ark., 1978.

Institute on Rehabilitation Issues. Implementations of independent living center programs in rehabilitation. Arkansas Rehabilitation Research and Training Center, Hot Springs, Ark. 1981.

Means, B., & Roessler, R. *Personal Achievement Skills.* Arkansas Rehabilitation Research and Training Center, Hot Springs, Ark., 1976.

Pflueger, S. *Independent living.* Institute for Research Utilization, Washington, D.C., 1977.

Roessler, R., & Means, B. *Personal Achievement Skills for the visually handicapped.* Arkansas Rehabilitation Research and Training Center, Hot Springs, Ark., 1977.

Varella, R. *Participating citizens.* American Coalition of Citizens with Disabilities, Washington, D.C., 1980.

Walton, K., Schwab, L., Cassatt-Dunn, M., & Wright, V. Independent living: Perceptions by professionals in rehabilitation. *Journal of Rehabilitation,* 1980, *46*(3), 57-63.

CHAPTER 11

PLACEMENT PERSONNEL—A GRADUATE PROGRAM CONCEPT

WILLIAM M. USDANE

T HE REHABILITATION ACT OF 1973 clearly notes an emphasis upon comprehensive services to severely handicapped individuals; these services are aimed at the eventual *employability* of this group. While there may have been many reasons in the past for avoidance of special priority with the most severely handicapped persons and their employability, their placement prospects have in many ways been mainly hindered by a *lack of well-trained rehabilitation placement personnel* to assist them in entering the labor market.

The current functional job demands of the state rehabilitation counselor are multiple. His coordinator activities, those of counseling, evaluation, and community relationships have all contrived to make it difficult for him to spend much time on the job development, job solicitation, job placement, and post-employment counseling areas.

Until placement work is given professional recognition and training on the graduate level equal to that of rehabilitation counseling and work evaluation, the severely handicapped individual will continue to lack professional assistance in attaining the dignity of an appropriate job.

The focus of the Rehabilitation Services Administration on vocationally rehabilitating the handicapped person for over fifty years has never included a sustained and distinct university training program for someone specifically called the *placement worker*. RSA has exhibited interest in the placement process from a training standpoint primarily through emphasis over the past thirty-five years on short-term training programs, state, regional and national placement institutes, and an employment accountability system.

Reprinted by permission from Volume 40 (1974), *Journal of Rehabilitation*, pp. 12-13.

CREATIVE DEVELOPMENTS & CHANGING TIMES

The rehabilitation process has undergone considerable change from the time when severely disabled individuals, now considered good prospects for industrial placement, were maintained in sheltered workshop settings. Creative developments in innovative assessment and evaluation techniques involving the severely disabled person have culminated in graduate training programs in vocational evaluation and work adjustment. These graduates along with the rehabilitation counselor training program graduates have provided types of professional assistance in counseling and assessment that prepare the severely disabled for proper placement.

As yet, unfortunately, the third member of the triumvirate, the placement worker, has neither graduate training programs to launch him, nor a clear recognition by the field of rehabilitation that he is needed as the third member of that triumvirate: rehabilitation counselor, work evaluator, and placement worker.

THE WORK-DEPRIVED ADOLESCENT

Erikson[1] notes a principle called a "sense of apprenticeship." This can be obtained through a paper route, an after-school job, a Saturday job, or any involvement in which the adolescent finds his general aptitudes and competencies adequate for the job. But the severely disabled, especially the congenitially severely disabled, do not go through this youth identification with any type of work sequence. Instead, the time of these individuals is taken up with physical medicine activities, or frequent lengthy hospitalizations. There is a tendency for them to have a deep sense of the inadequacy of their work competencies — a lack of confidence in their work "equipment."

The placement worker can assist in providing the severely disabled individual with a certain status of apprenticeship. For the past three years, RSA's experience with *Projects With Industry* has given many severely handicapped persons a "sense of apprenticeship" and a true sense of identification with work. This identification with work is an important aspect of growth and development. Erikson[1] states that though all children need time to play alone, time to spend in fantasy games, a child will never be completely satisfied unless he/she learns to make things well. Erikson labels this need as the "sense of industry." He feels further that this need must be met before the person can assume the role of parenthood.

A GRADUATE PROGRAM

A trisemester graduate program is suggested leading to the M.A. degree in placement work. This is not to imply that rehabilitation counselors cease to include placement functions along with other duties. Just as work evaluators and workers in work adjustment services have strengthened the role and function of the rehabilitation counselor, the development of a program to train individuals in placement work, is intended to complement the role and function of rehabilitation counseling.

Conceptually, the curriculum should be based upon the rehabilitation facility as an educational co-partner in the training process. In the first semester, four courses should be taught in the milieu of a halfway house, a rehabilitation center, a sheltered workshop, or a work evaluation and adjustment facility. Full graduate credit should be given to all off campus courses. The second semester should involve full-time fieldwork directly related to the placement process and within the milieu of a rehabilitation setting. The third semester should be conducted on the university campus, bringing together fieldwork experiences with final course content.

FIRST SEMESTER

Labor Economics and Job Development for the Severely Handicapped: (3 Units)

Labor market analysis; public policies and programs; theories and problems of economic growth; causes of unemployment; analysis of business cycles; transitional employment for the severely disabled; economic cycle forecasting.

Personnel Management and Industrial Relations Policy and Practice for the Severely Disabled: (3)

Labor management relations; personnel management practices and procedures; theories of managerial leadership; collective bargaining and the conduct of labor relations under agreements, unionism and job engineering; minimum wage law.

Medical-Social-Vocational Preparation of the Severely Handicapped for Job Readiness:

Medical orientation and use of medical information in the placement process; medical lectures in various diagnostic areas; consideration of psychiatric problems of the deinstitutionalized mental patient, and job analysis and modifications for the severely handicapped; use of consultation. Assembling, evaluating, and summarizing social and vocational information. Teamwork aspects of rehabilitation. Sources of information about occupations and their functional, physical, and intellectual requirements.

Organization and Administration of Community Services for Job Placement Process of the Severely Disabled:

Understanding the mandates of laws, regulations, and guidelines pertaining to the disabled; Rehabilitation Act of 1973, Social Security Act, Wagner O'Day Act, Randolph Sheppard Act, Housing and Transportation provisions; nature, scope and responsibilities of rehabilitation, health, and welfare agencies from a local, regional, and national standpoint; translation of professional skills in placement process to effective interaction with agencies and community for client advocacy.

SECOND SEMESTER (15 Units)

Field Internship in the Placement Process

The entire semester should be an agency involved with the placement of the severely disabled in gainful employment, transitional employment, or extended employment; job development and job solicitation; understanding and use of a job bank; development of specialized techniques in placement of blind persons; development of specialized techniques in placement of deaf persons; short-range and long-range placement plan development; techniques of job interview for client preparation; post job assistance with clients for client adjustment; differentiating problems of client employability and client placement potential; supervision for integration of course work and clinical practice; criteria and methods for student evaluation; procedures and techniques to assist students to evaluate their progress as an aid to professional self-development.

THIRD SEMESTER

(Only Semester Taken on Campus)

Small Business Management for Severely Handicapped Persons: (3)

Sources of assistance to small business management; essentials of operating a small business; workmen's compensation laws and principles; community resources for the disabled as assists in small business management; records and reports; research and demonstration findings (the DHEW/Social and Rehabilitation Research Reports); role of disabled individual's family in small business management; Randolph Sheppard Vending Stand Program.

Psycho-dynamics of Job Development and Job Solicitation: (3)

Techniques in employer contacts and job opportunities; role of placement work in employer relations; use of advisory committees and community consultants; development of on-the-job training programs; interaction with chambers of commerce in job development; job objectives for the homebound in data processing and information services.

Post-Job Adjustment of Severely Disabled Persons in Workshops or Industry: (3)

Follow-along and follow-up processes and techniques; group placements in job site evaluations; use of apartment and other housing approaches conjointly with job adjustment; use of transportation solutions to job adjustment problems.

Special Study (1-3)

Arising out of problems encountered during the internship, students should develop and plan a special study under supervision of the faculty; written report of study should be shared with facility in which problem arose.

SUMMARY

With new legislation emphasizing high priority for the severely disabled individual's eventual gainful employment, we must recognize that all legislation is experimental. We must recognize that rehabilitation service is a dynamic process — not a finished article. There are evidences of progress in our quest for a higher profile of the placement process, and the *Job Placement Division* is providing leadership on both national and local levels. There is literature already accumulated over the past decade that can provide a base for professional training in placement work.

Publications are available on placement techniques for blind persons and deaf persons — the result of specialized short-term training conferences of the past. The RSA Institute of Rehabilitation Services has published two documents on the placement process, and currently RSA has established a placement task force at the national level. The upcoming JPD national conference on placement is even more evidence that it is time to build upon these data for the careful development of a new professional individual whose responsibility for and with the severely handicapped individual provides the capstone of the rehabilitation process.

Selected Abstracts

Disability and Counselor Education

G.A. Lafaro (1982, p. 200)

Mainstreaming legislation is an impetus for social change in relation to treatment of individuals with disabilities. This change requires that counselor educators include content areas related to aspects of disability to prepare counselors to serve clients with disabilities. The author makes recommendations for curricular change for experiential and didactic training to increase a counselor trainee's sensitivity, skills, and knowledge regarding disability. Also, counselor educators are urged to team trainees from school and rehabilitation counseling training programs so that these professionals can work cooperatively for the benefit of the client with a disability.

Traditional Versus Experiential Model for Counselor Education

W.M. Holbert and J.H. Miller (1970)

Following a discussion of alternative models of rehabilitation counselor education, the experimental approach used at the University of Tennessee is presented with foci on the counseling practicum, the internship, and sensitivity training. A discussion of "the mystique of counseling and education" is presented along with concluding recommendations for the field.

A Training Model for Rehabilitation Counseling Education

W.A. Anthony, A.E. Dell Orto, R.G. Lasky, R.P. Marinelli, P.W. Power, and L.J. Spaniol (1977, p. 218)

This article describes and evaluates the development of a rehabilitation training model (RTM) that has been used in the Department of Rehabilitation Counseling at Boston University for the past three years. The article (a) focuses on the need for developing a rehabilitation training model, (b) identifies the specific skills, knowledge, and values of the RTM and provides examples as to how these are integrated into the RTM, (c) examines the context in which the RTM developed and grew, (d) presents a program evaluation model designed to assess the capability of the RTM in achieving its objectives, and (e) reflects on the implications of the RTM for the future development of the profession of rehabilitation counseling.

The Realities of Competency-Based Rehabilitation Counselor Education: A Response to Diamonti and Murphy

W.A. Anthony, A.E. Dell Orto, R.G. Lasky, P.W. Power, D.E. Shrey, and L.J. Spaniol (1977)

In response to Diamonti and Murphy's (1977) critique, the authors discuss the value of science, conceptual creativity, and the relationship between evaluation and objectivity. Their conclusion suggests that a competency-based RCE program does not encourage passivity on behalf of students but rather it energizes creativity.

The Realities of Competency-Based Rehabilitation Counselor Education: A Reply

M.C. Diamonti and S.I. Murphy (1977)

The author's reply to Anthony et al. (1977) includes discourse on rehabilitator competency, course content, evaluation and objectivity, screening procedures, and student passivity. (Ed.)

Rehabilitation Counselor Training: A Program Evaluation

G.O. Geist, D.B. Hershenson, and M. Hafer (1975, p. 305)

With the profession of rehabilitation counseling presently focusing on such major issues as ethics, certification, and accreditation, accountability becomes a key word. This study was conducted to meet the accountability issue for one graduate training program. The program was investigated in three different areas of outcome, using all available graduates from the program. The three areas entailed general background information on the graduates, their satisfaction with their training and current employment, and supervisors' reports on satisfactoriness of the graduates' functioning on the job. Discussion of results concerns attraction and selection of students, processing the students through the program, and the eventual product produced by the program.

A Point of Convergence in the Evaluation of Rehabilitation Counselor Education (RCE) Program

D.J. Dellario (1980, p. 128)

The current state of the art of Rehabilitation Counselor Education (RCE) program objectives and evaluative criteria presents a picture of ambiguity. A point of convergence that ties together competency-based, performance-based, professionally-based and accountability-based criteria is necessary so that RCE programs can be judged fairly and equitably. An RCE meta-objective is proposed that can serve as this point of convergence.

New Developments in Rehabilitation Counselor Education

Arkansas Rehabilitation Research and Training Center (1975, p. 330)

The eight brief articles which comprise this Special Feature include: (1) an overview of the Arkansas model for translating research into practice; (2) an outline of a comprehensive inservice case management training package designed to improve the rehabilitation counselor's skills in five areas of functioning; (3) a description of an interpersonal skills training package designed to improve the counselor's ability to facilitate client self-exploration; (4) an outline of a research training manual consisting of ten units covering basic topics in the interpretation of rehabilitation research; (5) an overview of a group counseling approach designed to improve the personal adjustment of rehabilitation clients; (6) a description of a physical fitness training package that can be used to improve the health habits and physical condition of clients; (7) an outline of the Arkansas Continuing Education Program, which has focused on upgrading counselor knowledge and skills in dealing with four severe disability groups; and (8) an overview of a new modeling strategy for training rehabilitation counselors to be more effective helping professionals.

Local and National Availability and Accessibility and Training Materials in Rehabilitation Education

W.G. Emener and J.D. Rasch (1982, p. 40)

Two-hundred and thirty-five rehabilitation educators (51.2% return rate) responded to survey items designed to assess: (a) their local accessibility to rehabilitation resource and training materials; (b) national availability of rehabilitation resource and training materials; and (c) the primary distributors of education and training resource materials (exclusive of textbooks) and the competency area(s) within which the distributors' materials were used. Results, discussions of findings, and specific recommendations for future research and the continued development of information, resource materials, and dissemination programs are included.

An Interdisciplinary Program For Preparing Professional Leaders

Philip Browning (1982, p. 57)

An interdisciplinary doctoral program in rehabilitation is described. Also presented is the short- and long-range impact of this professional training program, which was implemented during the decade of the seventies.

References and Suggested Additional Readings for Part II

Ames, T.R., & Boyle, P.S. (1980). The rehabilitation counselor's role in the sexual adjustment of the handicapped client: The need for trained professionals. *Journal of Applied Rehabilitation Counseling, 2*(4), 173-178.

Anthony, W.A., Dell Orto, A.E., Lasky, R.G., Marinelli, R.P., Power, P.W., & Spaniol, L.J. (1977). A training model for rehabilitation counseling education. *Rehabilitation Counseling Bulletin, 20*(3), 218-235.

Anthony, W.A., Dell Orto, A.E., Lasky, R.G., Power, P.W., Shrey, D.E., & Spaniol, L.J. (1977). The realities of competency-based rehabilitation counselor education: A response to Diamonti and Murphy. *Rehabilitation Counseling Bulletin, 21*(1), 58-62.

Arkansas Rehabilitation Research and Training Center (1975). New developments in rehabilitation counselor education. *Rehabilitation Counseling Bulletin, 19*(1), 330-343.

Atkinson, D.A. (1981). Selection and training for human rights counseling. *Counselor Education and Supervision, 21*(2), 101-108.

Berven, N.L., & Scofield, M.E. (1980). Evaluation of professional competence through standardized simulations: A review. *Rehabilitation Counseling Bulletin, 24*(2), 178-202.

Berven, N.L., & Wright, G.N. (1978). An evaluation model for accreditation. *Counselor Education and Supervision, 17*(3), 188-194.

Berven, N.L., McCracken, N., Jellinek, H.M., & Doran, E.A. (1983). Contributions of a rehabilitation counselor education advisory committee. *Journal of Applied Rehabilitation Counseling, 14*(2), 23-25.

Bitter, J.A. (1978). Continuing education for new rehabilitation counselors. *Rehabilitation Counseling Bulletin, 22*(1), 74-77.

Browning, P. (1982). An interdisciplinary program for preparing professional leaders. *Journal of Rehabilitation, 48*(4), 57-59, 79.

Bruyere, S.M., & Elliot, J.K. (1979). RRCEPs and continuing education for rehabilitation personnel. *Rehabilitation Counseling Bulletin, 23*(2), 131-135.

Chiko, C.H., Tolsma, R.J., Kahn, S.E., & Marks, S.E. (1980). A model to systematize competencies in counselor education. *Counselor Education and Supervision, 19*(4), 283-292.

Clowers, M.R., & Belcher, S.A. (1978). A service-delivery model for the severely disabled individual: Accountability data-collection system. *Rehabilitation Counseling Bulletin, 22*, 53-59.

Council on Rehabilitation Education. (1978). *Accreditation manual for rehabilitation counselor education programs*. Chicago, IL: Author.

Crystal, R.M. (1981). An integrative model for rehabilitation training and practice. *Journal of Applied Rehabilitation Counseling, 12*(4), 191-194.

Dellario, D.J. (1980). A point of convergence in the evaluation of rehabilitation counselor education (RCE) program. *Journal of Applied Rehabilitation Counseling, 11*(3), 128-131.

Diamonti, M.C., & Murphy, S.T. (1977). Behavioral objectives and rehabilitation counselor education: A critique. *Rehabilitation Counseling Bulletin, 21*(1), 51-57. (b)

Diamonti, M.C., & Murphy, S.T. (1977). The realities of competency-based rehabilitation counselor education: A reply. *Rehabilitation Counseling Bulletin, 21*(1), 63-66. (a)

Division of Counseling Psychology (1963). *The role of psychology in the preparation of rehabilitation counselors.* Washington, D.C.: American Psychological Association.

Dowd, E.T., & Emener, W.G. (1978). Lifeboat counseling: The issue of survival decisions. *Journal of Rehabilitation, 44*(3), 34-36.

Downes, S.C., McFarlane, F.R., & Alston, P.P. (1974). Survey of the NRCA membership regarding the basis for evaluating counselor performance. *Journal of Applied Rehabilitation Counseling, 5*(4), 196-200.

Emener, W.G. (1980). Professional literature in rehabilitation: Areas of concern. *Journal of Rehabilitation, 46*(3), 70-77. (b)

Emener, W.G., & Ferrandino, J.A. (1983). A philosophical framework for rehabilitation: Implications for clients, counselors, and agencies. *Journal of Applied Rehabilitation Counseling, 14*(1), 62-67.

Emener, W.G., & Koonce, G.B. (1978). Categorical sources of articles in the *Journal of Rehabilitation, :* 1959-1975. *Journal of Rehabilitation, 44*(3), 25-27.

Emener, W.G., & McFarlane, F.R. (in press). A futuristic model of rehabilitation education. *Journal of Applied Rehabilitation Counseling.*

Emener, W.G., & Placido, D. (1982). Client feedback: A valuable source of counselor development. *Journal of Applied Rehabilitation Counseling, 13*(1), 18-23. (a)

Emener, W.G., & Placido, D. (1982). Rehabilitation counselor evaluation: An analysis and critique. *Journal of Rehabilitation Administration, 6*(2), 72-76. (b)

Emener, W.G., & Rasch, J.D. (1982). Local and national availability and accessibility and training materials in rehabilitation education. *Journal of Rehabilitation, 48*(4), 40-44.

Emener, W.G., Rasch, J.D., & Spector, P.E. (1983). Knowledge adequacies and training needs of rehabilitation educators. *Counselor Education and Supervision, 22*(3), 242-249.

Engram, B.E. (1981). Communication skills training for rehabilitation counselors working with older persons. *Journal of Rehabilitation, 47*(4), 51-56.

Feinberg, L.B., & McFarlane, F.R. (1979). Setting-based factors in rehabilitation counselor role variability. *Journal of Applied Rehabilitation Counseling, 10*(2), 95-101.

Geist, C.S. (1980). Development of an independent living rehabilitation program curriculum. *Journal of Rehabilitation, 46*(2), 53-55.

Geist, G.O., & Emener, W.G. (1981). Rehabilitation counseling and rehabilitation counselor education: Implications for social work and social work education. In Browne, J.A., Kivlin, B.A., & Watt, S. *Rehabilitation services and the social work role: Challenge for change.* Baltimore: Williams & Wilkins.

Geist, G.O., & McMahon, B.T. (1981). Pre-service rehabilitation education: Where graduates are employed. *Journal of Rehabilitation, 47*(3), 45-47.

Geist, G.O., Hershenson, D.B., & Hafer, M. (1975). Rehabilitation counselor training: A program evaluation. *Rehabilitation Counseling Bulletin, 19*(1), 305-314.

Hanna, C., Mullinax, J., & Sadler, V. (1983). Rehabilitation nurse or vocational reha-bilitation counselor: Competency-based selection. *Journal of Rehabilitation, 49*(4), 75-78.

Harrison, D.K. (1980). Competency evaluation in rehabilitation (CEIR): Toward a competency-based client-outcome system. *Journal of Applied Rehabilitation Counseling, 2*(1), 18-24.

Holbert, W.M., & Miller, J.H. (1970). Traditional versus experiential model for coun-selor education. *Journal of Applied Rehabilitation Counseling, 1*(3), 21-30.

Hollingsworth, D.K., & Reagles, K.W. (1980). Confronting barriers to the utilization of program evaluation. *Journal of Rehabilitation Administration, 4*(3), 94-98.

Hutchinson, J., & Cogan, F. (1974). Rehabilitation manpower specialist: A job description of placement personnel. *Journal of Rehabilitation, 40*(2), 31-33.

Jones, G.B., & Dayton, C.W. (1977). A competency-based staff development ap-proach for improving counselor education. *Counselor Education and Supervision, 17,* 107-115.

Kunce, J.T., & Vales, L.F. (1984). The Mexican American: Implications for cross-cultural rehabilitation counseling. *Rehabilitation Counseling Bulletin, 28*(2), 97-108.

Livingston, R. (1979). The history of rehabilitation counselor certification. *Journal of Applied Rehabilitation Counseling, 10*(3), 111-118.

Lofaro, G.A. (1982). Disability and counselor education. *Counselor Education and Super-vision, 21*(3), 200-207.

Matkin, R.E. (1980). The rehabilitation counselor in private practice: Perspectives for education and preparation. *Journal of Rehabilitation, 46*(2), 60-62.

McFarlane, F.R., & DiPaola, S.M. (1979). Rehabilitation counselor, vocational eval-uator and work adjustment specialist: Are these professionals different? *Journal of Applied Rehabilitation Counseling, 10*(3), 142-147.

McMahon, B.T., & Matkin, R.E. (1983). Preservice graduate education for private sector rehabilitation counselors. *Rehabilitation Counseling Bulletin, 27*(1), 54-60.

McMahon, B.T., Geist, G.O., Geist, C.S., & Berry, D.J. (1981). The desirability of weighted standards in CORE accreditation. *Rehabilitation Counseling Bulletin, 25*(1), 38-40.

McMahon, B.T. (1979). Private sector rehabilitation: Benefits, dangers, and implica-tions for education. *Journal of Rehabilitation, 45*(3), 56-58.

Mosher, F.C. (1978). The public service in a temporary society. In J.M. Shafritz & A.C. Hyde (Eds.), *Classics in public administration*. Oak Park, IL: Moore.

Olshanksy, S. (1967). An evaluation of rehabilitation counselor training. *Vocational Guidance Quarterly, 5,* 164-167.

Patterson, C.H. (1957). Counselor or coordinator? *Journal of Rehabilitation, 23*(3), 13-15.

Patterson, C.H. (1965). Specialization in rehabilitation counseling. In W. Holbert (Ed.): *Proceedings of a conference on vocational rehabilitation counselor specialization: Cause and effects.* Atlanta, GA: April 29-30, 1965, pp. 11-20.

Patterson, C.H. (1967). Specialization in rehabilitation counseling. *Rehabilitation Coun-seling Bulletin, 10*(4), 147-154.

Pipes, R.B., Buckhalt, J.A., & Merrill, H.D. (1983). Counselor education and the psychology of more. *Counselor Education and Supervision, 22*(4), 282-286.

Porter, T.L., Rubin, S.E., & Sink, J.M. (1979). Essential rehabilitation counselor diagnostic, counseling, and placement competences. *Journal of Applied Rehabilitation Counseling, 10*(3), 158-162.

Rimmer, S.M. (1981). A systems approach model for counselor education program development and redefinition. *Counselor Education and Supervision, 21*(1), 7-15.

Roessler, R.T. (1981). Training independent living rehabilitation specialists. *Journal of Rehabilitation, 47*(2), 36-39.

Rubin, S.E., & Puckett, F.D. (1984). The changing role and function of the rehabilitation counselor. *Rehabilitation Counseling Bulletin, 27*(4), 225-231.

Scalia, V.A., & Wolfe, R.R. (1984). Rehabilitation counselor education. *Journal of Applied Rehabilitation Counseling, 15*(3), 34-38.

Smits, S.J., & Emener, W.G. (1980). Insufficient/ineffective counselor involvement in job placement activities: A system failure. *Journal of Rehabilitation Administration, 4*, 147-155.

Stephens, J.E., & Kniepp, S. (1981). Managing human resource development in rehabilitation. In W.G. Emener, R.S. Luck & S.J. Smits. *Rehabilitation administration and supervision*. Baltimore: University Park Press.

Sussman, M.B., & Haug, M.R. (1967). *The practitioners: Rehabilitation counselors in three work settings*. Cleveland, Ohio: Western Reserve University.

Thomas, K.R. (1982). A critique of trends in rehabilitation counselor education toward specialization. *Journal of Rehabilitation, 48*(1), 49-51.

Thomason, B., & Saxon, J.P. (1973). A reality model for rehabilitation counselor education. *Journal of Applied Rehabilitation Counseling, 4*(1), 23-31.

Townsend, O.H. (1970). Vocational rehabilitation and the black counselor: The conventional training situation and the battleground across town. *Journal of Rehabilitation, 36*(6), 16-18.

Usdane, W.M. (1974). Placement personnel—a graduate program concept. *Journal of Rehabilitation, 40*(2), 12-13.

Wright, G.N. (1982). Contemporary rehabilitation counselor education. *Rehabilitation Counseling Bulletin, 25*(4), 254-256.

Wright, G.N. & Reagles, K.W. (1973). RCE—Duly accredited. *Journal of Rehabilitation, 39*(6), 33-35.

Wright, G.N., Reagles, K.W., & Scorzelli, J.F. (1973). Measuring the effectiveness and variations of rehabilitation counselor education programs. *Journal of Applied Rehabilitation Counseling, 4*(2), 76-87.

PART III

REHABILITATION COUNSELOR EDUCATION: KEY CONTENTS AND CONSTRUCTS

PART III. REHABILITATION COUNSELOR EDUCATION: KEY CONTENTS AND CONSTRUCTS

Introduction Commentary

THERE ARE NUMEROUS critical issues regarding the contents and constructs of rehabilitation counselor education programs such as their historical and future developments (Emener, 1984; Emener & McFarlane, 1985), minimally necessary content and construct areas (Council on Rehabilitation Education, 1978), and the extent to which they are related to program effectiveness (Wright, Reagles & Scorzelli, 1973). Experience has demonstrated repeatedly over time that there are two basic questions underlying rehabilitation education programming: (1) *What contents and constructs should be included in a rehabilitation counselor education program?* and (2) *How should such contents and constructs be determined?* From a process or developmental point of view, it would appear to address this latter question first.

In addition to calling upon their own professional experiences, rehabilitation counselor educators also rely upon results of needs assessment surveys (e.g., Freeman, 1978; McFarlane & Sullivan, 1979) and solicited input from practicing counselors (e.g., Joiner & Roberts, 1982) in the identification of the contents and constructs of their rehabilitation counselor education programs. Program advisory committees have also been found to be extremely helpful (see Berven, McCracken, Jellinek & Doran, 1983). Solicited, structured feedback from program graduates can be very useful: (a) a program can survey its own graduates (e.g., see Kauppi, Ballou, Jaques, Gualtieri & Blum, 1983; Scorzelli, 1975, 1979; Sullivan, 1982) and (b) graduates of numerous programs can be surveyed (for example, Janes & Emener, 1983, analyzed data from 194 recent graduates of eight cooperating rehabilitation counselor education programs). In Chapter 12, Scorzelli (1979) analyzed task analysis data from all graduates ($N = 54$) of the rehabilitation counselor education program at Northeastern University; his task analysis methodology has much utility and would appear to be an excellent approach. As stated earlier, rehabilitation educators' experiences as professional practitioners, and their values and preferences, weigh heavily in the determination of program contents and constructs. Emener and Rasch (1984), in Chapter 13, analyzed data from a response sample of 235 rehabilitation educators regarding actual and preferred instructional areas in rehabilitation education. Individual rehabilitation counselor education programs can find it quite beneficial to compare their own program's instructional areas (actual and preferred) to the national findings reported by Emener and Rasch (1984). Each of these approaches to determining the contents and constructs of a rehabilitation counselor education program has differential benefits, pro's and con's, and limitations. Thus, it is suggested that programs utilize all or combinations of these approaches to make the best determinations for their own individual programs.

Historically, the clinical construct of rehabilitation counselor education (viz. practica and internship) has been considered exceptionally important (Joint Liaison Committee, 1963; Lanning, 1971; Miller & Mulkey, 1975; Patterson, 1964; Warren, 1957). Fittingly, Atkins (1981), in Chapter 14, recently stated: "Clinical practice in rehabilitation education represents an essential component in the graduate student's course of study and serves as a transition between the didactic learning of the classroom and the employment of the student as a professional counselor." In a generic sense, the "clinical" component of a rehabilitation counselor education program is frequently considered to encompass many preparation constructs—for example, the development of initial interviewing skills (Sawyer & Allen, 1976), foci on the process dimension of counseling (MacGuffie & Henderson, 1973), and enhancement of self-awareness through sensitivity training experiences (Downes, 1971). Field-based clinical components (practica and internship) also include the systematic design and implementation of activities to prepare and enhance the skills of the students' field-based supervisors (see Berven, Possi, Doran, Ostby & Kaplan, 1982), and the development and refinement of coordination and administrative procedures (such as in the developmental use of a field training manual—see Trotter, Kult & Atkins, 1980). There are numerous critical issues regarding the clinical component of rehabilitation counselor education, and those relevant to "paid internships" are very important ones. Geist (1977), in Chapter 15, addresses many of these issues and specifically comments on "why should interns be paid?" The clinical area involves numerous issues regarding ethics, and it is incumbent upon students, educators, and field-based supervisors to be keenly cognizant of them (see Scofield & Scofield, 1978). The clinical component of a rehabilitation counselor education program is clearly very demanding, important, and critical; among other considerations, it requires a deep sense of *commitment* on behalf of students and their professors and field-based supervisors if the clinical experience is to realize the benefits and outcomes which it can potentially produce.

The academic curricular contents of a rehabilitation counselor education program can focus on numerous areas of knowledge, for example, rehabilitation content (Rubin & Roessler, 1978; Wright, 1980) and rehabilitation process (Phillips, 1980). Quite frequently, content areas are consistent with the developments of materials available in professional literature (see Emener & Koonce, 1978; Emener & Rasch, 1982) and guidelines provided by professional accrediting bodies (e.g., Council on Rehabilitation Education, 1978). Indeed, there are numerous specific content areas that a well-rounded, diverse rehabilitation counselor education program could include. The following alphabetized list is merely a partial, selected listing of examples:

1. *Administration and Supervision* (Emener, Luck & Smits, 1981; Matkin, Sawyer, Lorenz & Rubin, 1982; Riggar & Matkin, 1984)
2. *Cancer* (Sachs & Hansen, 1981)
3. *Communications skills with/for specific populations* (e.g., Engram, 1981)
4. *Conflict management* (Klein & Scofield, 1984)
5. *Ethics* (Hawley & Capshaw, 1981; Scofield & Scofield, 1978)
6. *Human rights* (Atkins, 1981)
7. *Independent living* (Roessler, 1981)
8. *Medical aspects* (e.g., Felton, 1963; Zelle, 1972)
9. *Philosophy and social ethics* (Dowd & Emener, 1978; Emener & Ferrandino, 1983; Gilbert, 1973)
10. *Placement* (Hutchinson & Cogan, 1974; Mulhern, 1980; Porter, Rubin & Sink, 1979; Usdane, 1974; Zadny & James, 1977)
11. *Program evaluation* (Struthers & Miller, 1981)
12. *Psychiatric rehabilitation* (Weinberger & Greenwald, 1982)
13. *"Real world" considerations* (see Morgan, 1982)
14. *Sexual adjustment* (Ames & Boyle, 1980; Walker, Sawyer & Clark, 1975)
15. *Vocational evaluation* (Sink & Porter, 1978)
16. *Work adjustment* (Coffey & Ellien, 1979; McFarlane & DiPaola, 1979)
17. *Writing behavioral objectives* (Hinman & Marr, 1984)

New content areas, in most instances, are initially developed and tested in the inservice training and continuing education arenas. Readers are urged to study Chapter 16 by Hinman and Marr (1984) because their project demonstrated that as a result of their training program "significant change in counselor behavior" was observed. It could be argued that rehabilitation counselor education students "should" be taught to write behavior-based client objectives, and if that is true, *where* (within the curriculum) *and how* should it be done? Questions of *where?* and *how?* could be raised with regard to any content area (including the 17 examples above), and professional rehabilitation counselor preparation programs are continuously challenged by content oriented questions such as these.

It has been suggested that modern technology is increasingly producing a growing population of disabled individuals in need of rehabilitation services.

Moreover, modern technology is also producing means by which disabled individuals can be served more effectively and more efficiently. For example, Chan and Questad (1981) stated: "In rehabilitation, microcomputers are now used to increase the functional capacities of disabled persons, but rehabilitation professionals could benefit from this technology also" (p. 153). Fittingly, Nave and Browning (1983) convincingly "encourage rehabilitation educators to take a major role in preparing future leaders to work with this [computer] technology" (p. 364). Students and faculty are strongly encouraged to study Chapter 17 by Crimando and Baker (1984). They provide compelling evidence in support of computer-assisted instruction in rehabilitation education, and, since the day is nearing (or already upon us) when every practicing rehabilitation counselor will use a computer in his or her work, what better place is there to use the computer than in the classroom!

In conclusion, the reader is again reminded that the content and construct areas of a rehabilitation counselor education program addressed in this part of this book indeed are not all inclusive. They are examples. It is hoped that they serve to illustrate the critical issues surrounding content and construct development, and it is trusted that they highlight the importance of the two major content/construct questions facing rehabilitation counselor education: (1) *What should be taught?* and (2) *How should this be determined?* Issues such as how subject matter should be taught and academic freedom are not within the scope of this book. Nonetheless, it would appear that the readings in this part of this book (and the suggested additional readings) provide exciting challenges to those students, educators, and practicing professionals in the continuing processes of reviewing and developing the contents and constructs of rehabilitation counselor education programs.

W.G. Emener

CHAPTER 12

ASSESSING THE CONTENT
OF A REHABILITATION
COUNSELING PROGRAM

JAMES F. SCORZELLI

Abstract

In order to comply with the standards for accreditation, the rehabilitation counseling program at Northwestern University was increased in length from one to two years. During this transitional phase of development, a job task outline was utilized to identify curriculum deficient areas of the program. Although this research indicated that the curriculum was fairly representative of the content areas in the job task outline, it was found that there was little opportunity for specialization. The implications of the research for newly formed rehabilitation counseling programs are discussed.

DURING THE DEVELOPMENT of the Rehabilitation Counselor Education (RCE) program at Northeastern University, a job task analysis was conducted to assist the program in curriculum and instructional planning (Scorzelli, 1975). The results of this research supported the counselor-coordinator training model (Ayer, Wright & Butler, 1968) and were in agreement with the previous research conducted on the roles and functions of the rehabilitation counselor (Muthard & Salamone, 1969). The use of the job task outline, supplemented with the guidelines on RCE program content (Hall & Warren, 1956; Joint Liason Committee, 1963), provided valuable information during this stage of program development.

Recently, there has been renewed interest in professional training models for rehabilitation counselors (Anthony, et al., 1977; McCauley, 1976; Steger, 1977). This appears to be a response to the accreditation movement in the field and to the current emphasis being placed on evaluation and accountability.

Reprinted by permission from Volume 9 (1979), *Journal of Applied Rehabilitation Counseling*, pp. 184-186.

Accordingly, the RCE program at Northeastern has found itself in transition in reassessing its curriculum and program objectives. The primary reason for reassessment is that the program has been increased in length from one to two years to comply with the standards for accreditation consideration (Council on Rehabilitation Education, 1974). In implementing this change, the job task outline was used with graduates to identify deficiencies in the program.

METHODOLOGY

The job task outline consisted of 87 job tasks categorized under 17 general rehabilitation counselor functions. Items were based on a review of the literature on the roles and functions of the rehabilitation counselor and on input from counselors and supervisors in New England (Region I). Each respondent was asked to rate each task as to its importance (four point scale) based on his/her knowledge of the roles and functions of the rehabilitation counselor.

SAMPLE

The sample consisted of all graduates ($N=54$) of the RCE program at Northeastern University since its formation (1974-1977). After the initial mailing, and two subsequent follow-up letters, 33 or 61 percent of the graduates replied. The perceptions of other employed rehabilitation counselors and supervisors, henceforth referred to as the employed-non-graduates, who were surveyed during the formation of the program, were used as a comparison group. This group included 55 individuals employed at 32 VR agencies, and 36 rehabilitation facilities in Region I (Scorzelli, 1975).

RESULTS

The graduates who responded were employed in a wide variety of work settings and, except for one, were employed in rehabilitation work. Four of the graduates indicated that they were supervisors, while the remainder indicated that they were practitioners. The graduates were slightly younger ($X=26$ years vs. $X=28$ years), and had a higher proportion of women (45% vs. 26%) than the employed-non-graduates.

The majority of the 17 general rehabilitation counselor functions (Table 12-1) were rated high by both groups, with the only exception being for: "group counseling;" "follow-up;" and "supervision of rehabilitation personnel." The graduates tended to give slightly higher ratings than did the employed-non-graduates, but overall an agreement between the groups with respect to the

Table 12–1

Mean Ratings* and Ranks of Functional Categories
as Rated by Employed-non-Graduates and Graduates Categories

	Employed-non-Graduates (n=55)		Graduates (n=33)		Total (n=88)	
	Mean	Rank	Mean	Rank	Mean	Rank
Utilization of Community Agencies & Professionals	3.74	1	3.90	1	3.80	1
Training Services	3.73	2	3.71	2.5	3.72	2
Vocational Counseling	3.66	3	3.71	2.5	3.68	3
Client Eligibility	3.57	4	3.64	5	3.59	4
Restoration Services	3.56	5	3.19	11	3.42	5
Work Adjustment Counseling	3.21	8	3.65	4	3.36	6
Vocational Evaluation	3.25	7	3.40	8	3.30	7
Therapeutic Counseling	3.12	11	3.54	6	3.27	8
Medical Eval./Referral	3.26	6	3.18	12.5	3.23	9
Psychol. Eval./Referral	3.08	12	3.44	7	3.21	10
Job Placement	3.16	9.5	3.22	10	3.18	11
Coordination/Case Management	3.16	9.5	3.18	12.5	3.17	12
Community Organization & Planning	3.03	13	3.28	9	3.12	13
Case Finding	3.01	14	3.13	14	3.05	14
Follow-up	2.69	15	3.00	15	2.80	15
Supervision Rehab. Personnel	2.44	16	2.87	17	2.59	16
Group Counseling	2.10	17	2.90	16	2.38	17

*Ratings: Extremely-4; Moderately-3; Slightly-2; Not at all-1

rankings of the functions were substantial (Kendall Tau Correlation Coefficient .66; $p<.01$).

Ratings of specific job tasks paralleled the trend observed for the general rehabilitation counselor functions. The tasks rated as most important involved evaluation, information giving, and vocational counseling (Table 12-2). Group work, supervision of rehabilitation personnel, and therapeutic counseling were rated as least important by both groups.

Table 12–2

Mean Ratings* of Job Tasks Rated
the Highest and Lowest by Employed-non-Graduates and Graduates

HIGHEST	Employed-non-Graduates (n=55)	Graduates (n=33)
Evaluates vocational and educational training needed	3.86	3.70
With client, determines what type of training is most feasible	3.86	3.69
Assists client in appropriate goal setting and decision making	3.82	3.81
Helps client accept vocational limitations of disability	3.80	3.86
Evaluates client's progress at regular intervals	380	3.72
Develops full knowledge of community and vocational resources	3.80	3.90
Assists client in determining most suitable vocational objectives	3.79	3.95
Inform client of agencies that can provide assistance	3.74	3.90
LOWEST		
Administers psychological tests	1.50	2.33
Group work, personal and social adjustment	1.93	2.68
Group work, clients with similar disabilities	1.94	2.70
Evaluates work performance of other professionals	2.05	2.52
Conducts in-service training for rehab. personnel	2.12	2.71
Performs therapeutic counseling on a regular basis	2.32	2.57

*Ratings: Extremely-4; Moderately-3; Slightly-2; Not at all-1.

DISCUSSION AND IMPLICATIONS

The results of the study indicated that there was moderate agreement between the graduates and employed-non-graduates about the importance of the

rehabilitation counseling tasks. This finding suggests that both groups perceived their roles similarly. However, the similarity in perceived roles may have
been due to having been exposed to the rigors of practice, and not necessarily
because of the training they received. Therefore, the use of students or recent
graduates would have been a better sample. Nevertheless, in spite of these limitations, the job task outline can be extremely useful in the development of rehabilitation counseling course objectives. This is especially true for newly formed
programs or those in the process of expanding their curricula to comply with
accreditation standards. Task-analyses can help insure that the content of
training is consistent with the roles and functions of those employed in the profession and help eliminate the "reality shock" that often confronts graduates of
professional training programs. In addition a job task outline can be useful to
practitioners and supervisors as a means of evaluation, and such evaluations
conducted on a periodic basis can provide valuable information for in-service
training programs.

To appreciate how the results of this survey assisted the program at Northeastern University, it is necessary to describe the dilemma surrounding increasing the length of the program. First, the program was initially developed to
meet the in-service training needs of the state VR personnel. Because these
employees had had extensive practical experience, a one year program was
deemed sufficient to meet their training needs. Secondly, the original program
was comparable with other one year programs in Region I. Therefore, there
was a fear that increasing the program's length would cut enrollments. However, the importance of the accreditation movement and the substantial growth
of the RCE program, which involved a wider range of prospective candidates,
set these concerns to rest. Although this program change was initiated by
the RCE coordinator, it was fully supported by the department and college
faculty.

In reviewing the results of the job task outline, it became apparent that the
basic core curriculum was representative of the content areas emphasized by
the respondents. Although the research helped to support the emphasis of the
curriculum, the program was still faced with the problem of increasing its
length. Although not directly obtained from the study, discussions with students and a C.O.R.E. consultant revealed that the program offered little opportunity for specialization. In fact, the only way a student could specialize was
to do so during his/her practicum experience. Therefore, the program has developed specializations in deafness, corrections, and special needs populations
and is actively exploring other areas of concentration. It is felt that this change
has made the program more attractive to prospective candidates, has provided
an opportunity for practitioners to enhance their professional growth by
obtaining training in areas of specialization, and has greatly improved the
quality of training received.

REFERENCES

Anthony, W.A., Dell Orto, A.E., Lasky, R.G., Marinelli, R., Power, P., Spaniol, L.J. A training model for rehabilitation counseling education. *Rehabilitation Counseling Bulletin,* 1977, *20*(3), 218-235.

Ayer, M.J., Wright, G.N., & Butler, A.J. Counselor orientation: Relationship with responsibilities and performance. Wisconsin Studies in Vocational Rehabilitation, University of Wisconsin Regional Research Institute, Madison, 1968, 1, X.

Council On Rehabilitation Education, Commission on Standards and Accreditation of Rehabilitation Counselor Education. *Manual of Accreditation,* Author, 1974.

Hall, J.H. & Warren, S.H. Rehabilitation counselor preparation. Washington, D.C.: National Rehabilitation Association and National Vocational Guidance Association, 1956.

Joint Liaison Committee of the Council of State Directors of Vocational Rehabilitation and the Rehabilitation Counselor Educators. Studies in rehabilitation counselor training: Experiences of state agencies in hiring VRA trainees. No. 2, Washington, D.C.: Author, 1963.

McCauley, W.A. *Whither rehabilitation education?* (A state-of-the-art report). Natresources, Inc., 1815 North Fort Myer Drive, Arlington, Virginia, 1976.

Muthard, J.E. & Salamone, P.R. Roles and functions of the rehabilitation counselor. *Rehabilitation Counseling Bulletin,* 1969, *13*(1), 81-168.

Scorzelli, J.F. Reactions to program content of a rehabilitation counseling program. *Journal of Applied Rehabilitation Counseling,* 1975, *6*(3), 172-177.

Steger, J.M. Rehabilitation counselor education and competency-based instruction. *Rehabilitation Counseling Bulletin,* 1977, *20*(4), 260-266.

CHAPTER 13

ACTUAL AND PREFERRED INSTRUCTIONAL AREAS IN REHABILITATION EDUCATION PROGRAMS

WILLIAM G. EMENER AND JOHN D. RASCH

Abstract

Based on a literature review, twelve critical instructional areas in rehabilitation education were identified: (a) Basic Principles; (b) Counseling Theories and Techniques; (c) Medical Aspects; (d) Psychosocial Aspects; (e) Occupational Information and Job Analysis; (f) Evaluation; (g) Case Management; (h) Community Organization and Resources; (i) Job Development and Placement; (j) Fieldwork; (k) Research; and (l) Professional Issues. A response sample of 235 rehabilitation educators (a 51.2% return) rated the extent to which each of the instructional areas were and should be emphasized across four levels of rehabilitation education programming—bachelor's, master's, doctoral, and continuing education levels. Results revealed that educators preferred most of the instructional areas to receive their greatest emphasis at the master's level. Educators did not indicate a desire for bachelor's level practitioners to be trained as counselors and indicated a preference for a strong research rather than clinical practice focus in doctoral programs.

THE PAST SIX DECADES of formal rehabilitation service delivery in America has witnessed the emergence of professional rehabilitation service providers—especially the rehabilitation counselor. A major concern in the professional preparation of rehabilitation counselors has been the changing roles and functions of rehabilitation counselors (Emener & Rubin, 1980). Evidence of significant role changes has been provided in several recent studies (e.g., Fraser & Clowers, 1978; Parham & Harris, 1978; Rubin & Emener, 1979; Zadny & James, 1977). Collectively, these studies suggested that, compared to their time allocations across job tasks in the middle 1960s, rehabilitation

Reprinted by permission from Volume 27 (1984), *Rehabilitation Counseling Bulletin,* pp. 269-280.

counselors are currently spending less time on counseling and guidance activities, more time on case recording, and more time on arranging and coordinating services. With continuously changing roles and functions of rehabilitation counselors, compounded by differential expectations of rehabilitation counselors (Emener & Rubin, 1980), two critical questions facing professional preparation programs have emerged: (a) what is actually being taught at different programming levels?; and (b) what should be taught at different programming levels? The purpose of this study was to survey rehabilitation educators to identify their perceptions of *actual* and *preferred* instructional emphases in bachelor's, master's, doctoral, and continuing education programs.

METHOD

This study was conducted as a component of *The 1981 Rehabilitation Education Survey,* which was endorsed by the National Council on Rehabilitation Education (NCRE).

SUBJECTS

The survey population consisted of all 459 NCRE members identified in the *1980 NCRE Directory.* Usable surveys were returned by 235 respondents, representing a 51.2 percent response rate. The respondents' demographic data revealed that: (a) 191 (84%) were male and 36 (16%) were female; (b) their mean age was 42.2 ($SD=9.0$); (c) they had master's degrees primarily in rehabilitation (55%), counseling (17%), or psychology (12%), and doctoral degrees primarily in rehabilitation (42%), counseling (33%), or psychology (11%); (d) they were predominantly assistant professors (31%), associate professors (24%), or professors (29%); (e) their Rehabilitation Services Administration (RSA) regional (geographic) distribution was commensurate with that of the NCRE survey population; (f) they were employed for an average of 13.3 years ($SD=6.9$) in the field of rehabilitation and for an average of 8.6 years ($SD=5.2$) as rehabilitation educators; and (g) they worked with master's students (84%), bachelor's students (54%), doctoral students (46%), and continuing education students (54%).

Instrumentation

In order to study actual and preferred instructional emphases in rehabilitation education, it was necessary to delineate a manageable number of instructional areas. This was accomplished through a synthesis of findings from earlier studies by Harrison (1980), Harrison and Lee (1979), Porter, Rubin,

FIGURE 13-1

Operational Definitions of 12 RC Competency Areas

1. *Basic Principles:* Knowledge of principles and concepts underlying rehabilitation, including history, philosophy, structure, and legislation.

2. *Counseling Theories and Techniques:* Knowledge of historical and current approaches to individual and group counseling with application to the field of rehabilitation. Training in basic counseling skills used in relationship building, problem/need identification, and action on rehabilitation problems.

3. *Medical Aspects:* Knowledge of the structure of medicine in the United States, medical specialties, medical terminology, and the medical examination. Knowledge of body systems, basic functions, common malfunctions, therapeutic services, restorative techniques, and disability evaluation. Knowledge of the unique characteristics of various disability groups, especially the severely disabled.

4. *Psychosocial Aspects:* Knowledge of behavioral and psychodynamic principles underlying personal adjustment to disability. Knowledge of adjustment issues in the family and community at large.

5. *Occupational Information and Job Analysis:* Knowledge of the vocational structure of society, including skill requirements of occupations, entry level requirements, and physical and emotional demands. Ability to effectively use occupational information and to analyze jobs.

6. *Evaluation:* Ability to determine diagnostic and assessment procedures needed, analyze and synthesize information, interpret data to client, and determine eligibility. Includes knowledge of psychometric tests, work samples, on-the-job evaluation, and situational assessment procedures.

7. *Case Management:* Ability to move and monitor clients through the rehabilitation process. Includes knowledge of case finding, rehabilitation plan development, service delivery/coordination, and follow-up.

8. *Community Organization and Resources:* Knowledge of community (local) organization and resources. Knowledge of service delivery systems, issues in linking and coordinating services with other agencies, and interagency cooperation.

9. *Job Development and Placement:* Knowledge of job development and placement procedures, including methods for contacting and interfacing with employers, and job modification.

10. *Fieldwork:* Ability to arrange practicum and internship placements in suitable agencies, monitor fieldwork, maintain a working relationship with field supervisors, and supervise students on an individual or group seminar basis.

11. *Research:* Knowledge of research methodology, including design, sampling, data analysis and interpretation, and familiarity with rehabilitation research literature.

12. *Professional Issues:* Knowledge of professional issues and current developments in rehabilitation, including ethics, legal issues, certification, program accreditation, and professional associations.

and Sink (1979) and the training content recommendations of the Council on Rehabilitation Education (CORE's) Commission on Standards and Accreditation for Rehabilitation Counselor Education (1978). Twelve instructional areas were chosen. It was felt that these twelve areas (operationally defined in Figure 13-1) represented the essence of current rehabilitation education programming and provided a manageable number of categories for data analysis and interpretation.

The Rehabilitation Education Survey consisted of a total of 23 items, 14 of which focused on educators' demographic characteristics. Other areas the survey investigated were: (a) local and national availability of rehabilitation resource and training materials and the sources from which educators access materials; and, (b) educator knowledge adequacy, need for in-service training, and willingness to attend in-service training. The Rehabilitation Education Survey was used to collect educator ratings on actual and preferred emphasis for each of the twelve instructional areas across four specific levels of rehabilitation education programming: bachelor's, master's, doctoral, and continuing education. On a seven-point bipolar scale educators rated: (a) the extent of emphasis actually given to each of the twelve instructional areas at each of the four programming levels; and (b) the extent of emphasis which should be given to each of the twelve instructional areas at each of the four programming levels. Adjectives anchoring each point of the seven-point scale were: 1 = very low; 2 = low; 3 = slightly low; 4 = average; 5 = slightly high; 6 = high; and 7 = very high.

Procedures

After presenting the proposal for this project to the National Council on Rehabilitation Education (NCRE), permission was obtained from NCRE to survey its membership (i.e., faculty with rehabilitation education responsibilities at member institutions and individual sustaining members). NCRE members were sent an introductory letter informing them that the NCRE-endorsed Rehabilitation Education Survey would soon arrive in the mail. Members were asked to complete and return the survey promptly. The survey was mailed with a cover letter and prepaid return envelope one week after the introductory letter was mailed. National leaders in rehabilitation education who were consulted strongly recommended that respondents and nonrespondents be assured of complete anonymity. Accordingly, no questionnaire-numbering procedure, which would have allowed for additional mailings to nonrespondents, was used. A follow-up letter was mailed to all NCRE members two weeks after the survey, encouraging them to complete and return the survey if they had not already done so.

Data Analyses

Data analyses included: (a) categorical frequencies and measures of central tendency, basically for descriptive purposes; (b) one-way ANOVAs to test for significant differences among mean ratings on actual emphasis for each instructional area across the four programming levels; (c) one-way ANOVAs to test for significant differences among mean ratings on preferred emphasis for each instructional area across the four programming levels; (d) Duncan Multiple Range Tests to evaluate differences among pairs of means following significant F tests; and (e) t tests to evaluate differences between actual and preferred competency emphases for each instructional area at each of the four programming levels. Statistical significance was set at $p < .05$.

RESULTS

Results are presented separately for actual emphasis ratings, preferred emphasis ratings, and statistical comparisons between actual and preferred ratings.

Actual Emphasis

The educators' mean ratings of the extent to which the twelve instructional areas are actually emphasized across the four levels of rehabilitation programming, and the significance testing of differences ($p < .05$), indicated that:

1. Only one instructional area received a "very high" actual emphasis rating ($\overline{X} = 6.0 - 7.0$) — Research ($\overline{X} = 6.3$) at the doctoral level.
2. Nine of the twelve instructional areas received "high" actual emphasis ratings ($\overline{X} = 5.0 - 5.9$): (a) two at the bachelor's level — Basic Principles ($\overline{X} = 5.4$) and Fieldwork ($\overline{X} = 5.2$); (b) seven at the master's level — Fieldwork ($\overline{X} = 5.8$), Counseling Theories and Techniques ($\overline{X} = 5.7$), Basic Principles ($\overline{X} = 5.4$), Psychosocial Aspects ($\overline{X} = 5.4$), Medical Aspects ($\overline{X} = 5.3$), Evaluation ($\overline{X} = 5.1$), and Occupational Information and Job Analysis ($\overline{X} = 5.0$); (c) three at the doctoral level — Professional Issues ($\overline{X} = 5.9$), Counseling Theories and Techniques ($\overline{X} = 5.2$), and Psychosocial Aspects ($\overline{X} = 5.0$); and (d) one at the Continuing Education level — Case Management ($\overline{X} = 5.0$).
3. Six of the twelve instructional areas received "slightly low" actual emphasis ratings ($\overline{X} = 3.0 - 3.9$): (a) three at the bachelor's level — Professional Issues ($\overline{X} = 3.7$), Counseling Theories and Techniques ($\overline{X} = 3.8$), and Job Development and Placement ($\overline{X} = 3.9$); (b) three at the doctoral level — Job Development and Placement ($\overline{X} = 3.5$), Medical Aspects ($\overline{X} = 3.9$); and Case Management ($\overline{X} = 3.9$); and (c) one at the continuing education level — Fieldwork ($\overline{X} = 3.4$).
4. One instructional area received a "low" actual emphasis rating ($\overline{X} = 2.0 - 2.9$) — Research at the bachelor's ($\overline{X} = 2.3$) and continuing education ($\overline{X} = 2.5$) levels.
5. All instructional areas except Community Organization and Resources and Basic Principles were rated significantly higher at the master's level than at the bachelor's level. Community Organization and Resources was rated highest at the bachelor's level ($\overline{X} = 4.7$). Basic Principles was rated equally high at both the bachelor's ($\overline{X} = 5.4$) and master's ($\overline{X} = 5.4$) levels.

6. Seven of the twelve instructional areas were rated significantly higher at the master's (M) level than at the doctoral (D) level: Basic Principles ($M\overline{X}=5.40$, $D\overline{X}=4.23$); Medical Aspects ($M\overline{X}=5.23$, $D\overline{X}=3.94$); Occupational Information and Job Analysis ($M\overline{X}=5.00$, $D\overline{X}=4.04$); Case Management ($M\overline{X}=4.59$, $D\overline{X}=3.96$); Community Organization and Resources ($M\overline{X}=4.51$, $D\overline{X}=4.00$); Job Development and Placement ($M\overline{X}=4.70$, $D\overline{X}=3.53$); and Fieldwork ($M\overline{X}=5.82$, $D\overline{X}=4.96$). Research and Professional Issues was rated significantly higher at the doctoral level ($\overline{X}=6.3$ and 5.9, respectively) than at any other level.

7. Eight of the twelve instructional areas were rated significantly higher at the master's (M) level than at the continuing education (CE) level: Basic Principles ($M\overline{X}=5.40$, $CE\overline{X}=4.33$); Counseling Theories and Techniques ($M\overline{X}=5.67$, $CE\overline{X}=4.08$); Medical Aspects ($M\overline{X}=5.23$, $CE\overline{X}=4.39$); Psychosocial Aspects ($M\overline{X}=5.37$, $CE\overline{X}=4.63$); Community Organization and Resources ($M\overline{X}=4.51$, $CE\overline{X}=4.06$); Fieldwork ($M\overline{X}=5.82$, $CE\overline{X}=3.40$); Research ($M\overline{X}=4.21$, $CE\overline{X}=2.48$); and Professional Issues ($M\overline{X}=4.75$, $CE\overline{X}=4.04$). The Case Management instructional area was rated significantly higher at the continuing education level ($\overline{X}=5.0$) than at any other level.

Preferred Emphasis

The educators' mean ratings of the extent to which the twelve instructional areas should be emphasized across four levels of rehabilitation programming and the significance testing of differences ($p<.05$), indicated that:

1. Six instructional areas received a "very high" preferred emphasis rating ($\overline{X}=6.0-7.0$): (a) four at the master's level—Counseling Theories and Techniques ($\overline{X}=6.1$), Fieldwork ($\overline{X}=6.1$), Psychosocial Aspects ($\overline{X}=6.0$), and Job Development and Placement ($\overline{X}=6.0$); (b) two at the doctoral level—Research ($\overline{X}=6.8$) and Professional Issues ($\overline{X}=6.5$); and (c) one at the continuing education level—Job Development and Placement ($\overline{X}=6.0$).

2. Eleven of the twelve instructional areas received "high" preferred emphasis ratings ($\overline{X}=5.0-5.9$): (a) four at the bachelor's level—Basic Principles ($\overline{X}=5.8$), Fieldwork ($\overline{X}=5.3$), Community Organization and Resources ($\overline{X}=5.2$), and Job Development and Placement ($\overline{X}=5.0$); (b) four at the master's level—Medical Aspects ($\overline{X}=5.9$), Occupational Information and Job Analysis ($\overline{X}=5.9$), Basic Principles ($\overline{X}=5.7$), and Community Organization and Resources ($\overline{X}=5.6$); (c) five at the doctoral level—Counseling Theories and Techniques ($\overline{X}=5.8$), Psychosocial Aspects ($\overline{X}=5.7$), Evaluation ($\overline{X}=5.6$),

Fieldwork ($\overline{X}=5.3$), and Medical Aspects ($\overline{X}=5.0$); and (d) eight at the continuing education level — Occupational Information and Job Analysis ($\overline{X}=5.7$), Case Management ($\overline{X}=5.6$), Community Organization and Resources ($\overline{X}=5.4$), Professional Issues ($\overline{X}=5.4$), Medical Aspects ($\overline{X}=5.4$) Psychosocial Aspects ($\overline{X}=5.4$), Evaluation ($\overline{X}=5.4$), and Counseling Theories and Techniques ($\overline{X}=5.2$).

3. Three of the twelve instructional areas received a "slightly low" preferred emphasis rating ($\overline{X}=3.0-3.9$); (a) two at the bachelor's level — Research ($\overline{X}=3.1$) and Counseling Theories and Techniques ($\overline{X}=3.9$); and (b) two at the continuing education level — Research ($\overline{X}=3.4$) and Fieldwork ($\overline{X}=3.9$).

4. None of the twelve instructional areas received a "low" ($\overline{X}=2.0-2.9$) or "very low" ($\overline{X}=1.0-1.9$) preferred emphasis rating at any level.

5. Preferred emphasis ratings indicated that: (a) at the bachelor's level none of the instructional areas were rated "very high" and two were rated "slightly low" (Research, $\overline{X}=3.1$; and Counseling Theories and Techniques, $\overline{X}=3.9$); (b) at the master's level four of the instructional areas were rated "very high" (Counseling Theories and Techniques, $\overline{X}=6.1$; Fieldwork, $\overline{X}=6.1$; Job Development and Placement, $\overline{X}=6.0$; and Psychosocial Aspects, $\overline{X}=6.0$), and none were rated below "average" ($\overline{X}<4.0$); (c) at the doctoral level two instructional areas were rated "very high" (Research, $\overline{X}=6.8$; and Professional Issues, $\overline{X}=6.5$), and none were rated below "average"; and (d) at the continuing education level one instructional area was rated "very high" (Job Development and Placement, $\overline{X}=6.0$), and two were rated "slightly low" (Research, $\overline{X}=3.4$; and Fieldwork, $\overline{X}=3.9$).

6. Eleven of the twelve instructional areas were rated significantly higher at the master's (M) level than at the bachelor's (B) level: Counseling Theories and Techniques ($M\overline{X}=6.07$; $B\overline{X}=3.96$); Medical Aspects ($M\overline{X}=5.88$, $B\overline{X}=4.67$); Psychosocial Aspects ($M\overline{X}=6.04$, $B\overline{X}=4.93$); Occupational Information and Job Analysis ($M\overline{X}=5.93$, $B\overline{X}=4.86$); Evaluation ($M\overline{X}=5.68$, $B\overline{X}=4.54$); Case Management ($M\overline{X}=5.57$, $B\overline{X}=4.71$); Community Organization and Resources ($M\overline{X}=5.60$, $B\overline{X}=5.23$); Job Development and Placement ($M\overline{X}=6.01$, $B\overline{X}=5.02$); Fieldwork ($M\overline{X}=6.12$, $B\overline{X}=5.28$); Research ($M\overline{X}=4.90$, $B\overline{X}=3.12$); and Professional Issues ($M\overline{X}=5.69$, $B\overline{X}=4.73$). There was no significant difference between the bachelor's level and master's level ratings for the Basic Principles instructional area.

7. Eight of the twelve areas were rated significantly higher at the master's (M) level than at the doctoral (D) level; Basic Principles ($M\overline{X}=5.69$, $D\overline{X}=4.52$); Medical Aspects ($M\overline{X}=5.88$, $D\overline{X}=5.05$); Psychosocial Aspects ($M\overline{X}=6.04$, $D\overline{X}=5.72$); Occupational Information and Job

Analysis (M$\overline{X}$=5.93, D$\overline{X}$=4.84); Case Management (M$\overline{X}$=5.57, D$\overline{X}$=4.32); Community Organization and Resources (M$\overline{X}$=5.60, D$\overline{X}$=4.71); Job Development and Placement (M$\overline{X}$=6.01, D$\overline{X}$=4.54); and Fieldwork (M$\overline{X}$=6.12, D$\overline{X}$=5.32). There were no significant differences between the master's and doctoral level ratings for the Counseling Theories and Techniques and the Evaluation instructional areas. Two of the instructional areas (Research, and Professional Issues) were rated significantly higher at the doctoral level than at any other level.

Actual Versus Preferred Emphasis

The educators' mean ratings of both actual and preferred emphasis for the twelve instructional areas across four levels of rehabilitation programming, and significance testing of differences ($p < .05$), indicated that:

1. Mean ratings for preferred emphasis were higher than those for actual emphasis for all twelve instructional areas across all levels of rehabilitation programming.

2. Across all twelve instructional areas and within each of the four levels of rehabilitation programming: (a) at the bachelor's level only in the Counseling Theories and Techniques and in the Fieldwork instructional areas were the actual and preferred emphasis ratings not significantly different; (b) at the master's level all preferred ratings were significantly higher than the actual ratings (least mean differences were in Basic Principles, 5.5 – 5.7, and in Fieldwork, 5.9 – 6.2; greater mean differences were in Community Organization and Resources, 4.6 – 5.6, Occupational Information and Job Analysis, 5.0 – 5.9, and Case Management, 4.6-5.5); (c) at the doctoral level all preferred ratings were significantly higher than the actual ratings (least mean differences were in Counseling Theories and Techniques, 5.4 – 5.9, Fieldwork, 4.9 – 5.4, and Research, 6.2 – 6.7; greater mean differences were in Occupational Information and Job Analysis, 3.9 – 5.1, and Job Development and Placement, 3.5 – 4.7); and, (d) at the continuing education level only in the Basic Principles and in the Fieldwork instructional areas were the actual and preferred emphasis ratings not significantly different (greatest mean differences were in Job Development and Placement, 4.4 – 6.0; Professional Issues, 3.9 – 5.3; and Community Organization and Resources, 4.0 – 5.3).

3. The *overall* actual and preferred average mean rating for each of the four programming levels indicated: (a) similar overall mean differences between actual and preferred emphasis at each of the four

programming levels; (b) highest ratings for overall actual ($\overline{X}=5.08$) and overall preferred ($\overline{X}=5.78$) emphasis at the master's level; (c) equal overall actual emphasis at the bachelor's ($\overline{X}=4.19$) and continuing education ($\overline{X}=4.19$) levels; and, (d) lowest overall preferred emphasis at the bachelor's level ($\overline{X}=4.79$).

DISCUSSION

This self-report survey was returned by 235 (51.2%) of the 459 NCRE members identified in the 1980 *NCRE Directory*. It contains all limitations commonly associated with survey research, particularly the problem of nonresponse bias. Furthermore, since many significance tests were run on the data, more than five percent of the significant results are likely to be spurious. It should be noted especially that ratings were made in relation to the twelve instructional areas and their definitions as provided by the researchers. Different instructional areas or definitions might have produced different results. It should also be noted that the respondents were more heavily involved in master's level education than with the other programming levels. Relatively few educators were directly involved with continuing education programs. The results may have been appreciably influenced by the limited number of respondents who had relevant experiences in continuing education programming. In fact, the subsets of some respondent categories were inspected, but the small subset cell sizes did not allow for appropriate analyses.

One of the most interesting results of this study was that in comparing bachelor's and master's level programming, all instructional areas were found to have received equal or greater actual emphasis ratings at the master's level. This result strongly suggests that rehabilitation education may be primarily oriented toward the preparation of master's level practitioners, and raises the question as to whether the respondents perceived a unique purpose or focus for undergraduate rehabilitation education. (It must be remembered, however, that the respondents reported a predominant emphasis of working with master's students, and thus this observation should be viewed with caution.) The undergraduate practitioner is apparently not being prepared, as indicated by the actual emphasis ratings, to the same general extent as master's level practitioners. The greatest discrepancies between the two levels were for ratings in Counseling Theories and Techniques and in Research, suggesting that bachelor's level practitioners are not being prepared as counselors or as consumers or producers of research. Moreover, the educators' preferred instructional emphasis ratings indicate a preference for bachelor's level practitioners to receive an emphasis in Basic Principles, Fieldwork, Community Organization and Resources, and Job Development and Placement rather than in Counseling Theories and Techniques or in Research. This would appear to be consistent with a generic model of undergraduate rehabilitation education (Feinberg, Sunblad, & Glick, 1974).

It is interesting, however, to contrast these results with Witten's (1980) findings that employers were generally satisfied with the preparation of bachelor's level practitioners and viewed them as being able to perform many of the tasks traditionally deemed appropriate for master's level staff. Witten (1980) also reported that "of those seniors (undergraduates) planning to work in rehabilitation after graduation, about half reported they would seek jobs as rehabilitation counselors" (p. 83). Although employers may be very satisfied with the job performance of bachelor's graduates, the results of this study suggest that caution should be taken when placing them directly into positions requiring high level counseling competencies. The apparent satisfaction of employers with bachelor's graduates who are not prepared as counselors may reveal the relative importance employers attach to the counseling function.

In comparing master's and doctoral level preparation, it is interesting to note that with the exception of Research and Professional Issues, every content area received a greater actual and preferred emphasis rating at the master's level. This result suggests that doctoral level programs are typically oriented toward the preparation of researchers (and by implication educators and possibly administrators as well) rather than toward the preparation of client service practitioners, and that educators indicate a preference for this orientation in doctoral level programs. The comparative lack of emphasis on counseling and fieldwork at the doctoral level is somewhat understandable because most doctoral programs require a master's degree and post-master's work experience as an admission requirement. The post-master's work experience requirement allows doctoral programs to emphasize training in nonclinical areas. The terminal degree for rehabilitation service delivery is clearly the master's and not the doctorate; this is reflected in the doctoral programming emphasis on research and professional issues rather than on direct client services.

The educators' actual emphasis ratings for continuing education programs suggest that Case Management is the most emphasized instructional area. This is probably related to the overriding importance attached to moving clients effectively through the rehabilitation process. Educators seem to be suggesting, however, that Job Development and Placement should receive the greatest emphasis at the continuing education level. This certainly reflects the importance attached to placement services and may indicate that educators are dissatisfied with the placement assistance currently provided by practitioners.

A comparison of the actual and preferred instructional ratings across all four programming levels indicates that, without exception, educators show a preference for every instructional area to receive greater emphasis at every programming level. This preference probably represents an appreciation of the importance of all the instructional areas and their relevance to rehabilitation education, and implies the related frustrations of wanting to prepare "fully functioning" practitioners within limited time constraints (i.e., a limited number of coursework hours).

Realistically, each programming level cannot be all things to all students. Unfortunately, that may be the ideal toward which rehabilitation education has been striving too long. It would seem more effective to have an educational model where a bachelor's degree in rehabilitation is required for admission to a master's program, and a master's degree for admission to a doctoral program (the latter is already generally followed). This would allow for generic rehabilitation services education at the bachelor's level, emphasizing rehabilitation concepts and case management, and for greater coverage of specialized knowledge areas such as counseling, vocational evaluation, and administration at the master's level. With the current cut-back environment in human services as well as in higher education, it behooves rehabilitation educators and the employers of their graduates to establish some consensus regarding instructional priorities at specific programming levels. Although this goal may presently seem somewhat idealistic, it nevertheless is the direction in which rehabilitation education should move.

ACKNOWLEDGMENT

Sincerest appreciation is extended to Doctor Thomas L. Porter, professor of rehabilitation counseling at Auburn University, for his encouragement and valuable assistance throughout the conduct of this project.

This study was part of a larger survey project endorsed by the National Council on Rehabilitation Education and supported by Quality Improvement Program Funds for Emphasis in the Human Services at the University of South Florida, Tampa. Persons interested in a copy of the broader survey *(The 1981 Rehabilitation Education Survey)* should contact the National Clearing House of Rehabilitation Training Materials, Oklahoma State University, 115 Old USDA Building, Stillwater, Oklahoma 74078 (Request Code 106-B).

REFERENCES

Council on Rehabilitation Education. (1978). *Accreditation Manual for Rehabilitation Counselor Education Programs*. Chicago, IL: Author.

Emener, W.G., & Rubin, S.E. (1980). Rehabilitation counselor roles and functions and sources of role strain. *Journal of Applied Rehabilitation Counseling, 2*(2), 57-69.

Feinberg, L.B., Sunblad, L.M., & Glick, L.J. (1974). *Education for the rehabilitation services: Planning undergraduate curricula*. Syracuse, NY: Syracuse University, School of Education.

Fraser, R.T., & Clowers, M.R. (1978). Rehabilitation counselor functions. Perceptions of time spent and complexity. *Journal of Applied Rehabilitation Counseling, 9*(2), 31-35.

Harrison, D.K. (1980). Competency evaluation in rehabilitation (CEIR): Toward a competency-based client-outcome system. *Journal of Applied Rehabilitation Counseling, 2*(1), 18-24.

Harrison, D.K., & Lee, C.C. (1979). Rehabilitation counseling competencies. *Journal of Applied Rehabilitation Counseling, 10*(3), 135-141.

National Council on Rehabilitation Education. (1980). *Membership directory.* Washington, D.C.: Author.

Parham, J.D., & Harris, W.M. (1978). *State agency rehabilitation counselor functions and the mentally retarded.* Lubbock: Texas Tech University, Resource and Training Center in Mental Retardation.

Porter, T.L., Rubin, S.E., & Sink, J.M. (1979). Essential rehabilitation counselor diagnostic, counseling, and placement competencies. *Journal of Applied Rehabilitation Counseling, 10*(3), 158-162.

Rubin, S.E., & Emener, W.G. (1979). Recent rehabilitation counselor role changes and role strain—a pilot investigation. *Journal of Applied Rehabilitation Counseling, 10*(3), 142-147.

Witten, B.J. (1980). *Preparation and utilization of undergraduate workers in rehabilitation: Comparative perceptions of respondents.* Unpublished doctoral dissertation, Syracuse University.

Zadny, J.J., & James, L.F. (1977). Time spent on placement. *Rehabilitation Counseling Bulletin, 21* (1), 31-35.

CHAPTER 14

CLINICAL PRACTICE IN MASTER'S LEVEL REHABILITATION COUNSELOR EDUCATION

Bobbie J. Atkins

Abstract

Clinical practice in rehabilitation education represents an essential component in the graduate student's course of study and serves as a transition between the didactic learning of the classroom and the employment of the student as a professional counselor. Although the value of clinical practice is well established in master's level rehabilitation education, a number of potential problems currently exist. The author examines several issues related to supervision in clinical practice and provides suggestions for clarification.

SINCE THE 1954 vocational rehabilitation legislation made funds available for partial teaching costs and student financial support in rehabilitation counseling, there has been a consistent expansion in the number of Rehabilitation Counselor Education (RCE) programs and in the basic curriculum. The curriculum for master's level education represents a broad spectrum of areas designed to equip graduates with the needed knowledges and skills to become effective rehabilitationists. Although it is difficult to isolate one aspect of the RCE master's curriculum as being the most important, all educators and practitioners agree that clinical practice is an essential component of the student's course of study.

Clinical practice represents the real-life experience in which the graduate student may test the theoretical and didactic learning of the classroom in an attempt to provide for the needs of disabled clients. As a result, this experience takes place in an environment in which the student can learn to deal with the

Reprinted by permission from Volume 21 (1981), *Counselor Education and Supervision*, pp. 169-175.

disabled clients' internal and external problems and the varied agencies that provide services to these consumers. Therefore, the major purpose of clinical practice is providing a transition between the university education program and placement as a professional rehabilitation counselor (Trotter, Kult, & Atkins, 1980). Additionally, the field placement (a) provides the student with a sense of relevancy and a testing environment for theoretical ideas, (b) affords the opportunity for observation of the use of various counseling models, and (c) allows the student to recognize the assets and limitations of counseling models for implementation as a rehabilitationist.

The importance of clinical practice in rehabilitation education curricula is further supported by the Council on Rehabilitation Education (CORE) and the American Rehabilitation Counseling Association (ARCA). Specifically, CORE requirements for the accreditation of RCE programs include 600 hours of supervised clinical practice. Similarly, ARCA, in *A Statement of Policy on the Professional Preparation of Rehabilitation Counselors* (1978) requires that clinical experience be provided in rehabilitation education. Although CORE requirements and ARCA's statements regarding the importance of clinical practice are clear and provide a guide for developing a graduated series of exposures for students, a number of problems are unresolved regarding practical experiences. This article will examine some of the important issues concerning supervision and supervisors in rehabilitation clinical practice.

DEFINING SUPERVISION

Although supervision is a key component in clinical practice in rehabilitation counseling, it lacks a standardized definition (Lanning, 1971). This deficiency represents a possible barrier to developing consistent field experiences for students. The following diverse definitions highlight the complexity of this dilemma. Kell and Mueller (1966) provided this definition: "A complex . . . inter-personal expression of qualities which enhance feelings of trust and security and . . . allows those being supervised the freedom to learn, grow, and change" (p. 99).

Patterson (1964) pointed out that the basis for defining supervision rested in its relationship component. It was his belief that supervision is therapeutic and is best performed when both teaching and therapy are involved. Although teaching and therapy represent the two boundaries of supervision, effective supervision should lie somewhere in between the two processes. A third definition of supervision was provided by the Joint Liaison Committee of the Council of State Directors of Vocational Rehabilitation and Rehabilitation Counselor Educators (1963): "Leadership in helping, guiding, and stimulating counselors to a critical appraisal and study of their own performance as affected by their individual attitudes and practices" (p. 3).

As evidenced by these definitions, supervision has varying meanings. The lack of a prototype for its definition in clinical practice will undoubtedly cause problems. First, the way in which the student's supervisor defines supervision will in part determine the structure for the experience. Second, the content of the experience will vary according to the accepted definition of supervision. Next, the definition of supervision will affect desired and expected goals and objectives for field experience. Finally, if the agency supervisor's, the educator supervisor's, or the students' definitions differ, inconsistencies in the practicum will occur and confusion for the student will be a likely result.

In spite of the diverse definitions and potential problems that may occur, we are reminded by Lanning (1971) that a common element — the nature of the interpersonal relationship — is usually found in all definitions of supervision. If Lanning's belief can be substantiated, rehabilitationists will be in a more advanced position to provide consistency in defining supervision. Consistency should serve to reduce confusion and provide structure for the development of specific purposes for clinical practice. The differences that exist in defining supervision relate closely to another problem in field placement, that is, defining the purposes of supervision.

PURPOSES OF SUPERVISION

The purpose of supervision relates to the objectives and expected outcomes for students involved in clinical practice. Hansen and Warner (1971) asserted that educators in RCE programs tend to disagree on the objectives of supervision for practical experience. Inherent in this situation is the negative effect that a lack of agreement could have on the quality and content of the field placement for RCE students. The current views in rehabilitation that serve as guidelines for delineating the purpose of supervision can be found in ARCA's statements regarding the professional preparation of counselors. These statements provide general instructions but do not provide the specificity required to ensure that graduates of RCE programs receive consistent experiences. The Joint Liaison Committee (1963) identified the purpose of supervision as focusing on assisting the student to develop professional attitudes and approaches to rehabilitation counseling. As with ARCA's guidelines, the committee's purpose lacks specificity.

Shorts (1978, p. 7) identified a set of purposes that have potential for providing needed clarity for the term supervision. The three main purposes include: (1) facilitating the supervisee's personal and professional development, (2) promoting competencies, and (3) promoting accountable counseling and rehabilitation services and programs. This statement of the purposes of supervision can be interpreted in a meaningful way by rehabilitation professionals.

Shorts's identification of the purposes of supervision are consistent with the opinions of authorities in the field (Combs & Super, 1963; Gaomi & Neumann, 1974; Patterson, 1971). Personal and professional development represent critical goals for supervisors and suggest that students' internal and external resources must interplay if effective development as a counselor is to occur. In addition, this purpose relates to Lanning's (1971) belief that the key to defining supervision is the development of a meaningful relationship between student and supervisor that allows for the creation of an environment where growth can occur. The second purpose described by Shorts provides support for the development of needed knowledge and skill to perform the duties of a rehabilitation counselor. This purpose also is related to ARCA's (1978) statement of policy concerning the role of the counselor, which reflects the belief that counselors must employ techniques of individual and group counseling to assist disabled clients in their adjustment.

The final purpose suggested by Shorts focused on accountability, which is clearly the "watch word" in human service programs. The emphasis that students' supervisors place on accountable behavior can be a positive force for ensuring quality services to clients. Developing meaningful rehabilitation plans, accurate case recording, and involvement in program development and change are examples of the roles supervisors play in promoting accountable actions in students (Shorts, 1978). It is expected that the learning of accountable behaviors as a student will transfer into the professional activities of that person as a professional counselor.

SELECTION, MOTIVATION, AND EVALUATION OF SUPERVISORS

Without the existence of a standardized definition of supervision, and without precise purposes for supervision, additional problems emerge. These problems are focused on selection, motivation, and evaluation of counselors who supervise students in clinical practice. Specific criteria for the selection of supervisors of students in field placements are lacking in the rehabilitation literature. It would appear that the prevailing opinion that agency supervisors should possess a master's degree in rehabilitation and be certified counselors (Wright, 1980) serves as the primary source of guidance for choosing counselor supervisors for clinical practice. If a consensus could be reached on the appropriate methods for supervisor selection, positive implications would follow for defining supervision, delineating the purpose(s) of supervision, and motivating and evaluating counselor supervisors.

With the ambiguous definition and purpose of student supervision, what motivates a rehabilitation counselor to assume a supervisory relationship with a student? Patterson (1971) believed that both the counselor and the agency have an obligation to provide clinical experience to students and that perhaps "the greatest contribution of the agency is in providing the opportunity for field experience" (p. 87). Although there is a lack of empirical evidence to support this hypothesis, a practical explanation for the counselor's willingness to supervise students may be found in the counselor's professional commitment to rehabilitation. With the increasing number of master's degree counselors employed in rehabilitation (counselors who have also been involved in supervised field experiences themselves), counselors are now recognizing and supporting the importance of student supervision.

Although the basic responsibility for student supervision rests with the faculty in RCE programs, the role of the professional rehabilitation counselor is indispensable. Yet, the additional time commitment often required to effectively supervise students, particularly at beginning levels, and the apparent lack of a precise prototype for supervision can be deterrents to the rehabilitationist's involvement in practicum supervision. These prohibitive aspects of field placement should stimulate educators to study the important clinical phase of rehabilitation education and develop consistent norms for practical implementation.

Evaluation of agency supervisors involved in clinical practice is the final problem to be addressed. The previously mentioned concerns regarding developing an acceptable definition for supervision, stating precise purposes for supervision, and specifying selection criteria for supervisors suggest that meaningful evaluation of supervisors will be difficult.

Several factors must be considered if meaningful evaluation methods for supervisors are to occur. As previously stated, rehabilitation educators will need to develop a more uniform definition of supervision and, once clarification is attained, this information will need to be communicated to potential agency supervisors. Also, there is the need for educators and practitioners to develop mutual objectives for student placement in rehabilitation agencies. Once mutual clarification occurs, evaluation would involve determining if and to what extent objectives were accomplished. Evaluation of supervisors should include self-reports and feedback from students. Therefore, meaningful evaluation requires that educators, rehabilitationists, and students work together in the evolution of outcome criteria.

Stoltenberg (1981) suggested that supervision is a developmental process and provided "The Counselor Complexity Model" (p. 59) for use in clinical supervision. The basic premise of the model is that development as a counselor requires a series of experiences, and specific stages of development can be identified. Although the model needs to be tested empirically, rehabilitationists could use selected aspects of the model as guidelines for developing evaluation data.

Since supervision is conceptualized as an influence process (Dodenhoff, 1981), determining the extent to which agency supervisors influence students in rehabilitation makes evaluation a critical area in clinical practice. Yet, before evaluation of agency supervisors can assume a significant role in the clinical practice area, the problems identified here must first be resolved. Ultimately, resolution of the supervisory problems discussed in this article will provide useful guidance in developing meaningful evaluation techniques.

SUMMARY

The importance of clinical practice in rehabilitation is well accepted in the profession (ARCA, 1978; Patterson, 1971; Trotter, Kult, & Atkins, 1980; Wright, 1980). Yet, field placement in rehabilitation represents a somewhat neglected area of empirical study. In particular, the areas involving definition and purpose(s) of supervision and selection, motivation, and evaluation of supervisors need consistent empirical exploration. Although considerable research has been conducted on clinical practice in related human service areas (e.g., counseling psychology, psychotherapy), research with a specific rehabilitation focus is limited. Since the primary responsibility for providing supervised clinical experience rests with the university faculty, rehabilitation educators must assume positive leadership in researching the entire spectrum of variables associated with field placement. A preliminary step could involve "inservice programs for current field counselor supervisors" (Shorts, 1978, p. 61). In addition to enhancing the supervising skills of participants, inservice training activities could be used for developing a data base for viable research investigation (e.g., knowledges gained, attitude change).

Scofield and Scofield (1978) reported that agency supervisors involved in student supervision were at best vaguely aware of their responsibilities and the goals of the student. This statement is not surprising based on this discussion of the ambiguous areas that exist in student supervision. Similarly, this type of confusion can be a deterrent to an effective field experience for the student, and ultimately reduce the quality of services provided for the disabled consumer. Consequently, the need for role and expectation clarification is crucial (Shorts, 1978).

In conclusion, the problems discussed in this article represent only a few of the concerns relating to clinical practice. Other issues include selecting and evaluating agencies for field experience, developing consistent terminology to identify the graduated series of practical experiences required in RCE programs, clarifying the role of communication between university and agency supervisors, and exploring students' expectations of the field work experience. Despite identifiable problems, rehabilitation students receive meaningful exposures in field work settings suggesting that the knowledge required to clarify issues concerning clinical practice currently exist. The challenge is to organize, document, and disseminate the resultant information to the profession. With the changing emphasis in rehabilitation and current financial constraints, the need for clarification and consistency in clinical experiences is paramount.

REFERENCES

A statement of policy on the professional preparation of rehabilitation counselors. In B. Bolton & M. Jaques (Eds.), *Rehabilitation counseling: Theory and practice.* Baltimore: University Park Press, 1978.

Combs, A.W., & Super, D.W. The perceptual organization of effective counselors. *Journal of Counseling Psychology,* 1963, *10,* 222-226.

Dodenhoff, J.T. Interpersonal attraction and direct-indirect supervisor influence on predictors of counselor trainee effectiveness. *Journal of Counseling Psychology,* 1981, *28,* 47-52.

Gaomi, B., & Neumann, M. Supervision from the point of view of the supervisee. *American Journal of Psychotherapy,* 1974, *28,* 108-113.

Hansen, J.C., & Warner, R.W. Review of research on practicum supervision. *Counselor Education and Supervision,* 1971, *10,* 261-271.

Joint Liaison Committee. *Studies in rehabilitation counselor training: Guidelines for supervised clinical practice.* Minneapolis: Author, 1963.

Kell, B.L., & Mueller, W.J. *Impact and change: A study of counseling relationships.* Englewood Cliffs, N.J.: Prentice-Hall, 1966.

Lanning, W.L. A study of the relationship between group and individual counseling supervision and three relationship measures. *Journal of Counseling Psychology,* 1971, *18,* 401-406.

Patterson, C.H. Supervising students in the counseling practicum. *Journal of Counseling Psychology,* 1964, *11,* 47-53.

Patterson, C.H. University and agency contributions to professional education. In H.A. Moses & C.H. Patterson (Eds.), *Readings in rehabilitation counseling* (2nd ed.). Champaign, Ill.: Stipes Publishing Co., 1971.

Scofield, M.E., & Scofield, B.J. Ethical concerns in clinical practice supervision. *Journal of Applied Rehabilitation Counseling,* 1978, *9,* 27-29.

Shorts, J.G. *A review of the role and function of field supervision as it relates to the professional preparation of student counselors.* Unpublished master's paper, University of Wisconsin-Milwaukee, 1978.

Stoltenberg, C. Approaching supervision from a developmental perspective: The counselor complexity model. *Journal of Counseling Psychology,* 1981, *28,* 59-65.

Trotter, A.B.; Kult, D.A.; & Atkins, B.J. *Field training supervisors manual.* Milwaukee: University of Wisconsin-Milwaukee, 1980.

Wright, G.N. *Total rehabilitation.* Boston: Little, Brown, & Co., 1980.

CHAPTER 15

INTERNSHIPS FOR REHABILITATION COUNSELORS: ON THE WAY TO A PROFESSIONAL CAREER

GLEN O. GEIST

R EHABILITATION COUNSELING has become recognized quickly as a viable professional career with a Code of Ethics, certification and training program accreditation process, thus taking its place alongside of the more established professions. The rehabilitation counseling student is required to spend some portion of his training working as an intern in a rehabilitation agency with the primary aim of enabling students to approximate the realities of a professional job. Under supervision, the internship involves progressively greater movement toward autonomous professional functioning whereby the student can apply classroom gained knowledge in practice.

Whereas many agencies are willing to provide internship experiences for students, very few are willing to provide remuneration for services performed. Many attractive applicants and potentially capable professionals, most notably those of minority groups and handicapped, are finding it impossible to acquire professional training without financial support. Paid internships is one evident means of providing such support and thus attracting and maintaining otherwise qualified personnel for the rehabilitation counseling profession.

Arguments against paid internships seem to be of three kinds. First, the agency budget will not allow this luxury. This argument, particularly in the present economic state of austerity, is difficult to refute. The second argument is that interns take up too much staff time. However, when the internship is set up efficiently, the time required for supervision and training is much less than the work performed independently by an intern with a caseload, and thereby

Reprinted by permission from Volume 43 (1977), *Journal of Rehabilitation*, p. 40.

can provide a means for more work to be accomplished. The third argument is that students are just students and, indeed, should pay for the privilege of doing an internship. However, students do pay for being an intern via the tuition costs at their universities.

WHY SHOULD INTERNS BE PAID?

There are a number of reasons, both professional and economic, as to why interns should be paid. Many agencies have in-service training programs for newly hired and untrained employees, which are more costly, both in terms of funds and staff time, than paying interns, much of whose training is already accomplished. Students work long and hard hours at the agencies; however students, like most people, are wont to provide according to their reward. Professionals have a moral obligation to train students in their discipline. With the advent of rehabilitation counselor certification, a criterion will be supervised experience under a certified counselor. To develop certified counselors, agencies will have to provide supervision. An internship program can provide the climate and opportunity for recruitment. Finally, such a program stimulates the progressional growth of the agency and provides a basis for continuous evaluation of the university training program.

Agencies which do not pay interns would have to upgrade their training programs to still attract interns. The effect this would have on improved services to clients is incalculable. It is noticeable that those agencies having paid internships generally have better training programs than those which do not pay. It is hardly likely that this is a coincidence.

Likewise, these agencies have the right to demand cooperation from the university programs in terms of seminars, courses in such areas as supervision and administration for agency personnel, and consultation on training program development and evaluation in the agency. Moreover, agencies would have a greater right to demand that the university curriculum reflect the needs of the rehabilitation counseling profession as it is practiced in the real life situation. To accomplish these things, agencies must provide for the training and payment of interns. This is most important for the development of the profession.

CHAPTER 16

TRAINING COUNSELORS TO WRITE BEHAVIOR-BASED CLIENT OBJECTIVES

Suki Hinman and John N. Marr

Abstract

A behavioral consultant was stationed at a large comprehensive vocational rehabilitation facility for the purpose of training counselors to write individual rehabilitation programs in terms of specific, behaviorally stated client objectives.
Individual training using modeling, shaping, immediate feedback with reinforcement, and fading was applied to actual cases. Use of a multiple-baseline design
showed replicated training-related increases as distinct from any other changes
occurring in the facility during the two-year period. The number of behaviorally
stated, client-centered objectives written per client increased significantly for
each of the twelve counselors as a function of training, whereas the number of
nonbehavioral objectives did not. On the average, counselors only wrote one behavioral objective for about every fifth client before training, compared to more
than four objectives *per* client after training. This represents a practical and statistically significant change in counselor behavior.

THE DEVELOPMENT of applied behavior analysis, or behavior modification, has been recognized by many rehabilitationists as the most significant single accomplishment in the discipline of psychology in this century
(Lorenz, 1981; McRae & Lutzker, 1982). In the past decade, behavior modification has been applied successfully in virtually all areas of education, health,

Reprinted by permission from Volume 27 (1984). *Rehabilitation Counseling Bulletin,* pp. 291-301.

This research was supported in part by a research and training center grant (G008200023, RT-13)
from the National Institute of Handicapped Research, Office of Special Education and Rehabilitation
Services, Department of Education, to the Arkansas Rehabilitation Research and Training Center.
The more detailed report of the method and results of this study, Training Counselors to Write Rehabilitation Programs in Terms of Behaviorally-Stated Client Objectives Via On-Site Consultation, is
available from the Dissemination Clerk, Arkansas Rehabilitation Research and Training Center, P.O.
Box 1358, Hot Springs, AR 71901, $2.00.

and human services (Lutzker & Martin, 1981), including a broad range of disabilities, vocational rehabilitation (VR) settings, and behavior problems. As Lorenz (1981) pointed out, the question is no longer whether these behavioral procedures are effective, but rather whether practitioners will use these proven techniques in a systematic fashion.

Because training in theory and application of behavior modification is still not required in most rehabilitation graduate education programs (Council on Rehabilitation Education, 1978; Wantz, Scherman, & Hollis, 1982), most VR practitioners have not been prepared to implement these techniques. Responsibility for training staff to use the procedures has generally fallen to the VR agency itself, and efforts to teach these skills have primarily used a short-term training approach. Follow-up data, however, consistently show low postworkshop utilization rates (Godley & Cuvo, 1981; Greene, Willis, Levy, & Bailey, 1978; Marr & Greenwood, 1979), indicating that short-term training alone is an ineffective means of promoting application of behavior management skills.

Several factors may contribute to this finding. For instance, even though large social institutions have been characterized as resistant to change (Fairweather, Sanders, Tornatzky, & Harris, 1974), arrangements for short-term training have often ignored the administrative commitment and middle-management support considered crucial to the adoption of new procedures (McRae & Lutzker, 1982; Soloff, Goldston, & Pollack, 1975). In addition, the three-day workshop without follow-up is antithetical to educators' conceptualization of skill development as an ongoing process. Participants who learn new techniques in a workshop context are seldom successful in applying them to new problems unless generalization is systematically programmed into the training (Stokes & Baer, 1977; Wehman, Abramson, & Norman, 1977). A three-day time period imposes limits on such programming, particularly when each application requires proficiency in several complex skills, as is the case with behavioral interventions.

A number of stategies for promoting the adoption of new procedures by practitioners have been suggested. For instance, Rogers (1971) noted the need to establish better communication links between the source of new information and the potential adopters, and Bozarth (1971) advocated the provision of on-site information and interpretation to practitioners as a means to improve such communication. Continued personal contact between innovator-researcher and practitioner has been stressed as important in facilitating application of new knowledge by practitioners (Glaser, 1978; Havelock, 1971; Muthard, 1980). In addition, the use of consultants has been found to increase staff receptivity to both internal and external communiction (Glaser, 1965; Glaser & Marks, 1966). Munro (1977) proposed that consultants to institutions be placed directly within front-line systems for extended periods of time. After reviewing the research on teaching behavioral procedures, Kazdin and Moyer (1976) strongly advocated both practical and instructional training in combination with a reinforcement system so that actual behavior in the situation results in positive consequences.

The approach selected for use in the present study was training by a consultant who was placed on-site at a large comprehensive VR facility and administratively assigned to the director. This provided personal contact between consultant and practitioner, allowed training to be performance-bound rather than time-bound, established administrative commitment to change at all levels of operation, and ensured that follow-up consultation would be available when needed.

The first steps in applied behavioral analysis are specifying the problem behavior on skill deficit as objectively as possible (Cone & Hawkins, 1977; Marr & Means, 1980) and formulating intervention program objectives in behavioral terms (Bergan, 1977; Leitenberg, 1976). Field counselors seldom state client objectives in performance terms on the Individualized Written Rehabilitation Program (IWRP) and frequently confuse services with objectives (Melia, 1978). Similarly, facility counselors seldom specify client objectives when writing programs and often list the means to an end (services) rather than the objective itself. Thus, the purpose of this study was to evaluate the effect of individual training of rehabilitation counselors on their ability to write specific behaviorally stated, client-centered objectives.

METHOD

Participants

All twelve master's-level counselors carrying vocational training cases at the Hot Springs Rehabilitation Center (HSRC) were trained by the consultant, a behavioral psychologist with several years experience.

Procedure

In cooperation with key facility staff the consultant first redesigned selected portions of the client program information-flow system. This accomplished three objectives: (a) to inform all relevant service-providing staff of a client's behavioral objectives; (b) to ensure that a specified target behavior would be dealt with in a consistent fashion across program areas; and (c) to facilitate the process of reporting progress toward those objectives back to the responsible counselor. The result was the Individualized Written Center Plan (IWCP) form, an amendment form, and a response document, which replaced all of the referral and reporting forms previously in use at the facility.

The IWCP was to be written by the counselor following a final program planning staffing and reflected the planning and decisions made on the basis of

FIGURE 16–1

**Mean Behavioral Objectives Written by Four Representative Counselors
Over Time as Training Occurred**

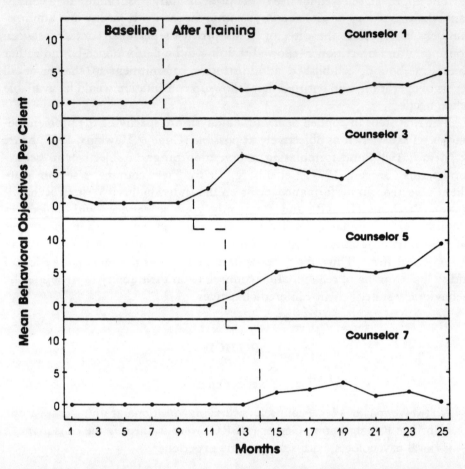

all available information from the client, the field counselor, and specialized medical, psychological, and vocational evaluations. The IWCP form was introduced to counselors individually, and provided the context for their training by the consultant.

COUNSELOR TRAINING. A multiple-baseline design was employed, whereby individual counselors were trained in a chronologically staggered fashion. Data were collected at two-month intervals over a two-year period (see Figure 16-1).

The consultant trained each counselor, using actual cases, until that counselor had demonstrated an acceptable level of proficiency. Individualized shaping and feedback were continued over whatever period of time (and number of cases) was necessary to train the counselor to write specific client-centered, behavioral objectives. The approach of learning by doing with actual cases provided counselors diversified practice, minimized the risk of their merely reproducing stock objectives from case to case, and ensured the opportunity for feedback and reinforcement in the work setting.

The consultant first met briefly with the counselor to review the IWCP process and the rationale for it, and to explain the training. She then familiarized herself with all written information concerning the counselor's clients admitted that week and attended both pre- and final staffings, participating when apparently relevant questions were not asked or nonbehavioral descriptions were reported (by counselor or evaluator).

Following the staffing, the consultant assisted the counselor in writing first a summary of relevant vocational evaluation information (i.e., vocational skill performance and behavioral assets and liabilities) and then the specific behaviorally stated objectives based on that information. The individualized training procedure consisted of modeling (demonstrating and describing explicitly the target counselor behavior), shaping (praising successive approximations to that target performance), and immediate feedback with reinforcement.

This procedure was then repeated for subsequent clients. After the first couple of cases, the consultant gradually but systematically withdrew her explicit directions as fast as the counselor demonstrated the desired results. In the course of writing IWCPs for a few clients, each counselor was trained to write both extremely explicit objectives specifying behavioral target levels, and less specific (but nonetheless behaviorally stated) objectives referring to classes of behaviors already broken down into their specific components elsewhere (i.e., established instructional curricula). Counselors were considered to have met criterion when each had written two plans with little or no corrective feedback from the consultant. Once the counselor had done so, the consultant continued to monitor IWCP performance. Counselors were provided corrective feedback as needed, and joint social reinforcement provided by the consultant and the counseling supervisor was gradually faded.

Responsibility for IWCP-related training, monitoring, and feedback was transferred from the consultant to the counseling supervisor in a systematic fashion. Following some objective-writing practice sessions, the counseling supervisor first took responsibility for training a new counselor. Next, he became the sole source of feedback to counselors on their IWCPs, although the consultant continued to meet with him weekly to review the documents. The transfer was complete when the consultant discontinued the weekly review sessions approximately six months after the last counselor was trained.

Dependent Variables and Scoring

All data were gathered from reports routinely generated by the counselor on the basis of the client's exit-from-evaluation staffing. From the population of clients who remained at the facility to receive additional services after completing vocational evaluation, the two cases completing evaluation nearest to each sampling period were drawn for each counselor every two months across 26 months. This resulted in an N of 306 case reports from which all data were gathered.

Using a multilevel classification system, frequency counts were taken on up to seven variables related to statement of client program objectives. First, each objective statement (as opposed to descriptions of past services rendered and global goal statements) was identified as either an institutional objective (implying something done to or for clients, e.g., "to provide . . .," "to train . . .") or a client objective (implying some client responsibility, e.g., "to acquire . . . skills," "to increase . . ."). If the statement was a client objective, it was then classified as either a nonbehavioral objective (vague, inexplicit) or a behavioral one. In order to meet the criterion for classification as a behavioral objective, the statement had to address either (a) a specific behavior and include the target level, or (b) a class of behavior or set of skills (e.g., welding skills) for which an established program with explicit curriculum existed.

Although counselor training focused on using explicit language to write client-centered behavioral objectives, emphasis was placed on the specification of additional information related to accomplishment of objectives that was considered crucial to effective communication of client programs to other service providers. This information included *who* was designated as responsible for working on the objective and reporting progress toward it, *how* the objective was to be accomplished, an effective date for *starting* the program, and the behavioral criterion for *ending* the program and declaring the objective accomplished. Accordingly, when a statement was classified as a behavioral objective, it was further noted whether the four procedural elements (who, how, start, end) were also present.

Two research assistants were provided written instructions for scoring the behavioral objectives variables and trained to a criterion of .90 accuracy (as compared to pre-established standard scoring) over a twenty-trial test set of actual cases not drawn in the sample to be scored. Both raters exceeded this criterion. After all identifying information had been removed and code numbers assigned, one case per counselor per sampling time was randomly assigned to each rater, and each rater's cases were put in random order. For the purpose of establishing the level of interrater reliability, twenty cases were randomly selected for scoring by both raters. Because the rater's task was in essence to make categorical judgments (i.e., was an objective present, and if so which kind was it?), Cohen's (1960) Kappa (K) was used to assess interrater reliability. The resulting K value for type of objective was .99. For each of the four additional variables (who, how, start, end) scored for objectives classified as behavioral, K was 1.00.

Table 16–1

Mean Numbers of Behavioral Objectives Written per Client by
Each Counselor Before and After Training

Counselor	All Sampling Periods		Immediate Pre-Post[a]	
	Before	After	Before	After
1	.00	3.00*	.00	4.50
2	.00	4.25*	.00	5.50
3	.20	5.25*	.00	5.00
4	.00	3.71*	.00	6.00
5	.00	5.57*	.00	3.50
6	1.21	4.83*	.50	5.25
7	.00	2.00*	.00	2.25
8	.14	5.10*	.00	6.00
9	.00	3.90*	.00	4.75
10	.00	3.33*	.00	3.25
11	.31	3.30*	.00	3.50
12	.00	4.83*	.00	6.25
Total	.16	4.10**	.04	4.65***

[a]Statistical tests not calculated for individual counselors.

 *$p < .05$ (Duncan's multiple range test).

 **$p < .001$ (correlated t-test).

 ***$p < .0001$ (orthogonal comparison).

RESULTS

The data collected on two cases per counselor were initially averaged for each sampling period, resulting in $N = 153$ for analysis. Group means were compared via correlated t tests. One-way (training) repeated measures analyses of variance (ANOVA) were employed for individual-level comparisons because the numbers of cases before and after training were often so unequal due to the multiple-baseline design. Means were further compared using Duncan's multiple-range test; all tests of significance were assessed at $p < .05$.

The primary goal of training was to teach the counselor to write client-centered behavioral objectives. The effect of training is reflected in the means presented in Table 16-1. When considering the data collected over the entire two-year study (all sampling periods), it is apparent that the number of behavioral objectives counselors wrote consistently increased as a function of training. Table 16-1 shows that whereas counselors as a group wrote one behavioral objective for about every fifth client before training, they wrote more than four per client after training, both a practical and a statistically significant increase, $t(11) = 13.11$. Although the increases for individual counselors varied in magnitude, all twelve counselors demonstrated a statistically significant increase in the number of behavioral objectives they wrote per client.

The short-term effects of training were analyzed by computing a one-way repeated measures ANOVA (four levels of sampling time) followed by planned comparisons of the four cases from the two sampling times immediately prior to training with the four cases from the two sampling times immediately after training for each counselor. These immediate pre-post comparisons, also presented in Table 16-1, showed a statistically significant increase of four and one-half behavioral objectives written per client by the group, $F(1, 44) = 79.86$, with each counselor demonstrating a substantial increase following training. This is a pattern similar to the long-term effects of training, but the short-term effects seem somewhat larger in magnitude. Examination of individual-level data over time indicated, however, that counselors continued to write behavioral objectives at a level substantially above their pretraining baselines up to eighteen months after training. Thus, the short-term effect of training was more pronounced, but the change in counselor performance was nonetheless an enduring one.

Analysis of the data on procedural elements (who, how, start, end) was carried out on the individual case level ($N = 162$ before, $N = 144$ after training), as opposed to the sampling of time means. Counselors only wrote twenty-four behavioral objectives before training: None were complete (i.e., all four elements present), and nearly one-sixth of them did not specify any information additional to the target behavior. In contrast, counselors wrote a total of 590 behavioral objectives after training, and of these seventy-eight percent were complete, only five percent omitted all four elements, and a scant six percent failed to specify the two time-frame elements. The overall figures indicated that of the behavioral objectives counselors wrote after training, an impressive eighty-eight percent were either complete or lacking just one element. Ten of the counselors exceeded that figure, with five at 100 percent. In short, training was quite successful in increasing not only the number of behavioral objectives written per client, but also the inclusion of information about the manner and time frame in which they were to be accomplished.

Another means of assessing the effect of counselor training on client-centered behavioral objectives was to analyze the other types of objectives that counselors wrote during the same period. Although optimally effective training should have produced an increase in behavioral objectives only, one could view the writing of more objectives of any type as a successive approximation to writing more objectives of the preferred type. Four counselors demonstrated a significant increase in institutional objectives, and the group increase from 0.98 per client to 1.96 per client was statistically significant, $t(11) = 2.88$. Conversion of these data to ratios, however, showed that the percentage of total objectives classified as institutional significantly decreased (from 73% to 32%) after training, $t(11) = 2.29$. In contrast, the percentage of behavioral objectives increased for every counselor as a function of training, and the overall increase in behavioral objectives (14% to 66%) was statistically significant, $t(11) = 9.08$. The decrease in the percentage of client-centered objectives that were nonbehavioral (12% to 2%) was not statistically significant.

DISCUSSION

The findings of this study, in conjunction with those from previous research, have implications that should be considered in planning future behavioral training for staff in facilities. For instance, because previous studies (e.g., Marr & Greenwood, 1979) suggest that short-term training (e.g., a three-day workshop) has little enduring effect on use of behavioral procedures, it is recommended that such workshops be used only to teach staff overall concepts and to familiarize them with procedures. As indicated by this study, one-on-one training by an expert is an effective method to initiate actual use of skills. The training employed response practice in the actual situation as advocated by Kazdin and Moyer (1976), followed by transfer of responsibility for monitoring objective writing from the consultant to the counseling supervisor. The programmatic transfer of that responsibility, paired with stated administrative expectations, was probably instrumental in maintaining the target behaviors of the counselors. It is suggested, however, that the process could be made more efficient via active involvement of the supervisor from the outset.

Kazdin and Moyer's review also suggests that contingency-based training and practice can be effectively conducted in small groups, which would be more cost-efficient than the approach used in the present study. The study did demonstrate, however, that implementation and maintenance of new procedures is in fact possible, contrary to the notion of generalized resistance to change as characteristic of institutions (Fairweather et al., 1974) when the administration and staff understand the need and actively cooperate to promote change, as was true in this situation.

The fact that the IWCP system is still operational a full twenty-eight months after complete withdrawal of the consultant seems to be conclusive evidence that the on-site training has had a significant and enduring effect on the service delivery system. Furthermore, the facility administrator has reported a positive reception of the IWCP system by both state field program and RSA Regional Office personnel.

The results of this study should be generalizable to other settings and to the other skills needed for rehabilitation professionals to implement the remaining components of comprehensive behavioral programming. The replicated changes in counselor behavior demonstrated through use of the multiple-baseline design indicate that the approach used in this study should be applicable wherever counselors are working. In addition, a preliminary analysis of data being collected under a research project in progress at a VR facility in Region IV (Marr, Hinman, & Ferritor, 1982) lends support to the notion that contingency-based training and practice in the work setting conducted for small groups of rehabilitation professionals can be effective in promoting implementation of a full range of behavioral skills. As in the present study, the researcher-consultants heeded the often heard admonishments (e.g., Zemke,

Standke, & Jones, 1981; Zimmerman & Tobia, 1978) to secure active, visible administrative support. In addition, the consultants were well-versed in behavioral methodology and rehabilitation, and met the other requirements for behavioral consultation advocated by Bergan (1977).

REFERENCES

Bergan, J.R. (1977). *Behavior consultation.* Columbus, OH: Charles E. Merrill.

Bozarth, J.D. (1971). Research dissemination and utilization. *Rehabilitation Research and Practice Review, 2,* 51-58.

Cohen, J. (1960). A coefficient of agreement for nominal scales. *Educational and Psychological Measurement, 20,* 37-46.

Cone, J.D., & Hawkins, R.P. (1977). *Behavior assessment: New directions in clinical psychology.* New York: Brunner/Mazel.

Council on Rehabilitation Education. (1978). *Accreditation manual for rehabilitation counselor education programs.* Chicago: Author.

Glaser, E.M. (1965). Utilization of applicable research and demonstration results. *Journal of Counseling Psychology, 12,* 201-205.

Glaser, E.M. (1978). If Mohammed won't come to the mountain . . . *Evaluation,* Special Issues, 48-53.

Glaser, E.M., & Marks, J.B. (1966). Putting research to use. *Rehabilitation Record, 7,* 6-10.

Godley, S.H., & Cuvo, A.J. (1981). Single-subject experimental designs: Applications to rehabilitation administration. *Journal of Rehabilitation Administration, 5,* 14-22.

Greene, B.F., Willis, B.S., Levy, R., & Bailey, J.S. (1978). Measuring client gains from staff-implemented programs. *Journal of Applied Behavioral Analysis, 11,* 395-412.

Havelock, R.G. (1971). *Planning for innovation.* Ann Arbor, MI: Institute for Social Research.

Kazdin, A., & Moyer, W.T. (1976). Training teachers to use behavior modification. In S. Yen & R.W. McIntire (Eds.), *Teaching behavior modification.* Kalamazoo, MI: Behaviordelia.

Leitenberg, H. (1976). Behavioral approaches to treatment of neuroses. In H. Leitenberg (Ed.), *Handbook of behavior modification and behavior therapy.* Englewood Cliffs, NJ: Prentice-Hall.

Lorenz, J.R. (1981). Behaviorally speaking: What is in it for rehabilitation managers? *Journal of Rehabilitation Administration, 5,* 2-3.

Lutzker, J.R. & Martin, J.A. (1981). *Behavior change.* Monterey, CA: Brooks/Cole.

Marr, J.N., & Greenwood, R. (1979). Utilization of behavioral knowledge from short-term workshops. *Evaluation and the Health Professions, 2,* 455-462.

Marr, J.N., & Means, B.L. (1980). *Behavior management manual: Procedures for psychosocial problems in rehabilitation.* Fayetteville; Arkansas Rehabilitation Research & Training Center.

Marr, J.N., Hinman, S., & Ferritor, D.E. (1982, October). Strategies to increase practitioner use of employment-related behavioral interventions (Project A-7). In

Application for the funding of a vocational rehabilitation research and training center under the National Institute of Handicapped Research (pp. 125-128). Fayetteville: Arkansas Rehabilitation Research and Training Center.

McRae, S., & Lutzker, J.R. (1982). Applied behavior analysis and rehabilitation administration: End of courtship, time for marriage. *Journal of Rehabilitation Administration, 6,* 105-112.

Melia, R.P. (1978). The IWRP and deaf individuals: A challenge to excel. *Journal of Rehabilitation of the Deaf, 12,* 3-8.

Munro, J.A. (1977). Avoiding front-line collapse within mental retardation facilities utilizing an alternative consultative approach. *Canada's Mental Health, 25*(3), 10-13.

Muthard, J.E. (1980). *Putting rehabilitation knowledge to use* (Rehabilitation Monograph No. 11). Gainesville, FL: Rehabilitation Research Institute.

Rogers, E.M. (1971). Research utilization. In W.S. Neff (Ed.), *Rehabilitation psychology,* Washington, D.C.: American Psychological Association.

SAS Institute, Inc. (1975). *SAS User's Guide: Statistical Analysis System, Version 79.6.* Cary, NC: Author.

Soloff, A., Goldston, L.J., & Pollack, R.A. (1975). *Innovation in vocational rehabilitation through research utilization* (Final Report). Chicago: Jewish Vocational Service.

Stokes, T.F., & Baer, D.N. (1977). An implicity theory of generalization. *Journal of Applied Behavioral Analysis, 10,* 349-368.

Wantz, R.A., Scherman, A., & Hollis, J.W. (1982). Trends in counselor preparation: Courses, program emphases, philosophical orientation, and experimental components. *Counselor Education and Supervision, 21,* 258-268.

Wehman, P., Abramson, M., & Norman, C. (1977). Transfer of training in behavior modification programs: An evaluative review. *Journal of Special Education, 11,* 217-231.

Zemke, B., Standke, L., & Jones, P. (1981). Insuring back-on-the-job performance. In R. Zemke, L. Standke, & P. Jones (Eds.), *Designing and delivering cost-effective training — and measuring the results: The best of training.* Minneapolis: Lakewood Publications.

Zimmerman, J.W., & Tobia, P.M. (1978). Programming your outside consultants for success. *Training and Development Journal, 32*(12), 14-19.

CHAPTER 17

COMPUTER-ASSISTED INSTRUCTION IN REHABILITATION EDUCATION

WILLIAM CRIMANDO AND RICHARD BAKER

Abstract

This study investigated the use of computer-assisted instruction in training rehabilitation personnel. Writing evaluation reports was the subject matter of the instructional program. It was hypothesized that students who learned the concepts of report writing with a computer-based tutorial would perform significantly better on a test of those concepts than students who had been provided with a lecture on the same material. The results supported this hypothesis, and implications for rehabilitation education are discussed.

TO TRAIN COMPETENT rehabilitation professionals, educators should make sure not only that the content they are teaching is relevant (i.e., representative of the content domain of professional practice) but also that their teaching methods are efficient and effective. In this study, computer-assisted instruction (CAI) was investigated as an instructional method in rehabilitation education. The CAI method has been used in teaching content in dentistry (Tira, 1977), research methods (Malamuth, Shure, & Johnston, 1975), medical topics (Deignan, Seager, Kimball, & Horowitz, 1980), and writing (Wresch, 1982). Furthermore, CAI has been found more effective than lectures on many occasions (Deignan et al., 1980; Tira, 1977).

One topic in a master's level vocational evaluation curriculum — writing evaluation reports — was used to test the effectiveness of CAI. Because of the demonstrated superiority of CAI in concept mastery over other teaching methods, it was hypothesized that students who learned report-writing concepts with a CAI tutorial would score significantly higher on a test of those concepts than students who had been provided with a lecture on the same material.

Reprinted by permission from Volume 28 (1984), *Rehabilitation Counseling Bulletin*, pp. 50-54.

Students' attitudes toward learning with CAI were also investigated so that their observations could be used in future development of educational software.

METHOD

Participants

Thirty students in a master's-level rehabilitation education program participated in this study—twenty students in an evaluation and adjustment services class and ten volunteers from other classes. The students were randomly assigned to one of two groups—a CAI group and a lecture group. Assignment was stratified so that the evaluation students (who might have had prior experience with the material) were equally represented in the two groups. The CAI group consisted of seven women and eight men, ranging in age from 21 to 59 ($M = 28.5$, $SD = 9.4$). The lecture group consisted of eleven women and four men, whose ages ranged from 21 to 61 ($M = 31.6$, $SD = 11.8$).

Training

The levels of the independent variable consisted of two types of instruction—regular lecture and computer-assisted. The lecture was a standard two-hour lecture on report writing used in previous classes, with detailed outlines on overhead transparencies. Frequent examples were incorporated for clarification, and students were encouraged to ask questions.

To help ensure consistency of content, the CAI unit was developed from lecture outlines, supplemented by standard texts and author experience. The CAI unit consisted of five subunits, each lasting approximately twenty minutes. Interspersed throughout the unit were review questions that the student had to answer before proceeding. Correct answers were followed by more text, praise, or both. Incorrect answers were followed either by the correct answer and more text or by the text from which the question had been drawn so that the student could review it before attempting the question again. The computer text was accompanied by a manual containing directions for using the microcomputer and examples for use during the lesson. Text, questions, and examples were validated for content by three expert raters: a vocational evaluator, an evaluation educator, and a licensed psychologist who had often provided vocational evaluations for rehabilitation agencies.

The program that controlled the presentation of text was developed using a CAI-authoring program, which allows the developer to concentrate on content rather than the format program. The unit was presented on Apple 2 Plus and Franklin Ace 100 microcomputers, equipped with five ¼-inch disk drives and twelve-inch green screen video monitors.

Instrumentation

The dependent measure was a thirty-point short answer posttest that assessed student mastery of concepts from both the lecture and CAI. Half of the points tested concept recall (e.g., "What is the purpose of the background summary?"). The remaining questions consisted of segments from an evaluation report in which students had to identify errors. For example, the segment, "Mrs. Smith evidenced poor personal hygiene and inappropriate social skills while in evaluation," required an answer of "vague," "specific behaviors undefined," or similar responses. The tests were rated blindly by one of the researchers who was following an answer guide.

An eight-item instrument was also devised to assess attitudes of participants toward instruction received. The instrument included items concerning participants' perceptions of the length, thoroughness, degree of detail, and degree of importance of the unit, as well as their enjoyment, interests, skill levels after completion, and desires to have more instruction delivered using the same method. The participants were asked to indicate their agreement to each item on a five-point Likert-type scale.

Procedure

The students were asked to review a standard text on report writing to equalize prior exposure to the material. Those in the lecture group received the standard lecture with examples and were allowed to ask questions. The students in the CAI group were given brief instruction on using the microcomputer, directions for completing the unit, and the manual. They were told they could proceed at their own pace and could reread any lesson. Total time of completion ranged from 51 to 107 minutes ($M = 93$ minutes, $SD = 25$). A brief attitude survey and the posttest were administered immediately following instruction. The students were told to identify themselves by a three-letter code to maintain blind rating. In the CAI group, these codes were automatically stored on disk by the program so as to distinguish the CAI group from the lecture group subsequent to scoring the tests.

RESULTS AND DISCUSSION

An independent samples t-test was used to test the hypothesis that students in the CAI group would score significantly higher on the posttest than their counterparts in the lecture group. Posttest scores for the CAI group ranged from 9 to 26 points ($M = 16.7$, $SD = 4.4$), while in the lecture group, they ranged from 5 to 18 points ($M = 13.5$, $SD = 3.6$), indicating a significant difference between groups: $t_{28} = 2.23$, $p < .05$. The students in the CAI group thus scored significantly higher than those in the lecture group.

Student reactions to the instruction were also examined using the brief attitude survey, and median tests were performed to compare the two groups on each of the eight items. The only item on which the two groups differed in their extent of agreement was: "I enjoyed this session." The CAI group indicated greater agreement: $X^2_1 = 5.22$, $p < .05$. An analysis of the written comments of the CAI students suggested that the difference was due to the novelty of using the microcomputer, self-pacing, and having to answer questions correctly before proceeding with text.

The implications of this study extend to both educators who want to develop CAI units and those who prefer more traditional approaches. Those features that the students liked and disliked about CAI might well be considered in developing all instructional approaches:

1. *Mandatory review.* One of the features that distinguishes CAI from ordinary programmed instruction is that users have to answer review questions before proceeding with text, without the opportunity to page back through the text, without the opportunity to page back through the text to find the answers (Avner, Moore, & Smith, 1980). The students are therefore forced to demonstrate mastery of one set of concepts before proceeding to another.

2. *Individualization* (Dean, 1977; Ross & Wasicsko, 1981). The opportunity to move at one's own pace, a feature of most CAI units, is not possible in lecture formats. But the instructor might want to build in other opportunities for individualized learning, by using contract grading, discussion groups, and hands-on demonstration.

3. *Structure.* The care and rigor with which CAI units are produced might be used when developing lectures, by specifying learning objectives, dividing lessons into smaller, well-defined sublessons, and providing frequent review and summary.

4. *Novelty.* Certainly, teachers have been advised to vary teaching styles and formats (Ross & Wasicsko, 1981). Novelty seems to increase attention to the subject matter. Software developers must make sure that the novelty does not wear off. Gagne, Wagner, and Rojas (1981) advised that CAI be developed using color, motion, and sound—capabilities that are available on many microcomputers—to provide selective emphasis of text and maintain attention to the important points.

Computer-assisted instruction will never replace human teachers, nor should it. Rehabilitation students need to interact with masters of the profession to discuss and synthesize what they learn and to integrate it into their practice. Lectures and demonstrations might better be used as vehicles of motivation rather than sources of critical information (Dean, 1977). If CAI and efficient formats like it are used for concept mastery, instructors and students will then have more time to critically examine the material, discuss its implications, and test its power in actual practice.

REFERENCES

Avner, A., Moore, C., & Smith, S. (1980). Active external control: A basis for superiority of CBI. *Journal of Computer-Based Instruction, 6* (4), 115-118.

Dean, P.M. (1977). Why CBI? An examination of the case for computer-based instruction. *Journal of Computer-Based Instruction, 4* (1), 1-7.

Deignan, G.M., Seager, B.R., Kimball, M., & Horowitz, N.S. (1980). *Computer-assisted, programmed text, and lecture modes of instruction in three medical training courses: Comparative evaluation* (Report No. AFHRL-TR-79-76). Lowry Air Force Base, CO: Air Force Human Resources Laboratory. (ERIC Document Reproduction Service No. 192717).

Gagne, R.M., Wagner, W., & Rojas, A. (1981). Planning and authoring computer-assisted instruction lessons. *Educational Technology, 21* (9), 17-26.

Malamuth, N.M., Shure, G.H., & Johnston, S.A. (1975). Teaching research methods with a computer-based model of group-induced shifts. *Journal of Computer-Based Instruction, 2* (1), 1-10.

Ross, S.M., & Wasicsko, M. (1981). *Models of adaptive instruction: A handbook for college and university teachers.* (Report developed for Freed-Hardeman College). Henderson, TN: Freed-Hardeman College. (ERIC Document Reproduction Service No. 209214).

Tira, D.E. (1977). Rationale for and evaluation of a CAI tutorial in a removable partial prosthodontics classification system. *Journal of Computer-Based Instruction, 4* (2), 34-42.

Wresch, W. (1982). *Prewriting, writing, and editing by computer.* Paper presented at the 33rd Annual Meeting of the Conference on College Composition and Communication, San Francisco.

Selected Abstracts

Counselor Input to Topics of Rehabilitation Education and Research
J. Joiner and D. Roberts (1982, p. 34)

> This study, encouraged by the past president of the National Rehabilitation Counseling Association and as a task of the association's Professional Development Council, was designed primarily to determine the perceptions of counselor input into decisions regarding topics of rehabilitation education and research. Counselors and representatives of education and research programs were surveyed with a research and training questionnaire. The results indicate some areas of disagreement between counselors and program representatives. Recommendations designed to resolve the disagreements are offered.

Graduates' Views of Instructional/Competency Areas in Rehabilitation Counselor Education Programs: A Hypothesis Generality Study
M.W. Janes and W.G. Emener (1983, p. 38)

> A response sample of 194 recent rehabilitation counselor education (RCE) graduates (24.4% return rate) from eight cooperating institutions rated the extent to which each of twelve RCE instructional/competency areas were and should be emphasized within RCE programs and are currently being utilized in their employment. The twelve RCE instructional/competency areas, from The 1981 Rehabilitation Education Survey (Emener & Rasch, 1981), were: (a) Basic Principles, (b) Counseling Theories and Techniques, (c) Medical Aspects, (d) Psychosocial Aspects, (e) Occupational Information and Job Analysis, (f) Evaluation, (g) Case Management, (h) Community Organization and Resources, (i) Job Development and Placement, (j) Fieldwork, (k) Research, and (l) Professional Issues. Results, comparing the RCE graduates' actual, preferred, and utility ratings across these twelve areas, and cross-comparisons with the Emener and Rasch (1981) RCE educators' actual and preferred ratings, are presented in the generation of critical research hypotheses in need of empirical investigation.

Microcounseling as a Training Model for the Rehabilitation Initial Interview
H.W. Sawyer and C.M. Allen (1976, p. 170)

> Two microcounseling variations (videotape modeling and reinforcement feedback) were compared in teaching undergraduate female students to respond to client cues that create difficulty in the initial interview. Results indicated that both variations produced significant learning of interviewer response content and learning retention on follow-up. In addition, videotape modeling produced significant learning generalization. The implications point to the effectiveness of utilizing these micro-counseling techniques

in teaching undergraduate students basic initial interviewing skills, with videotape modeling providing to the better of the two variations.

Training for Cooperating Agency Supervisors in Rehabilitation Counselor Education

N.L. Berven, M.E. Possi, E.A. Doran, S.S. Ostby, and S.P. Kaplan (1982, p. 47)

The authors describe a brief training program for cooperating agency supervisors providing field experience in a rehabilitation counselor education program.

Sexual Rehabilitation of the Spinal Cord Injured: A Program for Counselor Education

M.L. Walker, R.P. Clark, and H. Sawyer (1975, p. 279)

Counselor educators recognize the need for competency in counseling severely disabled clients toward sexual rehabilitation, but teaching strategies and materials have been slow in emerging. An instructional plan and sequence is specified, using existing media to evoke participant reaction to sexually laden topics. Through careful sequencing and with informed and relaxed discussion leaders, anxiety is reduced and avoidance of discussion of sexual topics lessened.

Training and Curricula in Psychiatric Rehabilitation: A Survey of Core Accredited Programs

J. Weinberger and M. Greenwald (1982, p. 287)

CORE-accredited rehabilitation counseling programs (RCE) ($N=59$) were surveyed to detail the nature of training available in the area of psychiatric rehabilitation. Results revealed considerable diversity in the coursework and field experience among programs. Only seven CORE-accredited RCE programs offer a distinct specialty in psychiatric rehabilitation. The authors recommend development of consistent curriculum guidelines in psychiatric rehabilitation.

The Development of Rehabilitation Counselor Competence in Conflict Management: The Need for an Experiential Training Approach

M.A. Klein and M.E. Scofield (1984, p. 302)

This study demonstrates that an experiential training program consisting of coping skills training, instruction and modeling of appropriate conflict management behaviors, and exposure/rehearsal is an effective method for teaching conflict management competence to rehabilitation counselor trainees. Both a lecture/discussion approach and an experiential method were effective in imparting information relative to delayed-training control group; however, only the experiential method was found effective in actual skills development. Results from standardized simulated provocations as well as from other measures indicated that trainees were totally unprepared for successful management of conflict in professional practice without specialized training.

Preparing Rehabilitation Leaders for the Computer Age

G. Nave and P. Browning (1983, p. 364)

Computer technology has become increasingly important in the lives of handicapped persons and in the work world of rehabilitation professionals. This article is intended to encourage rehabilitation educators to take a major role in preparing future leaders to work with this technology. A curriculum consisting of two courses is introduced as one step in this direction.

Microcomputers in Vocational Evaluation: An Application for Staff Training

F. Chan and K. Questad (1981, p. 153)

Today low-cost microcomputers are capable of performing many complex functions that once required large, costly computers. In rehabilitation, microcomputers are now used to increase the functional capacities of disabled persons, but rehabilitation professionals could benefit from this technology, also. Vocational evaluation planning is a complex process and is especially difficult for novice evaluators. To illustrate the potential applications of microcomputers to the vocational evaluation field, this article presents as an example a system that uses a microcomputer to approach the problems encountered by novice evaluators when planning an evaluation. This approach consists of two computer programs and a strategy for using them in a vocational evaluation facility. The basic features of the programs are described and the strengths and weaknesses of the total approach are discussed.

References and Suggested Additional
Readings for Part III

Ames, T.R., & Boyle, P.S. (1980). The rehabilitation counselor's role in the sexual adjustment of the handicapped client: The need for trained professionals. *Journal of Applied Rehabilitation Counseling, 2*(4), 173-178.

Atkins, B.J. (1981). Clinical practice in master's level rehabilitation counselor education. *Counselor Education and Supervision, 21*(2), 169-175.

Atkinson, D.A. (1981). Selection and training for human rights counseling. *Counselor Education and Supervision, 21*(2), 101-108.

Berven, N.L., McCracken, N., Jellinek, H.M., & Doran, E.A. (1983). Contributions of a rehabilitation counselor education advisory committee. *Journal of Applied Rehabilitation Counseling, 14*(2), 23-25.

Berven, N.L., Possi, M.E., Doran, E.A., Ostby, S.S., & Kaplan, S.P. (1982). Training for cooperating agency supervisors in rehabilitation counselor education. *Rehabilitation Counseling Bulletin, 26*(1), 47-51.

Chan, F., & Questad, K. (1981). Microcomputers in vocational evaluation: An application for staff training. *Vocational Evaluation and Work Adjustment Bulletin, 14*(4), 153-158.

Coffey, D., & Ellien, V. (1979). *Work adjustment curriculum development project: A summary.* Menomonie, WI: University of Wisconsin — Vocational Rehabilitation Institute, Research and Training Center.

Council on Rehabilitation Education. (1978). *Accreditation manual for rehabilitation counselor education programs.* Chicago, IL: Author.

Crimando, W., & Baker, R. (1984). Computer-assisted instruction in rehabilitation education. *Rehabilitation Counseling Bulletin, 28*(1), 50-54.

Dowd, E.T., & Emener, W.G. (1978). Lifeboat counseling: The issue of survival decisions. *Journal of Rehabilitation, 44*(3), 34-36.

Downes, S.C. (1971). The use of sensitivity training in the rehabilitation counselor education program. *Journal of Applied Rehabilitation Counseling, 2*(1), 22-26.

Emener, W.G. (in press). Rehabilitation counselor education: A state of the art perspective. In E. Pan, T.E. Backer, & C.L. Vash, 1984. *Annual review of rehabilitation.* New York: Springer.

Emener, W.G., & Ferrandino, J.A. (1983). A philosophical framework for rehabilitation: Implications for clients, counselors, and agencies. *Journal of Applied Rehabilitation Counseling, 14*(1), 62-67.

Emener, W.G., & Koonce, G.B. (1978). Categorical sources of articles in the *Journal of Rehabilitation:* 1959-1975. *Journal of Rehabilitation, 44*(3), 25-27.

Emener, W.G., & McFarlane, F.R. (in press). A futuristic model of rehabilitation education. *Journal of Applied Rehabilitation Counseling.*

Emener, W.G., & Rasch, J.D. (1984). Actual and preferred instructional areas in rehabilitation education programs. *Rehabilitation Counselor Bulletin, 27*(5), 269-280.

Emener, W.G., Luck, R.S., & Smits, S.J. (1981). *Rehabilitation administration and supervision.* Baltimore: University Park Press.

Engram, B.E. (1981). Communication skills training for rehabilitation counselors working with older persons. *Journal of Rehabilitation, 47*(4), 51-56.

Felton, J.S. (1963). A survey of medicine and medical practice. *Journal of Rehabilitation, 29*(1), 11-12.

Freeman, J.B. (1978). Rehabilitation counselor and supervisor perceptions of counselor training needs and continuing education. *Journal of Applied Rehabilitation Counseling, 10*(3), 154-157.

Geist, G.O. (1977). Internships program for rehabilitation counselors. *Journal of Rehabilitation, 43*(2), 40.

Gilbert, L.D. (1973). The changing work ethic and rehabilitation. *Journal of Rehabilitation, 39*(4), 14-17.

Hawley, I.D., & Capshaw, T.B. (1981). Professionalism and ethical responsibilities in rehabilitation. In W.G. Emener, R.S. Luck, & S.J. Smits (Eds.), *Rehabilitation administration and supervision,* Baltimore: University Park Press.

Hinman, S., & Marr, J.N. (1984). Training counselors to write behavior-based client objectives. *Rehabilitation Counseling Bulletin, 27*(5), 291-301.

Hutchinson, J., & Cogan, F. (1974). Rehabilitation manpower specialist: A job description of placement personnel. *Journal of Rehabilitation, 40*(2), 31-33.

Janes, M.W., & Emener, W.G. (1983). Graduates' views of instructional/competency areas in rehabilitation counselor education programs: A hypotheses generating study. *Journal of Applied Rehabilitation Counseling, 15*(2), 38-43.

Joiner, J., & Roberts, D. (1982). Counselor input to topics of rehabilitation education and research. *Journal of Applied Rehabilitation Counseling, 13*(1) 34-36.

Joint Liaison Committee (1963). *Studies in rehabilitation counselor training: Guidelines for supervised clinical practice.* Minneapolis: Author.

Kauppi, D.R., Ballou, M., Jaques, M.E., Gualtieri, J.J., & Blum, C.R. (1983). Job satisfaction predictors of rehabilitation counseling graduates. *Rehabilitation Counseling Bulletin, 26*(5), 336-341.

Klein, M.A., & Scofield, M.E. (1984). The development of rehabilitation counselor competence in conflict management: The need for an experiential training approach. *Rehabilitation Counseling Bulletin, 27*(5), 302-311.

Lanning, W.L. (1971). A study of the relationship between group and individual counseling supervision and three relationship measures. *Jounral of Counseling Psychology, 11,* 47-53.

MacGuffie, R.A., & Henderson, H.L. (1973). Process orientation: A dimension in counselor training. *Journal of Applied Rehabilitation Counseling, 4*(4), 234-238.

Matkin, R.E., Sawyer, H.W., Lorenz, J.R., & Rubin, S.E. (1982). Rehabilitation administrators and supervisors: Their work assignments, training needs, and suggestions for preparation. *Journal of Rehabilitation Administration, 6*(4), 170-183.

McFarlane, F.R., & DiPaola, S.M. (1979). Rehabilitation counselor, vocational evaluator and work adjustment specialist: Are these professionals different? *Journal of Applied Rehabilitation Counseling, 10*(3), 142-147.

McFarlane, F.R., & Sullivan, M. (1979). Educational and training needs of rehabilitation counselors: Implications for training. *Journal of Applied Rehabilitation Counseling, 10*(1), 41-43.

Miller, J.H., & Mulkey, S.W. (1975). Dual counselor-teacher model accommodates student-state agency need. *Journal of Rehabilitation, 41*(5), 15-18, 40, 42.

Morgan, C.A. (1982). An evolving practicum for the World of IS—one approach. Counselor survival and noncounseling skills. Preservice conditioning for "The World of IS." *Journal of Rehabilitation, 48*(2), 29-32, 72.

Mulhern, J.R. (1980). Introducing a job placement course in rehabilitation counseling master's program. *Rehabilitation Counseling Bulletin, 24*(2), 171-172.

Nave, G., & Browning, P. (1983). Preparing rehabilitation leaders for the computer age. *Rehabilitation Counseling Bulletin, 26*(5), 364-367.

Patterson, C.H. (1964). Supervising students in a counseling practicum. *Journal of Counseling Psychology, 11*, 47-53.

Phillips, J.S. (1980). A rehabilitation process model. *Journal of Rehabilitation, 46*(1), 42-45.

Porter, T.L., Rubin, S.E., & Sink, J.M. (1979). Essential rehabilitation counselor diagnostic, counseling, and placement competences. *Journal of Applied Rehabilitation Counseling, 10*(3), 158-162.

Riggar, T.F., & Matkin, R.E. (1984). Rehabilitation counselors working as administrators: A pilot investigation. *Journal of Applied Rehabilitation Counseling, 15*(1), 9-13.

Roessler, R.T. (1981). Training independent living rehabilitation specialists. *Journal of Rehabilitation, 47*(2), 36-39.

Rubin, S.E., & Roessler, R.T. (1978). *Foundations of the vocational rehabilitation process.* Baltimore: University Park Press.

Sachs, M.B., & Hansen, C.L. (1981). A model for workshops on cancer for vocational rehabilitation professionals. *Journal of Rehabilitation, 47*(1), 28-30.

Sawyer, H.W., & Allen, C.M. (1976). Microcounseling as a training model for the rehabilitation initial interview. *Journal of Applied Rehabilitation Counseling, 7*(3), 170-175.

Scofield, M.E., & Scofield, B.J. (1978). Ethical concerns in clinical practice supervision. *Journal of Applied Rehabilitation Counseling, 9* 27-29.

Scorzelli, J.F. (1975). Reactions to program content of a rehabilitation counseling program. *Journal of Applied Rehabilitation Counseling, 6*(3), 172-177.

Scorzelli, J.F. (1979). Assessing the content of a rehabilitation counseling program. *Journal of Applied Rehabilitation Counseling, 9*(4), 184-186.

Sink, J.M., & Porter, T.L. (1978). Convergence and divergence in rehabilitation counseling and vocational evaluation. *Journal of Applied Rehabilitation Counseling,* 1978, *9*(1), 5-20.

Smits, S.J., & Ledbetter, J.G. (1979). The practice of rehabilitation counseling within the administrative structure of the state-federal program. *Journal of Applied Rehabilitation Counseling, 10*(2), 78-84.

Struthers, R.D., & Miller, J.V. (1981). Program planning, program evaluation, and research utilization in state vocational rehabilitation agencies. In W.G. Emener, R.S. Luck, & S.J. Smits (Eds.): *Rehabilitation administration and supervision.* Baltimore, Maryland: University Park Press.

Sullivan, M. (1982). A follow-up study of rehabilitation counseling graduates. *Journal of Applied Rehabilitation Counseling, 13*(1), 6-10.

Szuhay, J.A. (Ed. 1980). *The history of CRCE/NCRE.* Washington, D.C.: National Council on Rehabilitation Education.

Trotter, A.B., Kult, D.A., & Atkins, B.J. (1980). *Field training supervisors manual.* Milwaukee: University of Wisconsin — Milwaukee.

Usdane, W. (1974). Placement personnel: A graduate program concept *Journal of Rehabilitation, 40*(2), 12-13.

Walker, M.L., Clark, R.P., & Sawyer, H. (1975). Sexual rehabilitation of the spinal cord injured: A program for counselor education. *Rehabilitation Counseling Bulletin, 18*(4), 279-285.

Warren, S.L. (1957). Internship program for rehabilitation counselors. *Journal of Rehabilitation, 13*(3), 4-5, 20-22.

Weinberger, J., & Greenwald, M. (1982). Training and curricula in psychiatric rehabilitation: A survey of core accredited programs. *Rehabilitation Counseling Bulletin, 25*(5), 287-290.

Wright, G.N. (1980). *Total rehabilitation.* Boston: Little, Brown, and Company.

Wright, G.N., Reagles, K.R., & Scorzelli, J.F. (1973). Measuring the effectiveness and variations of rehabilitation counseling programs. *Journal of Applied Rehabilitation Counseling, 17,* 76-87.

Zadny, J.J., & James, L.F. (1977). Time spent on placement. *Rehabilitation Counseling Bulletin, 21*(1), 31-35.

Zelle, J.A. (1972). Introducing rehabilitation counseling to medical education. *Journal of Rehabilitation, 38*(5), 16-18.

PART IV
STUDENT/TRAINEE ISSUES

PART I

STUDIES IN MANAGEMENT ISSUES

PART IV. STUDENT/TRAINEE ISSUES

Introduction Commentary

AMONG REHABILITATION counselor educators' commitments is the development of specific skills and knowledge of the rehabilitation counselor (see Anthony, Slowkowski & Bendix, 1976). Fittingly, rehabilitation counselor education is also committed to the continued investigation of the effects of its educational and training activities on students and trainees (Anthony & Carkhuff, 1970; Parloff, Waskow & Wolfe, 1978). The term "training" connotes preparation for tasks, duties, roles and functions, etc. as they currently exist; the term "education" connotes preparation beyond this immediate focus and includes learning designed to accommodate and facilitate future change and development. In his talk to a group of rehabilitation counselor education students preparing to leave the academic environment, Nadolsky (1977), in Chapter 18, addressed this important futurism notion of rehabilitation counselor *education:* "As each of you leave the academic environment and enter your chosen career, it is *true* that the educated rehabilitation counselor possesses the potential to play a significant part in establishing and shaping the future direction of human services in this country." In view of these above missions and important attributes and considerations of rehabilitation counselor *education,* the student/trainee issues in this part of this book take on added, special meaning.

The recruitment and selection of students into a rehabilitation counselor education program encompasses numerous important issues. During the earlier years of rehabilitation counselor education, especially in the late 1950s and 1960s and for reasons consistent with rehabilitation counselor education's manpower development mission, the typical student was chronologically older than at present and was frequently a second careerist (Olshansky, 1967; McGowan & Porter, 1967; Wrenn, 1952; Wright, 1980). Graduate rehabilitation counselor education programs consider a number of applicant criteria in their selection processes such as undergraduate grade point average, standardized test scores (e.g., Graduate Record Examination, Miller Analogies Tests), previous experience, personal philosophy, and interpersonal qualities (Kunce,

Thoreson & Parker, 1975; Patterson, 1962). Moreover, it is not uncommon for applicants to have a variety of disabilities. Thus, it is suggested that admissions committees be familiar with the mandates of Section 504 of the Rehabilitation Act and sensitive to relevant recruitment/selection issues such as those addressed by Iovacchini and Abood (1981): When is a student considered handicapped? Are alcoholics and drug addicts considered handicapped? When is a handicapped student a "qualified handicapped" student? What admissions policies must be followed? Must modifications be made in academic requirements? What actions must be taken to assure program accessibility? Additional student recruitment issues in the 1980s are discussed by Rasch, Hollingsworth, Saxon and Thomas (1984) in Chapter 19. Their 1982 National Council on Rehabilitation Task Force on Student Recruitment reports data from a return sample of 159 students, and they conclude with fourteen recommendations and recruitment activities that the task force felt should be considered in rehabilitation education programs. The importance of good recruitment and selection cannot be overemphasized. Moreover, it should be considered from a lifelong, developmental perspective and with a philosophical appreciation of a life-style of learning. Emener (1975), in Chapter 20, articulates this philosophical approach: "The purpose of rehabilitation is the restitution of the process of life in the face of disability . . . Rehabilitation counselors, counselor educators, administrators, and supervisors can never dismiss their roles as students— students of life." If a rehabilitation counselor education program is designed to model and facilitate this developmental, lifelong learning approach, it would appear most appropriate for it to pervade recruitment and selection activities.

Investigations of counselor education students' characteristics and attributes have been quite extensive (see Parloff, Waskow & Wolfe, 1978). Studies of rehabilitation counseling students' and rehabilitation counselors' characteristics and attributes have also been conducted. For example, Thomas, Carter and Britton (1982), in Chapter 21, surveyed fifty graduate students in a rehabilitation counseling program regarding their attitudes toward the Protestant Work Ethic (PWE) and, among other conclusions, stated: "The students were more likely to endorse those aspects of the PWE reflecting the intrinsic value of work than those dealing with earnings, social status, and advancement." The work ethic value is central to the field of rehabilitation (see Gilbert, 1973; Thomas, Britton & Kravetz, 1974; Thoreson, 1964), and the assessment of students' attributes regarding it is important. Theoretical and empirical investigations of students' (and student counselors') attitudes toward rehabilitation-relevant phenomena include those toward mainstreaming (Filar, 1982), obesity (Kaplan, 1984; Kaplan & Thomas, 1981), euthanasian issues (Dowd & Emener, 1978), state rehabilitation agency processes (Emener & Andrews, 1977) and goals (Emener, 1978), disabled persons (Krauft, Rubin, Cook & Bozarth, 1976), and attitudes toward themselves (Clark, 1978). Employees' preferences regarding graduates' characteristics have been studied (e.g., Culberson, 1979; Witten, 1980); however, they have been conducted mostly on graduates of undergraduate rehabilitation education programs. Personal characteristics of rehabilitation counseling students (and counselors) have been studied — for example, their locus of control (Pinkard & Gross, 1984) and the relationship between locus of control and other phenomena such as attitudes toward economically poor individuals (Majumber, McDonald & Greever, 1977) and discrimination ability (Martin & Shepel, 1974). Given the importance for attending to personal attributes that are detrimental to rehabilitation counselor service delivery such as the Zeigarnik effect (Miller & Roberts, 1979) and burnout (Churniss, 1980; Emener, 1979; Emener, Luck & Gohs, 1982), it indeed would appear critical for rehabilitation counselor education programs to attend to the personal attributes of their students — especially those relevant to their functioning as professional rehabilitation counselors.

Studies regarding the graduates of undergraduate rehabilitation education programs have been conducted (e.g., Gandy, 1983; Witten, 1980); likewise, studies regarding rehabilitation counselor education graduates have also been conducted. For example, Kunce, Thoreson and Parker (1975), in Chapter 22, analyzed academic ability and occupational outcome data of 100 graduates from two university master's-level rehabilitation counselor education programs and, in their discussion of their findings, they concluded: "From a negative standpoint, counselor educational programs seem to prefer the academically elite. . . . From a positive perspective, the counselor programs are, in fact, selecting students with varied abilities — some who have a high probability of electing counseling roles and some who will tend to choose rehabilitation-related positions in teaching and administration." While this study was on the graduates of two rehabilitation counselor education programs, follow-up studies have been conducted on the graduates of one program (Crisler & Eaton, 1975; Crisler & Fowler, 1981; Kauppi, Ballou, Jaques, Gualtieri & Blum, 1983), eight programs (Janes & Emener, 1983, 1985), and ten programs (Sullivan, 1982). The primary focus of these studies was on employment trends of the graduates. It should also be noted that Geist and McMahon (1981) surveyed 106 pre-service rehabilitation education program directors to determine the demand for and employment patterns of 3,389 graduates. Janes and Emener (1985) studied graduates' perceptions of their employment and career satisfaction. In Chapter 23, Kauppi, Ballou, Jaques, Gualtieri and Blum (1983) discuss the results of their job satisfaction study on the seventy-two graduates from their rehabilitation counselor education program, and among their conclusions they stated, "Sex was found to be the only significant predictor of job satisfaction, with females more satisfied than males." Not only are readers urged to study their procedures, results, and discussions but also to consider their study as a good example of student follow-up!

As indicated at the outset of this Introduction Commentary, rehabilitation counselor education programs should be committed to the continued investigation of the effects of their educational and training activities on students and trainees—not only on the students while they are in the program but after they graduate, as well. Essentially, a rehabilitation counselor education program should honor its continued, developmental obligation to maximize its potential contributions to the rehabilitation of disabled citizens through the recruitment, selection, education and training, placement, and follow-up of high functioning professional rehabilitation counselors. They should be committed not just to their students, in view of their students' jobs as rehabilitation counselors, but to their students, in view of their students' lifelong careers in the field of rehabilitation.

W.G. Emener

CHAPTER 18

THE EDUCATED COUNSELOR: RESPONSIBILITIES IN A SERVICE SOCIETY

Julian M. Nadolsky

RECENTLY, a group of graduate students in rehabilitation counseling assembled for the final class session with a professor who had served as their advisor, confidant, and instructor during the campus-based phase of their master's degree program. Upon entry into the classroom, the professor overheard some students discussing their probable future as rehabilitation counselors. The students seemed to be primarily concerned with the types of contributions that they would be permitted to make within a state rehabilitation agency. They were also uncertain about being accepted by their more experienced peers. Realizing that the students' concerns were of the variety which mitigate against effective professional practice, the professor decided to gear his presentation toward some of the more subtle responsibilities that are expected of, but rarely assumed by, educated rehabilitation counselors. In this final presentation, the professor attempted to provide some direction to the students by explaining the critical relationship that exists between the actions of educated rehabilitation personnel and the survival of their discipline.

It should be noted that this is a hypothetical paper. However, it is intentionally presented in a format that, hopefully, will enable the educated rehabilitation counselor (both student and practitioner) to identify with its content and to assume the responsibility for acting upon its implications. The professor's remarks in this hypothetical situation are presented below.

Reprinted by permission from Volume 43 (1977), *Journal of Rehabilitation*, pp. 30-32.

DIRECTION

As the majority of our students complete their course work requirements and embark upon an internship experience, it seems fitting to offer each of you a personal note of gratitude for your patience in allowing me and other faculty members to enter your lives during a sometimes painful, but always rewarding and challenging experience. We have tried to make an impression on you concerning the importance and seriousness of both rehabilitation and counseling. We have also tried to equip you with the knowledge and skill essential to your functioning as effective rehabilitation counselors. Finally, and perhaps most important, we have tried to instill within each of you an attitude that emphasizes the primacy of the individual in any service process. The extent to which we (and our colleagues in other universities) have succeeded in our efforts will be reflected by the nature and quality of rehabilitation service programs that become available to handicapped individuals during future years.

At this point it also seems fitting to remind each of you that the career you are about to enter is part of a complex and continually growing human service process in our society. It is part of a process that is unfolding as our society changes its emphasis from that of manufacturing to one of service. A decade or two ago, those individuals who entered a human service career were viewed by others with mixed opinions. On the one hand, they were viewed with envy since their daily activities were carried out in pleasant surroundings and involved some form of mysterious or miraculous interchange with others in a process which did not entail the completion of a finished product. On the other hand, the motives of these individuals were often misunderstood and mistrusted since their activities were non-competitive in nature, devoid of obvious physical exertion, and supported by tax funds or charitable donations.

HUMAN SERVICES — A NEW FIELD

In the recent past, our society was primarily geared toward the production and distribution of material goods. The majority of our citizens were employed in some phase of competitive private enterprise, mainly within the business or industrial sector of society. Since most of our citizens were needed to meet the demands of business and industry, they were encouraged to be competitive and rewarded for their aggressive efforts in the manufacturing or distribution process. Relatively few human service occupations were available, and most citizens were either unaware of their existence or would not give consideration to entering such a limited, and "self-limiting," field of endeavor.

Today, considerable emphasis is placed upon the provision of social or human services in our society. Many different types of social service programs exist and multitudes enter a human service occupation each year. As a result of technological efficiency, coupled with an expanded awareness of social problems and an emphasis upon consumerism, our society is rapidly evolving from an industrial or manufacturing society into a service society. In the not too distant future, the majority of individuals in our society will probably be employed in some phase of the human service process. Furthermore, if the present trend continues (and there is no reason to believe that it will not), the government will become, not only the primary *purchaser*, but also the major *provider* of human services. This means that the government will be in control of human service programs since it will both define the parameters of such programs and purchase only those services that fall within its defined boundaries.

MAINTAINING STANDARDS

The majority of you will be government employees. Although most of your colleagues in government will not possess the educational background that you now have, they will be fitted into slots within the bureaucratic human service structure which will enable them to carry out their position-defined duties. Needless to say, you will be much better equipped than most of your colleagues, but you will be outnumbered. Since there is strength in numbers, you may feel obligated or forced to fit yourself into a bureaucratic human service position which is essentially routine in nature, imposes minimal demands and maximal restrictions upon your mode of operation, and does not enable the skilled individual to use much of his or her expertise.

It will not be difficult to fit yourselves into such a mold since your daily obligations will be easier to fulfill and, by being compliant, you will become a definite candidate for promotion within the bureaucratic hierarchy. Of course, it will be necessary to suppress certain attitudes that have been developed (such as the primacy of the individual), but this is a feat that can be readily accomplished in a situation where opposing attitudes predominate. In fact, it may be difficult to view and treat your clients as individuals, rather than as members of a category, since research data will probably exist which gives wholehearted support to the fact that categorization is essential to the true understanding of individuals, their problems, and their needs. In other words, you will learn through experience that "truth" is a variable concept which changes in accordance with the demands of the specific situation.

As each of you leave the academic environment and enter your chosen career, it is *true* that the educated rehabilitation counselor possesses the potential to play a significant part in establishing and shaping the future direction of human services in this country. Hopefully, your education has provided the background which enables you to recognize that the problems encountered by humans are uniquely individual in nature and cannot be satisfactorily resolved through the application of a pre-conceived bureaucratic system which is entirely based upon and supported by rational methods. It is the irrational element that often plays a substantial part in problem resolution; unfortunately, bureaucratic systems cannot effectively incorporate such elements into their service delivery structure.

By focusing upon the knowledge gained through education and by maintaining the idealism that accompanies education, you possess the inner power and resources to transcend the bureaucratic system as you operate within it and to become a model for emulation by the other human service personnel. Since education is accompanied by responsibility, it is imperative that you use your resources to make positive changes of an *implosive* variety within the system, rather than registering chronic complaints about the system so that changes are forced upon the system from the outside. In most instances, these externally imposed changes are of an *explosive* variety and have a devastating effect upon the system and its personnel.

SUMMARY—GOVERNMENT INTERVENTION

In summary, it should be noted that you have chosen a career which is part of a growing, but accountable human service process in our society. Due to an increasing demand for service, the government has assumed responsibility for the major share of growth in this process. As inflation "bites" into tax dollars, both the government and the entire human service process itself will probably be severely questioned. Human service is a relatively new concept in our society, but so is government intervention. These two concepts seem to go hand-in-hand and in the future they may be more closely united and dependent upon one another than is now realized.

In a democratic and materialistically abundant society it is virtually impossible to limit a demand for service. Furthermore, one of the consequences of a technologically efficient society is a rise in unemployment within private manufacturing and business enterprises. Government intervention through the establishment of tax supported human service programs is viewed by many as a cure-all for our social ills since such intervention deals directly with the demand for service, while providing a non-competitive buffer against rising unemployment. However, many individuals seriously question the intervention of government into the private sector of our economy and especially question the increasing expenditure of tax dollars for the creation of jobs within the human service realm.

We are now experiencing only the beginning stages of government intervention into the economy. As government assumes a larger role in maintaining the economy, both government itself and the human service programs that it established and supports will probably become the target for severe criticism from individuals outside of government. This criticism and questioning could conceivably result in a demand for change from the outside. The ensuing changes might be of an explosive variety and could have a disasterous effect upon the prevailing human service structure and upon our entire system of government.

As education rehabilitation counselors (and as probable government employees), you must be aware of the interrelationship between events in our society. You must take the initiative to embark upon implosive changes that are positive in nature and designed to enhance the development of human services while upholding our democratic form of government. You must not only remain an effective clinician (and a competent bureaucratic servant), but also seek out, encourage, and support the development of meaningful human service programs within the confines of the competitive, profit-oriented, private sector of society. If our society is to maintain a large and effective human service component, it will be necessary to expand beyond the parameters of government and to "open the door" for the emergence of competition from private-based programs. It is through the commitment and involvement of both the public and the private sector of society that the human service concept will prevail and our government will continue to evolve along democratic lines.

CHAPTER 19

STUDENT RECRUITMENT ISSUES
IN THE 1980S

JOHN D. RASCH, DAVID K. HOLLINGSWORTH,
JOHN P. SAXON, AND KENNETH R. THOMAS

Abstract

In 1982, the National Council on Rehabilitation Education (NCRE) formed a
Task Force on Student Recruitment to study and report on recruitment issues in
the 1980s. This article summarizes the findings and recommendations of the task
force.

BEFORE THE 1980s, the recruitment of qualified students was not a serious challenge for most rehabilitation education programs. There were two
basic reasons for this: (a) employment opportunities within the state-federal rehabilitation program and other human service agencies were generally plenti-
ful, and (b) Rehabilitation Services Administration (RSA) traineeships served
as recruitment incentives, making rehabilitation studies both financially attractive and feasible for interested students. Student recruitment problems in the
1980s stem from decreased employment opportunities in publicly supported
human service agencies, and from a reduction in student training monies, including the availability of low interest guaranteed student loans. Although it is
not within the power of rehabilitation education programs to revitalize human
service labor markets or to restore lost traineeships and loans, certain actions
can be taken to facilitate the recruitment of qualified students while these conditions exist.

In order to clarify recruitment issues and identify recruitment strategies,
the NCRE Task Force on Student Recruitment: (a) contacted rehabilitation

Reprinted by permission from Volume 28 (1984), *Rehabilitation Counseling Bulletin*, pp. 46-49.

educators for their views, (b) reviewed program brochures and university cata-log descriptions, and (c) surveyed interests and career goals of students taking rehabilitation courses. The student survey was conducted with the assistance of the NCRE regional representatives, and consisted of a return sample of 159 students from nine of the ten regions. Students reported they were working toward master's degrees in rehabilitation counseling ($N=118$), vocational eval-uation ($N=7$), and rehabilitation administration ($N=4$); undergraduate de-grees in rehabilitation ($N=14$); doctoral degrees in rehabilitation ($N=12$); and miscellaneous other majors ($N=7$).

After reviewing survey data, written programmatic materials, and the per-sonally expressed views of educators, the task force concluded that rehabilita-tion education programs have highly variable recruitment needs. Some programs have no need to review their present student recruitment activities, whereas others need to increase and redirect their efforts. The following is a list of recommendations and recruitment activities that the task force felt should be considered in rehabilitation education programs:

1. In reviewing university/college catalogs and bulletins, it was noted that some schools with rehabilitation education programs had no program descrip-tions or only short ones. In some cases the word "rehabilitation" was not in-dexed in the catalog or bulletin, and course offerings were not fully described. It is therefore recommended that every rehabilitation education program re-view its university catalog or bulletin to ensure that the program and courses are accurately and fully described.

2. It is recommended that every program develop a brochure targeted to-ward student recruitment, and that the brochure be of a size that allows for easy mailing. Based on interests expressed in the student survey, the availabil-ity of training in counseling skills and in psychosocial aspects of disability should be emphasized. Graduate career flexibility should also be emphasized by noting the variety of work settings and diverse client populations graduates may serve.

3. Results of the student survey indicated that more than half of the stu-dents surveyed were working or previously had worked full-time in a human service setting. Many students who enter rehabilitation education programs also have child-rearing responsibilities or need to work on a part-time basis while in school. Programs wishing to maximize their recruitment of students with work or child-rearing responsibilities should offer evening courses that meet for several hours once a week.

4. It was found that some rehabilitation education programs have, as the cornerstone of their recruitment activities, the task of identifying each graduat-ing class's psychology or related social and behavioral science majors. These graduates receive an introductory letter and program brochure. This tech-nique appears to be a highly effective way of announcing a rehabilitation edu-cation program to a large pool of potential applicants.

5. Recruitment materials should be available at the university counseling center, student admissions office, and dean's office. It may also be helpful to send these materials periodically to faculty in select undergraduate or community college programs (e.g., psychology faculty), because much informal vocational guidance and advising occurs through these faculty/student contacts.

6. Most rehabilitation education programs apparently have an introductory course open to undergraduates or students outside the program. This course is often the first and only rehabilitation course potential applicants take, and it is especially important that it be interesting and dynamic.

7. Universities often have freshmen and transfer student orientations, as well as orientations for juniors who have declared a specific major. Rehabilitation programs, whether graduate or undergraduate, should be represented at these orientations.

8. Prospective students often make their first contact by stopping by the rehabilitation office, rather than by calling in advance for an appointment. It may help recruitment if faculty office hours are coordinated so that at least one faculty member is available during normal university hours. When a faculty member is not present, office staff should have an established procedure for handling student inquiries (e.g., given the student a brochure or other materials and schedule an appointment with a faculty member).

9. It is recommended that faculty consider putting a "display" bulletin board or glass-enclosed exhibit on a wall outside their program office to increase visibility and attract student interest in rehabilitation counseling.

10. Materials descriptive of the program should periodically be mailed to local service agencies to increase community awareness of the program. In addition to possibly generating student applications, greater awareness of the program might facilitate the placement of practicum and internship students.

11. Programs without such arrangements may wish to explore the possibility of work-study arrangements with the state vocational rehabilitation agency, local rehabilitation facilities, and private-for-profit rehabilitation companies.

12. The survey suggested that students are interested in working with many different client populations. It may therefore be advisable to develop elective courses, if none exist, that address specific populations.

13. Faculty should be active in local chapters of professional associations (e.g., AACD, NRA, NRCA, and NARPPS) and should make presentations at these associations' and other meetings to increase the rehabilitation program's visibility. As part of their community service role, faculty members might develop an in-service training program that would be consistent with their expertise and would be available to local agencies.

14. Lastly, some programs may wish to consider "pre-professional" marketing services; that is, arrange for students from the marketing program at their university's business school to do independent studies or class projects with the rehabilitation education program as their client.

CHAPTER 20

THE REHABILITATION COUNSELOR:
A STUDENT OF LIFE*

WILLIAM G. EMENER

THE SUGGESTION that a rehabilitation counselor should be a student of *life* evokes numerous considerations. Initial deliberation may be to consider McGowan and Porter's[5] beliefs regarding rehabilitation counselors:

1. That counselors manipulate and/or control behavior . . .
2. That they need to establish commonly agreed upon goals in regard to desirable outcomes of counseling, from the frame of reference of the client and then to actively help the client reach these goals.
3. That a counselor's basic beliefs as to the nature of man influence his choice of counseling techniques, his goals, his choice of setting in which to operate, and his interest in a *process* versus a *product* orientation to counseling . . .
4. That each counselor enters into the counseling relationship with a learned predisposition (on the basis of home, school, religion, and social training) towards certain counseling techniques . . .

The historical emergence of the professional rehabilitation counselor uncovers divergencies from a specialized application of social case work[3] to a counseling psychologist.[8] Identification of *familial disciplines* has been confounded by the continuously growing number of similar disabilities with which rehabilitation counselors work. Rehabilitation has continued to broaden its "eligible for services" population. Nevertheless, we must never forget that in rehabilitation "we know that we must consider the whole man," and that "the purpose of rehabilitation is the restitution of the process of life in the face of disability."[13]

Reprinted by permission from Volume 41 (1975), *Journal of Rehabilitation*, pp. 16-17, 43.
* *"The unexamined life is not worth living for man"* Plato, Apology, 38a

It appears fitting, then, that one hypothetical ideal is for rehabilitation counselors to know everything there is to know about *life*. This is an ambitious goal, but we must keep in mind two things: (a) to encourage rehabilitation counselors to keep abreast of developing knowledge in the area of human behavior so we may pursue the ideal expressed (knowing everything there is to know about *life*); and, (b) to suggest the following hierarchy of four primary study areas for rehabilitation counselors who are self-enrolled as *students of life*.

BASIC NATURE OF MAN

In a hierarchy of discernible study areas, the pivotal foundation of rehabilitation counseling is a sound comprehension of the basic nature of man. McGowan and Porter[5] succinctly and cogently demonstrated this:

> That a counselor's basic beliefs as to the nature of man influence his choice of counseling techniques, his goals, his choice of setting in which to operate, and his interest in a *process* versus a *product* orientation to counseling. That he is incapable of giving to his clients more freedom than he allows himself. That if he believes in a humanistic explanation of man's nature, he will tend toward techniques that encourage the "emergence" of feelings, attitudes, and beliefs from within his clients, with full confidence that the counselee would make a "good" or correct decision. That if he believes in a naturalistic or scientific explanation of man's nature, he will prefer techniques of counseling which encourage reeducation and a general "containment" approach. By the same token if he believes man can best be explained in terms of culturalism, theism, or any other philosophical belief, that he will adopt a compatible philosophy with techniques which are consistent with it.

It is interesting, yet disturbing, to encounter a counselor who accepts a psychoanalytic view of man (being basically hostile and carnal) and yet professes to be a neoanalytic counselor from whom we could expect a more optimistic picture of man. Rogers once raised an intriguing question as to how a counselor could subtly demonstrate a basic innate tendency to destroy and be harmful and simultaneously verbalize deep feelings of caring for his clients? Thus, any studious investigation into the basic nature of man should be twofold: (a) a scholarly inquiry to possibly discover palatable alternatives and to temper one's present beliefs; and, (b) an avenue for facilitating deeper self-understanding (assuming that our ability to understand another is positively correlated with our ability to understand ourselves).

HUMAN BEHAVIOR

General agreement appears to be consistent with Schontz's[12] recommendation that it is unwise and not helpful to attempt to identify and attribute personality syndromes to respective disabilities. Nevertheless, it is imperative for rehabilitation counselors to be able to understand their clients in terms of "what effects do specific events have upon behavior?"[12]

Ideally, each rehabilitation counselor should have a functional understanding of *his own* theory of personality and human behavior — one that is comprehensive, explicit, parsimonious, and open to self-criticism and alteration. Each counselor should eclectically consider the pros and cons of a multitude of systems, and theories of personality (e.g., trait-factor, learning theory, psychoanalytic, neoanalytic, socioeconomic, topological field, interpersonal, client-centered, etc.) and thus further develop and temper *his own theory.*

Possibly the most important thing a counselor offers his client is himself. The rehabilitation counselors' roles and functions place heavy emphasis on the *vocational* aspects of their clients' lives. But as Osipow[7] has indicated, there exists a pervading explicit and implicit assertation from most current vocational choice and career development theory that an individual's work role is an expression of his personality, needs, and other characteristics.

Aside from the value of personal comfortableness that one is afforded by having a functional understanding of his own theoretical orientation to personality and human behavior, the rehabilitation counselor is in a much better position to be helpful to his client if he can understand and assess his client's motivation, self-confidence, impulsivity, reaction to peers and supervisors, frigidity, emotional stability and security, persistence, interpersonal relations, and adaptability. Basically, this suggests some attainment of functional and tentative answers to questions like: "How does my client think?" "How does he feel?" and, "Why does he do what he does?"

ALTERNATIVE HELPING MODALITIES

If an individual has a relatively firm understanding of the basic nature of man and a respectively congruent theory of personality and human behavior (specifically with regard to stress and disability), he is then in a tenable position to consider a personal and functional scheme or strategy for *helping.*

Most definitions of counseling, for example, contain an inherently explicit indication of *help.*[10,11,15] Rehabilitation counselors should formulate *their own* personality congruent *helping models.* Carkhuff[1] offers suggestions to facilitate comprehensiveness and parsimony:

Assumption I. Any comprehensive model of helping processes must include relevant dimensions concerning the helping person.

Assumption II. Any comprehensive model of helping processes must relate helper variables to indexes of helpee change.

Assumption III. Any comprehensive model of helping processes must relate helper variables to differential treatment approaches (p. 34).

Every rehabilitation counselor should initially digest Morgan's[6] article "I, The Client" as an embarkation into the study of *helping*. He initiates a gut level appreciation for considering the helping modalities in rehabilitation counseling by quoting George A. Michael: "Anyone who wants to make a living folding parachutes ought to be required to jump frequently." (p. 409).

REHABILITATION COUNSELING

To appreciate the suggestion that a rehabilitation counselor should *deal* with the basic nature of man, human behavior, and alternative helping modalities before considering rehabilitation counseling, consider the plausible quandary a counselor is in when he is confronted by a new client (or case folder) and asks himself, "what is the nature of the problem?"

Super suggests that this question breaks down into two parts: "one dealing with the presenting problem or the problem as the client sees it; the other, the underlying problem or the problem as the referring agent and perhaps the counselor himself sees it."[14] Then in order to determine "what to do" to help their clients, rehabilitation counselors attempt to marshall all of their knowledges and skills (twenty-four are discussed by Hall and Warren, 1956[2]) in order to operationalize an appropriate differential treatment approach personally relevant for each client. Nonetheless, a counselor's conceptualization of the basic nature of man, his theoretical assumptions regarding human behavior, and his approach to helping people, all directly affect how he deals with clients — "as a case finder, caseworker, determiner of legal eligibility, clerk, research worker, compensation expert, artificial appliance expert, and an employment and placement specialist, among other things."[8]

To summarize this suggests the following hierarchy:

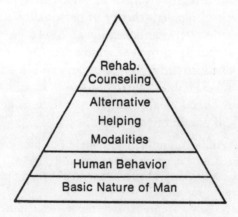

As a rehabilitation counselor continually investigates and studies these four hierarchial areas of life, his theoretical conceptualizations for each one individually and as an overall gestalt, should:

1. be *comprehensive* in scope and have some all-purpose utility;
2. be *explicit and precise* with clear meaning and denotative quality;
3. be *parsimonious* and not overly explanatory in nature;
4. be able to *withstand epistemological queries* and generate useful research;
5. be *fluid* and not rigidly opposed to inspection and potential alteration and change; and,
6. be *congruent with the counselor's life-style*. Rehabilitation counseling should not be a separate or unilateral component of a rehabilitation counselor's life: it should be a consistent and congruent part of his life.

To minimize becoming a tunnel-visioned technician and to maximize "becoming" closer to an ideal, a rehabilitation counselor's study of rehabilitation counseling is necessary but not sufficient. We must also investigate our assumptions and predispositions regarding the building blocks upon which rehabilitation counseling rests: basic nature of man, human behavior, and alternative helping modalities.

Rehabilitation counselors, counselor educators, administrators and supervisors can never dismiss their roles as students — students of life. Underneath our professional veneers, we are people; Jourard[4] suggests, "One measure of a man is the questions he raises, and another is the goals for which he uses his powers and talents."

REFERENCES

1. Carkhuff, R.R., *Helping and Human Relations*. Vol. I. *Selection and Training*. New York: Holt, Rinehart and Winston, 1969, p. 34.
2. Hall, J.H. and Warren, S.L., eds., *Rehabilitation Counselor Training*. Washington, D.C.: National Vocational Rehabilitation Association and National Guidance Association, 1956.
3. Hamilton, K.W., *Counseling the Handicapped in the Rehabilitation Process*. New York: Ronald Press. 1950.
4. Jourard, S.M., *Disclosing Man to Himself*. New York: Van Nostrand Reinhold Company. 1968, pp. 7, 8.
5. McGowan, J.T. and Porter, T.L., *An Introduction to the Vocational Rehabilitation Process*. U.S. Department of Health, Education, and Welfare. Vocational Rehabilitation Administration. Revised July, 1967, p. 108.
6. Morgan, C.A., "I, The Client." In J.G. Cull and R.E. Hardy eds., *Vocational Rehabilitation: Profession and Process*. Springfield, Ill.: Charles C Thomas. 1972, p. 409-420.
7. Osipow, S.H., *Theories of Career Development*. New York: Appleton-Century-Crofts. 1968.

8. Patterson, C.H., "The Interdisciplinary Nature of Rehabilitation Counselor Training." *The Personnel and Guidance Journal.* 1958, *36,* pp. 310-313.

9. Patterson, C.H., "The Counselor's Responsibility in Rehabilitation." *Journal of Rehabilitation.* 1958, *24*(1), pp. 7-8, 11.

10. Patterson, C.H., *Counseling and Guidance in Schools: A First Course.* New York: Harper. 1962.

11. Pepinsky, H.F. and Pepinsky, P.N., *Counseling Theory and Practice.* New York: Ronald. 1954.

12. Schontz, F.C., "Physical disability and personality." In W.S. Neff, ed., *Rehabilitation Psychology.* Washington, D.C.: American Psychological Association, Inc. 1971, pp. 33-73.

13. Spencer, W.A., "Rehabilitation—The Road to Independence. *Rehabilitation Record.* 1963, *4,* (3), 22-25.

14. Super, D.E., "The Appraisal Process in Counseling." In A. Jacobs, J.P. Jordaan and S. DiMichael, eds., *Counseling in the Rehabilitation Process.* New York: Teachers College, Columbia University. 1961, pp. 34-51.

15. Tyler, L., *The Work of the Counselor.* New York: Appleton-Century-Crofts. 1961.

CHAPTER 21

THE PROTESTANT WORK ETHIC, DISABILITY, AND THE REHABILITATION STUDENT

Kenneth R. Thomas, Sue A. Carter, and Jean O. Britton

Abstract

Fifty graduate students in rehabilitation counseling were surveyed regarding their attitudes toward the Protestant Work Ethic (PWE) using the original and a modified form of the *Bowling Green University Survey of Work Values*. Results indicated that the students were more likely to endorse those aspects of the PWE reflecting the intrinsic value of work than those dealing with earnings, social status, and advancement. In addition, the students were found to generally hold the same PWE orientation for themselves as they did for disabled persons.

IT IS FAIRLY well-established that the Protestant Work Ethic played a central role in shaping the industrial development and prevailing value system of America (Stefflre, 1966; Weber, 1958). More recent studies indicate that the ethic continues to influence the typical individual's attitude toward work and the meaning attached to the work role (Mirels & Garrett, 1971; Neff, 1968).

Several authorities in the field of rehabilitation counseling have noted that there also exists a close relationship between the Protestant Work Ethic and the rehabilitation movement in this country (DiMichael, 1964; Thoreson, 1964; Vineberg, 1958). According to Thomas, Britton, and Kravetz (1974), this relationship is evident in the eligibility criteria of public vocational rehabilitation agencies, in the definitions of what constitutes a successful rehabilitation, and in the economic and even philosophical arguments used by rehabilitation administrators to gain additional appropriations from state and federal legislative bodies.

Reprinted by permission from Volume 21 (1982), *Counselor Education Supervision*, pp. 269-273.

Since rehabilitation counselors are the primary providers of vocational and personal adjustment counseling services in virtually all rehabilitation agencies and facilities, it may be assumed that their work values and expectations for client behavior could considerably influence the outcome of the rehabilitation process. For example, as Kumar and Pepinsky (1965) pointed out several years ago, counselors have their own value systems and prejudices, and these biases can affect what they will do with and for the client.

In a study by Thomas and others (1974), 137 state agency rehabilitation counselors were found to endorse the Protestant Work Ethic for themselves and for disabled persons as measured by the original and a modified form of the *Bowling Green University Survey of Work Values* (Wollack, Goodale, Wijting, & Smith, 1971). Highly significant differences were found, however, in the degree to which the counselors endorsed the ethic for themselves as opposed to the degree to which they endorsed it for disabled persons (i.e., the counselors consistently endorsed the ethic more strongly for themselves than for disabled persons).

The purpose of the present study was to extend this earlier line of research by investigating the Protestant Work Ethic orientations of graduate students in rehabilitation counseling at a major midwestern university. Specifically, the researchers hoped to: (a) provide descriptive information on the work ethic orientations of graduate students in rehabilitation counseling; (b) determine whether these students hold the same patterns of work ethic orientation for themselves as they do for disabled persons; and (c) make recommendations for training to rehabilitation educators.

METHOD

Participants

The participants in this study were fifty graduate students in rehabilitation counseling at a major midwestern university. This group consisted of seventeen men and thirty-three women ranging in age from twenty-two to forty, with a mean age of 25.6. All fifty of the participants were pursuing graduate studies at the master's level, and each had completed at least one clinical practice experience with a disabled client at the time of the study.

Instruments

Two research instruments were used. The first was the *Bowling Green University Survey of Work Values* (SWV) (Wollack et al., 1971). The SWV is a fifty-four-item instrument that purports to provide an index of people's attitudes toward work in general rather than their feelings about specific jobs. It is based on the

Protestant Work Ethic and consists of six subscales containing nine items each. Three of the subscales, Pride in Work, Job Involvement, and Activity Preference, reflect the intrinsic value of work. Two others, Attitude toward Earnings and Social Status of Job, reflect the extrinsic rewards of work. The sixth subscale, Upward Striving, deals with the value a person places on advancing to a better job and to a higher standard of living. Wollack and others (1971) report alpha coefficient and test-retest reliabilities on the six subscales ranging from .53 to .71 in studies with industrial workers, government workers, and insurance employees.

The second instrument was adapted from the SWV to assess how the rehabilitation counseling students viewed the work ethic for disabled persons. The items on this instrument were essentially the same as those on the SWV except that terms such as man, worker, and person were changed to read man with a disability, worker with a disability, and person with a disability. For example, the item "Even if a man has a good job, he should always be looking for a better job" was changed to read "Even if a man with a disability has a good job, he should always be looking for a better job."

Procedure and Analysis

The fifty participants were randomly assigned to one of two groups by selecting alternate names from an alphabetized listing. Members of the first group were administered the SWV and members of the second group were administered the modified form of the instrument.

Data were analyzed by means of computing a one-way analysis of variance between groups for each of the six subscales on the SWV. Since Type 1 errors were additive in this study, the criterion value for establishing significance on these comparisons was set at .008 ($\frac{1}{6} \times .05$). This procedure maintained the significance level of the study as a whole at .05.

RESULTS AND DISCUSSION

Results from the analysis of variance comparisons between the groups on the six SWV subscales are presented in Table 21-1.

Inspection of this table reveals that the groups differed significantly in their ratings of the Protestant Work Ethic on only one SWV subscale (Job Involvement). According to Wollack and others (1971), *Job Involvement* refers to the degree to which a worker takes an active interest in coworkers and company functions and desires to contribute to job-related decisions. Items on this subscale included such statements as "A good worker (with a disability) is interested in helping a new worker learn his job," "If a worker (with a disability) has a choice between going to the company picnic or staying at home, he would

Table 21-1
Comparisons between the Groups on the Six Subscales

Subscale	SWV		Adapted SWV		
	M	SD	M	SD	F
Social Status	26.8	6.2	27.7	2.8	.45
Activity Preference	40.5	4.1	39.5	3.4	.89
Job Involvement	40.6	4.2	43.8	3.7	7.85*
Upward Striving	32.1	4.4	34.0	3.8	2.86
Attitude toward Earnings	25.6	4.9	25.0	3.7	.24
Pride in Work	44.7	4.3	43.8	3.7	.54

*$p < .008$.

probably be better off at home," and "A good worker (with a disability) would do his job and forget about such things as company meetings or company activities."

The finding that the students rated Job Involvement as being more important for disabled persons than for themselves could reflect a sympathetic or compensatory response to disability. For example, the students may have believed it especially appropriate or necessary for disabled persons to be involved in the job and with co-workers to compensate for other deficiencies. One way of preventing such responses from becoming excessive would be for rehabilitation counselor educators to emphasize that while many disabled persons require assistance and encouragement in pursuing social relationships at work and elsewhere, each client's needs in this area should be assessed on an individual basis.

Comparison of the results of the present study with those of the Thomas and others (1974) study reveals several interesting similarities and differences. For example, results from the earlier study suggested strong endorsement of the Protestant Work Ethic by practicing rehabilitation counselors on all six SWV subscales, whereas in the present study strong endorsement was assigned to only the three subscales reflecting the intrinsic value of work (i.e., Activity Preference, Job Involvement, and Pride in Work). Also, the counselors in the Thomas et al. study were found to differ significantly in their perceptions of the work ethic for themselves versus disabled persons on fifty-one of the fifty-three individual item comparisons reported. By contrast, the student sample in the present study was found to hold significantly different work ethic orientations for themselves versus disabled persons on only one of six subscale comparisons.

Based on a comparison of results from the two studies, at least two research hypotheses may be posited. First, it may be hypothesized that rehabilitation counseling students are less likely than practicing rehabilitation counselors to endorse all aspects of the Protestant Work Ethic. And second, it may be hypothesized that rehabilitation counseling students are less likely than practicing counselors to hold different work ethic orientations for disabled persons than they do for themselves. Since many of the counselors surveyed in the 1974 study did not possess graduate degrees, support for the second hypothesis might provide a positive indication that rehabilitation counselor education programs have been reasonably successful in eliminating for their students many of the stereotypic attitudes held toward disabled workers.

Support for either hypothesis is tempered, however, by the following considerations:

1. Data for the Thomas and others study were collected prior to implementation of the 1973 Rehabilitation Act that mandated client involvement in rehabilitation planning.
2. State agency counselors may have different work ethic orientations than rehabilitation counselors in other settings.
3. The designs and procedures used in the two studies were similar but not exactly the same. For example, in the Thomas et al. study all participants responded to both the SWV and modified instrument.
4. Actual clients may have responded differently to the SWV than either the students or counselors.
5. And finally, the students' perceptions of the Protestant Work Ethic, not only for themselves but also for disabled persons, might change significantly following a period of regular rehabilitation counseling employment.

REFERENCES

DiMichael, S.G. Vocational rehabilitation: A major social force. In H. Borow (Ed.), *Man in a world of work*. Boston: Houghton Mifflin, 1964.

Kumar, U., & Pepinsky, H.B. Counselor expectancies and therapeutic evaluations. *Proceedings of the 73rd Annual Convention of the American Psychological Association*, 1965, 357-358.

Mirels, W.S., & Garrett, J. The Protestant ethic as a personality variable. *Journal of Consulting and Clinical Psychology*, 1971, *36*, 40-44.

Neff, W.S. *Work and human behavior*. New York: Atherton Press, 1968.

Stefflre, B. Vocational development: Ten propositions in search of a theory. *Personnel and Guidance Journal*, 1966, *44*, 611-616.

Thomas, K., Britton, J., & Kravetz, S. Vocational rehabilitation counselors view the Judeo-Christian work ethic. *Rehabilitation Counseling Bulletin*, 1974, *18*, 105-111.

Thoreson, R.W. Disability viewed in its cultural context. *Journal of Rehabilitation*, 1964, *30*, 12-13.

Vineberg, S.E. Concerning job readiness. *Journal of Rehabilitation*, 1958, *24*, 9-10; 23.

Weber, M. *The Protestant ethic and the spirit of capitalism*. New York: Scribner, 1958.

Wollack, S., Goodale, J.G., Wijting, J.P., & Smith, P.C. Development of the survey of work values. *Journal of Applied Psychology*, 1971, *55*, 331-338.

CHAPTER 22

REHABILITATION COUNSELOR EDUCATION TRAINEE SELECTION FACTORS AND SUBSEQUENT OCCUPATIONAL OUTCOMES

Joseph T. Kunce, Richard W. Thoreson, and Randall M. Parker

Abstract

Occupational outcomes of 100 graduates from two university master's-level rehabilitation counselor training programs were investigated. Follow-up data regarding their present occupational role showed that approximately four-fifths of the females and two-thirds of the males from both programs had primarily counseling-related job responsibilities one to four years after graduation. The lower proportion of counseling occupational outcomes for males related to their scores on ability tests. About half of the males with graduate admission ability scores above the median had primarily administrative, teaching, or research positions at follow-up. Males with lower scores, however, had primarily counseling responsibilities (80 percent). Implications of these findings for trainee selection and program goals are discussed.

R EHABILITATION COUNSELOR education programs seek to obtain and educate academically capable students who are motivated to work in the rehabilitation field. Satisfactoriness of the subsequent vocational outcomes of such students is a controversial topic (e.g., ARCA Research Committee 1973; Brown et al. 1967; Haug & Sussman 1973; Miller & Muthard 1965; Muthard & Salomone 1969). Much of the controversy concerns the type of employment settings the graduates choose (e.g., state rehabilitation programs vs. public or private institutions) and the specific vocational roles they perform (e.g., counseling vs. teaching or administration).

Reprinted by permission from Volume 18 (1975), *Rehabilitation Counseling Bulletin,* pp. 176-180.

The authors wish to thank G.D. Carnes, Carl Hansen, George Nagle, and Susan Sleater for their help in making this report possible.

The present study examined rehabilitation counselor trainee occupational outcomes with respect to a frequently used selection factor—ability test scores. Two separate training programs were evaluated to determine the pervasiveness and implications of any obtained significant findings.

METHOD

Subjects

Subjects were 100 master's-level graduates of rehabilitation counseling programs: fifty from the University of Missouri—Columbia (Missouri) and fifty from the University of Texas at Austin (Texas). Follow-up data were collected to determine their present occupational roles. At the time of follow-up, students may have graduated anywhere from one to four years earlier.

Procedure

Various academic ability scores were available for the graduates. Most at Missouri had scores on the Millers Analogy Test (MAT), since this test was considered in the selection of students, and most had also taken the Ohio State Psychological Examination (OSPE) as part of an advisory test battery after admission to the rehabilitation counseling program. The Graduate Record Examination (GRE) was routinely administered and employed as a selection criterion by the Texas graduate school for all applicants, yielding a verbal score (GRE/V) and a quantitative score (GRE/Q).

Graduates from each training program were categorized using follow-up data to determine whether their major occupational function was as a counselor or as a noncounselor (student, teacher, or administrator). Noncounselors and counselors both worked in a wide array of rehabilitation work settings. Differences in ability scores for male and female graduates from both training programs according to occupational role were evaluated by analysis of variance procedures. Implications of differences were evaluated by an analysis of crossbreaks.

RESULTS

Graduates from both schools showed high academic ability scores. The mean raw score was 53 for the MAT and 111 for the OSPE. The mean standard score was 584 for the GRE/V and 547 for the GRE/Q.

Ability scores tended to relate to subsequent occupational roles for male graduates at both universities. The mean scores for the noncounselors on the

Table 22-1

Mean Ability Scores of Rehabilitation Graduates of the University of
Missouri–Columbia and the University of Texas at Austin

Group	Ability Test	n	Mean Scores		F
			Counselors	Noncounselors	
Males					
Missouri	MAT	39	51.4	58.7	2.86
	OSPE	36	108	122	6.59*
Texas	GRE/V	23	559	557	.00
	GRE/Q	23	519	584	4.30*
Females					
Missouri	MAT	8	44.0	68.0	insuff. data[a]
	OSPE	11	100	135	insuff. data[a]
Texas	GRE/V	27	606	606	.00
	GRE/Q	27	552	548	.00

[a]Only 2 female noncounselors in the Missouri group.
*$p < .05$.

Table 22-2

Role Outcomes of Graduates from the University of Missouri–Columbia
and the University of Texas at Austin

Group	n	Counselors		Noncounselors	
		%	n	%	n
Males					
Missouri	39	67	26	33	13
Texas	23	65	15	35	8
Females					
Missouri	11	82	9	18	2
Texas	27	81	22	19	5

Table 22-3

Role Outcomes of Male Graduates of the University of Missouri–Columbia
and the University of Texas at Austin According to Ability

Group	n	Counselors		Noncounselors	
		%	n	%	n
Missouri males[a]					
OSPE≥115	18	56	10	44	8
OSPE<115	18	83	15	17	3
Texas males					
GRE/Q≥550	13	54	7	46	6
GRE/Q<550	10	80	8	20	2

[a]No OSPE scores for 3 Missouri male subjects.

OSPE and the GRE/Q were significantly higher than those for the counselors. Scores on the MAT showed a similar, but nonsignificant, trend. Scores on the GRE/V were essentially identical for both groups of males (see Table 22-1).

No clearcut findings were found for female graduates regarding ability measures and vocational outcome (see Table 22-1). At Texas the mean GRE/V and GRE/Q scores were identical for female counselors and noncounselors. At Missouri there were only two female noncounselors, making statistical comparisons between the noncounselors and counselors infeasible. In both schools, however, the female graduates held counseling occupational roles (82% and 81%) more often than did the males (67% and 65%). These results are summarized in Table 22-2.

The relationship of intellectual attributes to male counselor role outcomes are illustrated in Table 22-3. Of the academically gifted males, fifty-six percent at Missouri and fifty-four percent at Texas had primary counseling occupational roles. In contrast, eighty-three percent and eighty percent of the graduates with more modest scores at Missouri and Texas, respectively, were also primarily engaged in counseling occupational roles.

DISCUSSION

Diverse and contradictory interpretations regarding the relationship between graduates' academic ability and outcome can readily be drawn. From a negative standpoint, counselor educational programs seem to prefer the academically elite. A bias of selecting such students may, therefore, increase the proportion of graduates who have a relatively low probability of choosing counseling positions after graduation. From a positive perspective, the counselor programs are, in fact, selecting students with varied abilities—some who have a high probability of electing counseling roles and some who will tend to choose rehabilitation-related positions in teaching and administration.

The relevancy of book-learning skills as a criterion for selecting counseling trainees has been challenged by practitioners and academicians. Schofield (1965), for example, speculated that in selecting counselors "modest intellectual endowment would perhaps prove a more positive qualification than extremely high intelligence" (p. 150). The present finding on counselor role deflection of high ability male graduates is consistent with Schofield's speculation. On the other hand, this role deflection could be indicative of special abilities (as inferred from higher quantitative skills tapped by the GRE/Q and the OSPE among male noncounselors) that enable a person to move more easily from counseling into other roles such as teaching or administration.

The greater adherence of female graduates to rehabilitation counseling roles from both schools was somewhat unexpected, since fewer women than men are employed in rehabilitation fields. Failure to find a clearcut relationship between intellective factors and noncounseling positions for women also suggest that alternative opportunities may have been less available (or less feasible) for female graduates at the time this study was conducted.

CONCLUSIONS

From a comparative analysis of occupational outcomes of graduates of two rehabilitation programs it was concluded that (a) male graduates with higher quantitative abilities were more likely to pursue administative or academic endeavors than their fellow graduates: (b) female graduates were less apt to deflect from rehabilitation counseling roles than were males; (c) restriction of selection of counseling students to those with exceptionally high ability may lead to selection of a greater proportion of individuals who choose to assume primary roles in teaching or administration; and (d) restriction of academic selection of graduate students with more modest ability may lead to a higher proportion of graduates seeking counseling roles but may also be professionally damaging since individuals with unique abilities to contribute to the rehabilitation field with regard to administration and teaching may be excluded.

REFERENCES

ARCA Research Committee. A critique of Sussman and Haug's working paper No. 7. *Rehabilitation Counseling Bulletin,* 1973, *16*(4), 218-225.

Brown, W.H.; Butler, A.J.; Thoreson, R.W.; & Wright, G.N. A factor analytic study of the rehabilitation counselor role dimension of professional counselors. *Rehabilitation Counseling Bulletin,* 1967, *11*(2), 87-97.

Haug, M.R., & Sussman, M.B. Rehabilitation counseling in perspective: A reply to the critics. *Rehabilitation Counseling Bulletin,* 1973, *16*(4), 226-238.

Miller, L.A., & Muthard, J.E. Job satisfaction and counselor performance in state rehabilitation agencies. *Journal of Applied Psychology,* 1965, *49*(4), 280-283.

Muthard, J.E., & Salomone, P.R. The roles and functions of the rehabilitation counselor. *Rehabilitation Counseling Bulletin,* 1969, *13*(2), 81-166.

Schofield, W. A modest proposal in W.D. Nunokawa (Ed.), *Human values and abnormal behavior.* Glenview, Ill.: Scott, Foresman & Co., 1965. Pp. 148-153.

CHAPTER 23

JOB SATISFACTION PREDICTORS OF REHABILITATION COUNSELING GRADUATES

Dwight R. Kauppi, Mary Ballou, Marceline E. Jaques, John J. Gualtieri, and Craig R. Blum

Abstract

This study evaluated the extent to which various demographic variables (i.e., sex, presence of disability, racial identification, and age) were effective in predicting the job satisfaction of rehabilitation counseling graduates. This research was based on the responses of seventy-two graduates (35 females and 37 males) who completed a follow-up instrument. Job satisfaction was conceptualized as multidimensional, and was measured by a discrepancy score composed of the summed differences between individuals' responses to fifteen job conditions or job reinforcers applied to their "ideal" and present jobs, with each response rated on a five-point scale. As an additional measure, participants were directly asked whether they would change jobs if given the choice. A MANOVA was performed, and sex was found to be the only significant predictor of job satisfaction, with females more satisfied than males. The discrepancy score was found to be the most effective measurement instrument.

THE CONSTRUCT of job satisfaction is an important component of vocational and career development theory (Lofquist & Dawis, 1969; Super, 1957; Wanous & Lawler, 1972). In most theories, job satisfaction is considered to be a function of the interaction between the characteristics of the job and the characteristics of the person. The job characteristics generally studied for their effects on satisfaction have been factors related to the job itself or to the work situation. Person characteristics have often focused on the importance of psychological variables, such as the vocational needs or interests of the worker. For

Reprinted by permission from Volume 26 (1983), *Rehabilitation Counseling Bulletin, pp. 336-341.*

some jobs, however, demographic characteristics may be important determiners of satisfaction. Rehabilitation counseling represents a job where demographic characteristics of disability, sex, age, and racial/ethnic background may be significantly related to satisfaction.

Though little studied, these variables were included in this study on a rational basis assuming that they would influence the job satisfaction of rehabilitation counselors. For example, the job experience of counselors with a disability is likely to be different from the job experience of those who are not disabled. Some data does indicate that sex has an influence on the job experience of rehabilitation counselors (Kunce, Thoreson, & Parker, 1975). The orientation of the rehabilitation profession has historically been male, and until recently there have been more men than women in the field. The vocational aspects of the counselor's task often require involvement with the male-dominated work climate of business and industry. Age also may influence the work ethos and the resultant job satisfaction of rehabilitation counselors in a number of ways. Generally, the older the graduates, the more years they have worked previous to entering graduate schools. The acculturation influence in the growing up process seems to differ with time. Therefore, older graduates may have a different orientation to work than younger graduates. Likewise, racial and ethnic backgrounds of individuals seem to be determiners of a wide variety of work-related perceptions and attitudes, including the effects of discrimination.

Any cultural or demographic factor that influences an individual's attitude toward work, disability, or the helping profession may influence satisfaction as a rehabilitation counselor. In this study, we will examine the specific influence of four selected demographic variables on the job satisfaction of rehabilitation counseling graduates.

Muthard and Salamone (1973) found few predictors of job satisfaction in a large sample of rehabilitation counselors. Positive attitudes toward the profession and satisfaction with counseling or placement tasks were slightly predictive of job satisfaction. No relationship was found between a wide array of personality traits and job satisfaction. This latter finding is in line with Katz and Van Maanen's conclusions (1977) following a study of the job satisfaction of public employees. Their findings implied that job satisfaction was explained by extrinsic aspects of the work setting rather than by complex psychological characteristics of employees.

Other studies have suggested, however, that certain intrinsic variables may be important in relation to job satisfaction. Kunce, Thoreson, and Parker (1975), in a study of selection factors and occupational outcomes of rehabilitation counseling graduates, found that highly qualified males tended to move into administrative positions but that highly qualified females tended to remain in counseling positions.

The State University of New York at Buffalo (SUNYAB) Rehabilitation Counselor Training Program (RCTP) has been gathering data on its students for the past decade. A study of the 1957-1971 graduates (Jaques, Kauppi, & Schoen, 1974) found that almost all of the graduates were successful in finding professional opportunities in the rehabilitation field. Further follow-up of SUNYAB graduates is reported here, testing the hypothesis that the demographic variables of disability status, sex, age, and minority/ethnic status may influence job satisfaction.

METHOD

Sample

Participants for the study were seventy-two respondents to a follow-up questionnaire sent to 113 graduates of the RCTP who graduated between 1972 and 1978. The seventy-two respondents did not differ from the population of the 113 graduates on the demographic variables studied. There were thirty-seven males (51%) and thirty-five females (49%). Of the participants, sixteen percent (six males and six females) were disabled. Examples of disabilities reported include amputation, quadriplegia, congenital heart defects, diabetes, drug and alcohol addiction, and visual impairment. The age range was from twenty-three to fifty-six, with a mean age of thirty. Six males and three females (13%) were non-white. Almost ninety percent of the graduates were employed in rehabilitation and rehabilitation-related positions. These titles included vocational rehabilitation counselor, rehabilitation counselor, substance abuse counselor, placement and evaluation worker, supervisor, administrator, and mental health counselor. About five percent were other human service jobs, such as social worker, psychologist, and feminist therapist. Four (5%) were unemployed, but had held previous rehabilitation jobs.

Procedure

A follow-up questionnaire was first sent to the 1972-1975 graduates in 1976, and has been sent every year thereafter to those who have graduated the prior year. Data for this study were drawn from structured responses to questions regarding demographic characteristics and items relating to issues of job satisfaction.

The demographic characteristics were determined from responses to direct questions regarding the presence or absence of disability, description of disabilities present, sex, racial/ethnic identification, and birthdate. Graduates were asked to check their salary level in nine $2,000 intervals from rank one (below $7,000) to rank nine (above $21,000). Those checking rank one were assigned a salary of $6,500 and those checking rank nine $21,500. Participants in other ranks were assigned the midpoint salary.

Two measures relevant to job satisfaction were included. The first measure asked participants to express their satisfaction with their job on a five-point scale from one ("not at all satisfied") to five ("extremely satisfied"). Responses to this question are referred to as the Expressed Satisfaction (ES) scale.

The second measure was derived from a list of fifteen job conditions or reinforcers. Each item represented an element that may contribute to job satisfaction. The graduates were first asked to rate each condition on a Personal Importance (PI) rating from one ("extremely important") to five ("not at all important"). They were then asked to describe their current job on a Current Job (CJ) scale using the same descriptors on a similar one to five scale. A Discrepancy Score (DS) was then derived by subtracting the PI rating from the CJ rating and summing discrepancy ratings without regard to sign across all fifteen conditions to give each participant a DS from zero, no discrepancy to sixty, maximum discrepancy. Participants were also asked whether they would continue in the same job, another job, or no job if they had the opportunity.

Data Analysis

Data were analyzed using the MULTIVARIANCE (Finn, 1977), in a two-way 2 × 2 fixed effects multiple analysis of covariance. Salary was used as a covariate. The independent variables were sex and disability status, with ES and DS the two dependent variables assessing the job satisfaction. A series of preliminary one-way ANOVAs were performed, with age and racial/ethnic background as independent factors to determine whether they had a significant effect on job satisfaction. These analyses were performed because a complete factorial design including them was not possible due to small-cell Ns. There were no statistically significant differences, and thus further analyses were performed collapsing over these factors.

RESULTS

The variable that showed the clearest relationship with job satisfaction was the sex of the graduates, significant in the MANCOVA, Mult $F(1, 67) = 5.27$, $p < .01$.

On expressed stated satisfaction, disabled and nondisabled graduates had the same mean scores ($\overline{X} = 3.75$). Males claimed only slightly more job satisfaction ($\overline{X} = 3.8$) than did females ($\overline{X} = 3.6$).

On the second measure (DS), males showed more discrepancy between their personal preference and the actual conditions of their job ($\overline{X} = 15.6$) than did females ($\overline{X} = 11.3$).

The salaries of males and females differed by $2,000, with males being paid a mean of $14,055 and females a mean of $12,157. Nondisabled males earned the highest salaries (a mean of $14,194), followed by disabled males ($13,916), disabled females ($12,417), and nondisabled females ($11,896).

A number of variables were found to be unrelated to ES and DS. These include disability, age, racial/ethnic status, previous work experience, and score on the Miller Analogies Test on entrance into the program. The possibility that time of graduation might be related to satisfaction was evaluated by comparing the group of students graduating from 1972 through 1974 with those graduating from 1975 through 1978. No difference was found.

SUMMARY AND CONCLUSIONS

Of the demographic variables, only sex was significantly related to satisfaction in the MANCOVA. In univariate analysis, only the DS showed a significant relationship with sex, with women having a lower DS than did men. It would seem that the expectations of women were met to a greater degree than were the expectations of the male graduates.

One explanation for the effect of sex is the sex-role stereotyping that has served to shape job expectations for women generally. In order to generate possible explanations for the effect of sex, the differences between men and women in their ranking of the personal importance of job conditions were examined. Of the top three conditions, men and women agree on two: "the chance to learn new things" and "the chance to make a contribution to important decisions." They differed with their third selection, with men choosing "the chance to use special abilities" and women selecting "the chance to benefit society." Men and women agreed on ranking "freedom from supervision," "high prestige and social status," and "the chance to engage in satisfying leisure activities" as the three least important job conditions. In addition, women had "high salary" tied for the third least important.

Of the three highest ranked current job descriptors, men and women agree on two, "chance to benefit society" and "working as part of a team," as descriptive of their current jobs. They differed, however, on the third ranking selection, with women rating "the chance to learn new things" and men rating "the chance to make a contribution to important decisions" as descriptive of their current jobs. Men and women agreed that "high prestige and social status" are not descriptive of their current jobs. Men also ranked "freedom from pressure to conform" and "the chance to engage in satisfying leisure activities" among the three least descriptive job conditions. For women, "freedom from supervision" and "having a high salary" were ranked as least descriptive. While these rankings reflect similarities between men and women, it is also clear that there are a number of important differences between men and women's perception of job-related factors. For example, women's ranking of "chance to benefit society" as a job condition of personal importance may be a reflection of the nurturance role often attributed to women and may also explain the greater satisfaction women expressed with rehabilitation counseling.

These findings are consistent with the sex differences on mean salaries and satisfaction. A cause-effect inference cannot be made as to whether women earn less because their expressed need for a high salary is lower or whether they report a lower need because they were earning less. Differences between men and women could also result from the different job obtained, selection factors that are different for men and women, or meaningful sex differences relative to the job of the rehabilitation counselor.

Although age, disability, and racial/ethnic background are often thought of as important determiners of work-related attitudes, the individuals in this sample did not perceive them as predictors of job satisfaction. Of the demographics studied, sex was the most influential, though complex in its effect. Sex difference may be expressed in differential needs patterns or different job experiences, but probably represents an interplay of these and other social-psychological forces. It seems clear that demographic variables are intricate in their influence and do not follow the simple hypotheses that are often constructed.

REFERENCES

Finn, D.D. *User's Guide, MULTIVARIANCE: Univariate and multivariate analysis of variance, covariance, and regression.* Chicago: National Educational Resources, 1977.

Finn, J.D., & Matteson, I. *Multivariate analysis in educational research: Applications of the MULTIVARIANCE Program.* Chicago: National Educational Services, 1978.

Jaques, M.E., Kauppi, D.R., & Schoen, S. Program profile: A follow-up study of rehabilitation counseling graduates from 1957 to 1971. *Rehabilitation Counseling Bulletin,* 1974, *17,* 223-231.

Katz, R., & Van Maanen, J. The loci of work satisfaction: Job, interaction, and policy. *Human Relations,* 1977, *30,* 469-486.

Kunce, J.T., Thoreson, R.W., & Parker, R.M. Rehabilitation counselor education trainee selection factors and subsequent occupational outcomes. *Rehabilitation Counseling Bulletin,* 1975, *18,* 176-180.

Lofquist, L.H., & Dawis, R.V. *Adjustment to work.* New York: Meredith Corporation, 1969.

Muthard, J.E., & Salomone, P.R. The roles and functions of the rehabilitation counselor. *Rehabilitation Counseling Bulletin,* 1973, *13,* (1-SP), 81-168.

Super, D.E. *The psychology of careers.* New York: Harper & Row, 1957.

Wanous, J.P., & Lawler, E.E., III. Measurement and meaning of job satisfaction. *Journal of Applied Psychology,* 1972, *56,* 95-105.

Selected Abstracts

A Look at Counselor Education Programs in Light of Section 504 of the Rehabilitation Act of 1973

E.V. Iovacchini and R.R. Abood (1981, p. 109)

The fundamental objective of Section 504 of the Rehabilitation Act of 1973 is to prohibit discrimination against all handicapped individuals attempting to participate in any program or activity that receives federal financial assistance. Therefore, this act has had a major impact on most institutions of higher education. Counselor education programs at these institutions are specifically affected in areas related to admission and treatment of handicapped students. A recent U.S. Supreme Court case is helpful in establishing guidelines for the application of Section 504 to these counselor education programs.

Counselor Trainees' Attitudes Toward Mainstreaming the Handicapped

P.S. Filer (1982, p. 61)

This study reports the results of a questionnaire on attitudes toward mainstreaming handicapped students administered to graduate counseling students at a Midwestern university. Implications for counselor education programs are suggested.

Modification of Locus of Control Among Rehabilitation Counseling Graduate Students

C.M. Pinkard and P. Gross (1984, p. 39)

Changes in locus of control orientation during graduate education in rehabilitation counseling were investigated. Shifts in the internal-external dimensions were compared between graduate students in a rehabilitation counseling program who received experiential training in counseling and a control group in gerontology program who received didactic training. The results indicated that movement toward internality was determined by the types of instruction and the level of the initial external score. Implications are discussed in the context of personality changes and rehabilitation counselor education.

A Ten-Year Follow-Up of Graduates of a Rehabilitation Counselor Training Program

J.R. Crisler and M.W. Eaton (1975, p. 35)

The purpose of this study was to conduct a ten-year follow-up of graduates of the University of Georgia Rehabilitation Counselor Training Program focusing on initial and current employment status. A survey questionnaire was sent to all graduates ($N=332$) and a eighty-three percent return was received. The survey indicated that ninety-five percent of the graduates were initially employed by state DVR agencies or closely related agencies. There was some attrition of graduates from the state DVR agencies for two primary reasons: (a) better salaries and (b) greater advancement opportunities. A substantial difference in mean salaries exists between those graduates who remained with state DVR agencies and those who were initially employed by DVR agencies and later became employed by closely related agencies. All graduates had mean salaries greater than the national average. The survey clearly indicates, based on one graduate training program results, that RCTP are preparing professional trained personnel for the rehabilitation profession.

A Follow-Up Study of Rehabilitation Counseling Graduates
M. Sullivan (1982, p. 6)

This study focused on graduates from graduate level rehabilitation counseling training programs located in Region IX (i.e., Arizona, California, Hawaii, & Nevada). The study involved administering a manpower questionnaire to a sixty-one percent random sample of graduates from 1977 through 1980 from ten Rehabilitation Counseling training programs. Questionnaire items addressed graduates' satisfaction concerning their training program, graduate employability, present employment status, and satisfaction level with their present rehabilitation occupational position. Results indicated that the master's degree in rehabilitation counseling is formidable, with ninety-two percent of the graduates employed and eighty-two percent of the graduates presently employed in the field of rehabilitation. The major employers of graduates were private rehabilitation agencies and non-profit rehabilitation facilities. Graduates were employed at an average of 1.3 months after graduation and were either immediately employed as supervisors/administrators or moved into these job categories very soon after employment. The importance of implementing and conducting cyclic rehabilitation manpower studies is discussed in terms of providing effective manpower information for planning and accountability.

Pre-Service Rehabilitation Education: Where Graduates Are Employed
G.O. Geist and B.T. McMahon (1981, p. 45)

With the cooperation of the National Council on Rehabilitation Education, a nationwide survey of 105 pre-service rehabilitation education program directors was conducted to determine the demand for and employment patterns of 3,389 graduates. Five types of programs are described in terms of graduates' characteristics, post-graduate activity, and commitment to rehabilitation. The needs assessment results submitted by selected programs are also described. The authors conclude that a strong need for pre-service training continues to exist and that such programs should not be neglected in austere times.

Employment Outcome of Graduates of a Rehabilitation Counselor Training Program: A Comparison of Graduate Employment Between 1965-1974 and 1975-1979

J.R. Crisler and N.L. Fowler, (1981, p. 28)

Graduates of the Rehabilitation Counseling Program at the University of Georgia were compared over two time periods (1965-1974 and 1975-1979) on employment setting. Both follow-up studies indicate a high percentage of graduates employed in rehabilitation settings. There is a significant trend away from employment in the state/federal programs toward related rehabilitation programs between the two time periods and from initial employment to subsequent employment.

References and Suggested Additional
Readings for Part IV

Anthony, W.A., & Carkhuff, R.R. (1970). Effects of training on rehabilitation counselor trainee functioning. *Rehabilitation Counseling Bulletin, 6*, 333-342.

Anthony, W.A., Slowkowski, P., & Bendix, L. (1976). Developing the specific skills and knowledge of the rehabilitation counselor. *Rehabilitation Counseling Bulletin, 19*, 456-462.

Cherniss, C. (1980). Staff burnout: *Job stress in the human services.* Beverly Hills, CA: Sage Publications.

Clark, W.D. (1978). *Relationships among certain attitudes and types and level of educational experiences in rehabilitation students.* Unpublished doctoral dissertation, Florida State University, Tallahassee.

Crisler, J.R., & Eaton, M.W. (1975). A ten-year follow-up of graduates of a rehabilitation counselor training program. *Journal of Applied Rehabilitation Counseling, 6*(1), 35-41.

Crisler, J.R., & Fowler, N.L. (1981). Employment outcomes of graduates of rehabilitation counselor training program: A comparison of graduate employment between 1965-1974 and 1975-1979. *Journal of Rehabilitation, 47*(3), 28-32.

Culberson, J.O. (1979). Undergraduate education for rehabilitation: Agency perceptions of training and characteristics preferred of job applicants. *Journal of Rehabilitation, 45*(2), 39-43.

Dowd, E.T., & Emener, W.G. (1978). Lifeboat counseling: The issue of survival decisions. *Journal of Rehabilitation, 44*(3), 34-36.

Emener, W.G. (1975). The rehabilitation counselor: A student of life. *Journal of Rehabilitation, 41*(1), 16-17, 43.

Emener, W.G. (1978). Reconciling personal and professional values with agency goals and processes. *Journal of Rehabilitation Administration, 2*(4), 166-173.

Emener, W.G. (1979). Professional burnout: Rehabilitation's hidden handicap. *Journal of Rehabilitation, 1979, 45*(1), 55-58.

Emener, W.G., & Andrews, W. (1977). The individualized written rehabilitation program: Perceptions from the field. *Journal of Applied Rehabilitation Counseling, 7*(4), 215-222.

Emener, W.G., Luck, R.S., & Gohs, F.X. (1982). A theoretical investigation of the construct burnout. *Journal of Rehabilitation Administration, 6*(4), 188-196.

Filer, S.P. (1982). Counselor trainees' attitudes toward mainstreaming the handicapped. *Counselor Education and Supervision, 22*(1), 61-69.

Gandy, G.L. (1983). Graduates of an undergraduate rehabilitation curriculum. *Rehabilitation Counseling Bulletin, 26*(5), 357-359.

Geist, G.O., & McMahon, B.T. (1981). Pre-service rehabilitation education: Where graduates are employed. *Journal of Rehabilitation, 47*(3), 45-47.

Gilbert, L.D. (1973). The changing work ethic and rehabilitation. *Journal of Rehabilitation, 39*(4), 14-17.

Iovacchini, E.V., & Abood, R.R. (1981). A look at counselor education programs in light of Section 504 of the Rehabilitation Act of 1973. *Counselor Education and Supervision, 21*(2), 109-118.

Janes, M.W., & Emener, W.G. (1983). Graduates' views of instructional/competency areas in rehabilitation counselor education programs: A hypotheses generating study. *Journal of Applied Rehabilitation Counseling, 15*(2), 38-43.

Janes, M.W., & Emener, W.G. (in press). Rehabilitation counselor education graduates' perceptions of their employment and career satisfaction. *Rehabilitation Counseling Bulletin.*

Kaplan, S.P. (1984). Rehabilitation counseling students' perceptions of obese male and female clients. *Rehabilitation Counseling Bulletin, 27*(3), 172-181.

Kaplan, S.P., & Thomas, K.R. (1981). Rehabilitation counseling student perceptions of obese clients. *Rehabilitation Counseling Bulletin, 25*(2), 106-109.

Kauppi, D.W., Ballou, M., Jaques, M.E., Gualtieri, J.J., & Blum, C.R. (1983). Job satisfaction predictors of rehabilitation counseling graduates. *Rehabilitation Counseling Bulletin, 26*(5), 336-341.

Krauft, C., Rubin, S., Cook, D., & Bozarth, J. (1976). Counselor attitudes toward disabled persons and client program completion: A pilot study. *Journal of Applied Rehabilitation Counseling, 7,* 50-54.

Kunce, J.T., Thoreson, R.W., & Parker, R.M. (1975). Rehabilitation counselor education trainee selection factors and subsequent occupational outcomes. *Rehabilitation Counseling Bulletin, 18*(3), 176-180.

Majumber, R.K., McDonald, A.P., & Greever, K.B. (1977). A study of rehabilitation counselors: Locus of control and attitudes toward the poor. *Journal of Counseling Psychology, 24,* 137-141.

Martin, R.D., & Shepel, L.F. (1974). Locus of control and discrimination ability with lay counselors. *Journal of Counseling and Clinical Psychology, 42,* 741.

McGowan, J.F., & Porter, T.L. (1967). *An introduction to the vocational rehabilitation process.* Washington, D.C.: Department of Health, Education, and Welfare, Vocational Rehabilitation Administration.

Miller, L.A., & Muthard, J.E. (1965). Job satisfaction and counselor performance in state rehabilitation agencies. *Journal of Applied Psychology, 49,* 280-283.

Miller, L.A., & Roberts, R.R. (1979). Unmet counselor needs from ambiguity to the Zeigarnik effect. *Journal of Applied Rehabilitation Counseling, 10*(2), 60-66.

Muthard, J.E., & Morris, J.D. (1976). Predicting long-term job satisfaction and persistence among rehabilitation counselors. *Journal of Applied Rehabilitation Counseling, 7*(1), 27-33.

Nadolsky, J.N. (1977). The educated counselor: Responsibilities in a service society. *Journal of Rehabilitation, 43*(4), 30-32.

Olshansky, S. (1967). An evaluation of rehabilitation counselor training. *Vocational Guidance Quarterly, 5,* 164-167.

Parloff, M., Waskow, I., & Wolfe, B. (1978). Research on variables in relationship to process and outcome. In S. Garfield & A. Bergin (Eds.): *A handbook of psychotherapy and behavior changes.* 2nd Ed. New York: John Wiley.

Patterson, C.H. (1962). Test characteristics of rehabilitation counselor trainees. *Journal of Rehabilitation, 18*(5), 15-16.

Pinkard, C.M., & Gross, P. (1984). Modifications of locus of control among rehabilitation counseling graduate students. *Rehabilitation Counseling Bulletin, 28*(1), 39-45.

Rasch, J.D., Hollingsworth, D.K., Saxon, J.P., & Thomas, K.R. (1984). Student recruitment issues in the 1980s. *Rehabilitation Counseling Bulletin, 28*(1), 46-49.

Section 504 of the Rehabilitation Act of 1973, 29 USC §794 (Supp. IV 1974).

Sullivan, M. (1982). A follow-up study of rehabilitation counseling graduates. *Journal of Applied Rehabilitation Counseling, 13*(1), 6-10.

Thomas, K., Britton, J., & Kravetz, S. (1974). Vocational rehabilitation counselors view the Judeo-Christian work ethic. *Rehabilitation Counseling Bulletin, 18,* 105-111.

Thomas, K.R., Carter, S.A., & Britton, J.O. (1982). The protestant work ethic, disability, and the rehabilitation student. *Counselor Education and Supervision, 21*(4), 269-273.

Thoreson, R.W. (1964). Disability viewed in a cultural context. *Journal of Rehabilitation, 30,* 12-13.

Witten, B.J. (1980). *Preparation and utilization of undergraduate workers in rehabilitation: Comparative perceptions of respondents.* Unpublished doctoral dissertation, Syracuse University.

Wrenn, G.C. (1952). The selection and education of personnel workers. *Personnel and Guidance Journal, 31,* 9-14.

Wright, G.N. (1980). *Total rehabilitation.* Boston: Little, Brown, and Company.

PART V

INSERVICE TRAINING AND
CONTINUING EDUCATION

PART V. INSERVICE TRAINING AND CONTINUING EDUCATION

Introduction Commentary

HUMAN SERVICE organizations are constantly changing (Bennis, 1966; Nadler, 1979; Stephens & Kniepp, 1981). Moreover, practitioners' roles, functions, responsibilities and job tasks are also changing and becoming more specialized (Smits, Emener & Luck, 1981; Thomas, 1982). Concomitantly, accountability of human service organizations is continuing to be demanded by the public (Stretch, 1978). For reasons such as these, the rehabilitation counselor has been expected to participate in inservice training and continuing education—from the earlier years of professional rehabilitation counselor service delivery (see National Rehabilitation Association, Committee on Training, 1951; Ninth Annual Workshop on Guidance, Training and Placement, 1956; Shipman, 1961) to the present (Bruyere & Elliot, 1979; Godly, Hafer, Vieceli & Godly, 1984). From a historical perspective, the inservice training and continuing education of rehabilitation counselors has responded to: (a) state-federal vocational rehabilitation agency manpower development needs (see Porter & Settles, 1968); (b) the continuing development of "new" rehabilitation counselors (Bitter, 1978); (c) new knowledge and competency needs (for example, in the areas of technology, Browning & McGovern, 1974, and assertive behavior, Luck & Lassiter, 1978); (d) specific training needs within a particular state vocational rehabilitation program (Emener & Placido, 1982) as well as within a particular geographic region (see Bruyere & Elliot, 1979; RRCEP Directors, 1975); and (e) the continuing professional development needs of rehabilitation counselors in the private sector (Lynch & Martin, 1982). It is important to note, however, that the inservice training and continuing education of the rehabilitation counselor essentially is sine qua non to the continuing professionalism of the practice of rehabilitation counseling.

One of the major cornerstones of rehabilitation counseling's development *as a profession* includes the important components of inservice training and continuing education, and the professional life-style of continuing growth and development Brubaker, 1977; Hawley & Capshaw, 1981; Hershenson, 1982; Lynch & McSweeney, 1981; Parker & Thomas, 1981). Commensurate with the development of professionalism, inservice training and continuing education for rehabilitation counselors is also critical to professional and statutory credentialing developments (e.g., certification—Gianforte, 1976; Hansen, 1977; licensure—Newman, 1979; and credentialing—Scofield, Berven & Harrison, 1981). Thus, inservice training and continuing education is a critical aspect of rehabilitation counseling's continuing emergence as a professional, human service, health care component of American society (see Hawley & Capshaw, 1981). Pivotal to the provision of inservice training and continuing education, nonetheless, is the identification and determination of the rehabilitation counselor's inservice training and continuing education needs.

It has been strongly suggested that rehabilitation counselors' inservice training and continuing education should be related to their knowledge and performance deficiencies (Emener & Placido, 1982; McAlees & Corthell, 1972; McFarlane & Sullivan, 1979). Unfortunately, survey research results have suggested that the evaluation of rehabilitation counselor competence and performance is frequently inadequate and at times irrelevant (Bolton, 1978; Downes, McFarlane & Alston, 1974; Emener & Placido, 1982; Lorenz, 1979). It is hereby suggested, therefore, that the assessment, identification and determination of rehabilitation counselors' inservice training and continuing education needs be conducted specifically for such purposes and not determined solely or predominately upon counselor performance evaluations. In spite of the numerous efforts to enhance and improve inservice training and continuing education programs, many criticisms of them abound. For example, McAlees and Corthell's (1972) survey of 2672 National Rehabilitation Counseling Association members concluded: "While the respondents as a whole believe inservice training is effective and relevant, counselors were less positive in their evaluation [and] counselors did not perceive their agency as strongly supporting their in-service training" (p. 31). McFarlane and Sullivan (1979), in Chapter 24, analyzed needs assessment survey data from 330 rehabilitation counselors and reported that, while the counselors' perceived training needs focused on refinements in individual counseling techniques and placement, the training they had received over the previous past two years had focused on administrative/agency structure and placement activities. Thus, one of the many critical issues that should challenge the reader is the extent to which inservice training and continuing education should focus on needs perceived by the counselors, the counselors' supervisors and employers, and/or both?

Richardson and Obermann (1972) reported that counselors and supervisors perceive different needs for inservice training. Moreover, they reported that counselors and supervisors differ in their perceptions on the helpfulness of in-service training needs (they surveyed 104 rehabilitation counselors and nineteen rehabilitation supervisors), and among other findings they reported that more inservice training needs differences were obtained when the counselors were compared by state than by education, age, or gender. Differences were also found between groups; for example, supervisors felt case recording, knowledge of state/federal regulations and case management were more important training needs than did the counselors.

Emener, Mars and Schmidt (1984), in Chapter 26, describe a "counselor evaluation — client feedback" activity which practicing rehabilitation counselors and their supervisors are encouraged to use. Among the stated benefits of this systematic, client-feedback evaluation activity, the authors state that it "can provide valuable information for rehabilitation counselors and their professional development." If rehabilitation counselors are going to continually assess their inservice training and continuing education needs, they are urged to temper their self-assessments with their supervisors' assessments of them as well as evaluative feedback from their clients.

In comparison to inservice training and continuing education needs assessments using response samples predominately from the public sector (e.g., Freeman, 1979; McFarlane & Sullivan, 1979), Lynch and Martin (1982), in Chapter 27, reported interesting findings from their study of 147 members of the National Association of Rehabilitation Professionals in the Private Sector. For example, Lynch and Martin (1982) concluded: "With respect to training needs, of primary importance were tangible skill areas related to assessment, job analysis and placement, communication, and organization. Of least importance were those areas typically associated with generic interpersonal counseling." A comparative analysis of inservice training and continuing education needs assessment studies reveals numerous differences within states, between states, within groups of professionals, and between groups of professionals. Thus, it would appear fitting to conclude that to a large extent the inservice training and continuing education of the professional rehabilitation counselor should be approached idiographically — each counselor has differing needs! Moreover, it is suggested that each counselor should feel ethically and personally committed to being in charge of, and responsible for, his or her own continuing professional development!

Program planning and *evaluation* are critical to the field of rehabilitation — within agencies and facilities (see Struthers & Miller, 1981), within rehabilitation counselor education programs (see Wright, Reagles & Scorzelli, 1973), and within inservice training and continuing education (see Ferritor & Le-Land, 1982; Godly, Hafer, Vieceli & Godly, 1984; Moore, 1981). The planning and implementation of inservice training is important (see Stephens & Kniepp, 1981); evaluation planning and evaluation implementation are also important (Kirkpatrick, 1975). Programs designed to enhance the effectiveness and efficiency of the professional rehabilitation counselor should model the professionalism they are designed to enhance.

In conclusion, readers are encouraged to study the materials presented in this part of the book. And while professional trainers and professional educators are challenged to assess, plan, develop, implement, and evaluate their programs to maximize their potentials, the professional rehabilitation counselor is reminded that the one person who is ultimately responsible for the continuing education and development of the rehabilitation counselor is the individual rehabilitation counselor!

W.G. Emener

CHAPTER 24

EDUCATIONAL AND TRAINING NEEDS
OF REHABILITATION COUNSELORS:
IMPLICATIONS FOR TRAINING

Fred R. McFarlane and Michael Sullivan

Abstract

This study assesses the educational and training needs of state agency vocational rehabilitation counselors in Region IX. The Field Research Survey (FRS) was administered to a sample of 360 case-carrying counselors. Ninety-one and six-tenths percent (91.6%) or 330 of the rehabilitation counselors adequately completed the FRS. The main findings of the study were: (1) 32.1% of the rehabilitation counselors had completed some graduate training in rehabilitation; (2) 20.3% were involved in formal continuing education; (3) 74.4% of the rehabilitation counselor's last work experience was in areas other than counseling; (4) training received over the past two years focused on administrative/agency structure and placement activities; and (5) perceived training needs focused on refinement in individual counseling techniques and placement.

ALL HUMAN SERVICE fields, including rehabilitation, are constantly encountering the phenomenon of obsolescence. Obsolescence is more acute in the human service professions than in the technical/trade professions because the human service professional works with concepts, ideas and knowledge that constantly undergo rapid changes (Dublin, 1972; Lindsay, Morrison, & Kelley, 1972). To keep pace with change and professional obsolescence many organizations have adapted continuing education requirements as a condition for professional association membership. Licensing boards in many states have taken an even firmer step by requiring a specific number of continuing education credits before relicensing.

When relating the need for continuing education to rehabilitation, the

Reprinted by permission from Volume 10 (1979), *Journal of Applied Rehabilitation Counseling,* pp. 41-43.

rehabilitation counselor becomes the logical focal point for initiating continuing education. It is the rehabilitation counselor who must maintain the balance between changing client needs and professional and organizational changes.

The Rehabilitation Continuing Education Program in Region IX (RCEP IX) conducted a comprehensive education and training needs assessment of rehabilitation counselors in Region IX. The primary objectives of this study were three-fold:

1. To assess the extent of prior training and perceived rehabilitation counselor strengths;
2. To determine perceived rehabilitation counselor training needs to meet professional and client mandates; and
3. To develop a comprehensive basis for determining relevant, responsive continuing education.

POPULATION AND SURVEY PROCEDURE

The population for this study involved state agency rehabilitation counselors in Arizona, California, Guam, Hawaii, and Nevada. The instrument used for this study to identify and evaluate perceived education and training needs of rehabilitation counselors was the Field Research Survey (FRS), (Sullivan and McFarlane, in press). This instrument is composed of the following sections:

1. Educational information;
2. Employment history;
3. Training received during the last two fiscal years related to specific professional development activities; and
4. Perceived training needs with regard to specific client populations and professional development.

In the distribution and collection of the FRS booklet, the RCEP IX Evaluator met with state vocational rehabilitation staff to define the sample and administration procedures. As a result of those meetings, Arizona and Nevada surveyed 100 percent of their rehabilitation counselors. Arizona assumed responsibility for distribution and collection of the FRS booklets, while Nevada had the RCEP IX Evaluator travel to field offices for direct supervision and administration of the FRS. The Pacific Rehabilitation Continuing Education Program, located at the University of Hawaii, conducted the administration and collection of data in the Pacific Basin (Hawaii and Guam). In California, the RCEP IX Evaluator worked with the Bureau of Statistics and Research, Department of Rehabilitation, to develop an acceptable sample size and the mechanism for subject selection. A thirty-three percent sample size for

California was used with the RCEP IX mailing out the FRS booklets with return envelopes.

RESULTS AND DISCUSSION

Distribution and collection of the FRS booklets was completed during a six-month period. The time periods were May 1975, for Nevada; June 1975, for Arizona and the Pacific Basin (Hawaii and Guam); and December 1975, for California. Of the total of 360 FRS booklets distributed, there were 330 completed FRS booklets. Of the 330 booklets completed, there were fifty-five (55) from Arizona, 209 from California, thirty (30) from Nevada, and thirty-six (36) from the Pacific Basin. The findings of this study were based on a sample of 330 rehabilitation counselors in Region IX. This represents forty-seven percent of the total population of case-carrying state agency rehabilitation counselors in Region IX. The following provides a brief summary of the data by each FRS section.

EDUCATIONAL INFORMATION. The results indicated that 92.1 percent of the sample population have at least a Bachelor's degree and 49.4 percent have Master's degrees. Of the individuals who hold a Master's degree, 65.2 percent of them have their degrees in Rehabilitation. Therefore, of the total population surveyed, 32.1 percent have completed graduate training in Rehabilitation.

EMPLOYMENT INFORMATION. The rehabilitation counselors reported a mean of 3.1 years at their present job title, and a mean of 4.0 years at their agency. However, the rehabilitation counselors reported a mean of 10.8 years of experience in human care services.

Past work experience was reported in relationship to nine (9) job categories. Of the sample of 330 individuals, 25.6 percent had previously worked as counselors, 16.5 percent worked in the area of social work, and 14.3 percent were students before taking a job with the state agency. The job category of 'Other' received the most responses with 25.6 percent.

PREVIOUS TRAINING RECEIVED. Table 24-1 contains the eleven (11) most frequently received training activities during the last two (2) fiscal years.

PERCEIVED TRAINING. Rehabilitation counselors were asked to select their first, second and third choices for training to meet state agency and professional responsibilities. Table 24-2 provides a summary of the perceived training needs by the rehabilitation counselors.

The results of perceived training needs indicated that the first priority is the maintenance and refinement of individual counseling skills. Four (4) of the first eight (8) priorities relate specifically to the development of skills in vocational placement activities. In essence, while the actual training received focused on basic skills and agency functioning (Table 24-1), the rehabilitation counselor is requesting skills which will provide more data in assisting the client to make career decisions (Table 24-2).

Table 24–1

Most Frequent Training Received
in Last Two Fiscal Years

Training Received	Number	Percentage
State/Federal Regulations	216	65.5
Placement	212	64.2
Medical Aspects of Disability	208	63.0
Agency Administration	205	62.1
Physical Disabilities	191	57.9
Case Management	186	56.4
Individual Counseling Techniques	160	48.5
Case Confidentiality	155	47.0
Counseling Theory and Application	152	46.1
Psychological Aspects of Disability	149	45.2
Alcoholism	148	44.8

The two most frequent training areas were:

1. administrative/agency structure and organization; and

2. general treatment skills and knowledge.

Table 24-2

Perceived Training Needs

Training	Total Number of Responses
Individual Counseling Techniques	77
Placement	73
Psychological Aspects of Disability	59
Education/Occupational Information	51
Medical Aspects of Disability	49
Economic/Labor Forecasting	45
Resource Development	45
Group Counseling Techniques	43

The above results are a compilation of the first, second and third choices by each rehabilitation counselor and are arranged in priority order.

IMPLICATIONS FOR REHABILITATION COUNSELOR CONTINUING EDUCATION

While the results are reflective of only one federal HEW region, the implications have relevance to rehabilitation counselors and their ongoing need for continuing education. First, the profile of the practicing state VR agency rehabilitation counselor is traditionally one of an individual with prior experience in rehabilitation, and with a multiplicity of previous work experiences. Second, it is not surprising to see that the most common training received is in administration/organization areas. Third, the training requested focuses on basic skill maintenance.

Therefore, if state VR agency training, university training, and continuing education is to be relevant and practical, consideration must be given to examining need for basic skills training. The state VR agency must examine the extent and method of presentation of administration/organization training.

Often this training is designed to implement new/revised regulations. Are not these regulations based on good rehabilitation practices? If so, why do rehabilitation counselors not view the training as improving basic rehabilitation practices?

The request by rehabilitation counselors for training in basic skills areas poses two obvious implications for university-based training. The first implication is that curriculum must be relevant, applied, and its effect should have "staying power" beyond the university setting. The second implication focuses on making graduate training accessible to not only potential rehabilitation counselors, but practicing rehabilitation counselors. This may require more part-time and work-study programs to upgrade the formal educational training of the practicing rehabilitation counselor.

Finally, the results pose definite implications for continuing education. There must be continuing assessment of the background of rehabilitation counselors and their perceived training. This must be updated and refined constantly. Further, however, is to assess not only immediate training, but the implications for longitudinal training. Sequencing of training is critical. However, to sequence training requires an accurate training needs assessment and knowledge of changing priorities. Professional obsolescence can be minimized, if training needs can be assessed and designed to provide ongoing professional development.

REFERENCES

Dublin, S.S. Obsolescence or lifelong evaluation, *American Psychologist,* 1972, *27,* 486-498.

Lindsay, C.A., Morrison, J., and Kelley E.J. Professional obsolescence: Implication for continuing professional education, *Adult Education,* 1974, *25*(1), 3-22.

Sullivan, M.B., and McFarlane, F.R. Training needs identification and assessment of rehabilitation counselor, *Rehabilitation Counseling Bulletin,* in press.

CHAPTER 25

REHABILITATION COUNSELOR AND SUPERVISOR PERCEPTIONS OF COUNSELOR TRAINING NEEDS AND CONTINUING EDUCATION

Jeanne B. Freeman

Abstract

The purpose of this study was to determine whether rehabilitation counselors and supervisors had different perceptions of (a) knowledge areas important for rehabilitation counselors, (b) the continuing education needs of rehabilitation counselors, and (c) the preferred methods of providing continuing education for rehabilitation counselors. This study also measured the differential effects of education, sex, and age on the selected knowledge areas, defined needs, and preferred training methods. A Training Needs Survey was administered to all of the counselors and supervisors in three western states. The main finding was that more differences were obtained when counselors were compared by state, than by education, age, or sex. More similarities were found between counselors and supervisors than differences on the important knowledge areas and training needs, however supervisors felt case recording, knowledge of state/federal regulations and case management were more important training needs than did the counselors. Overall, the workshop/seminar was the preferred method of inservice training.

TRADITIONALLY EDUCATION has been considered a life-long process; as people interacted with their environment they continued to learn, apart from any formal education they may receive. An individual's capacity to learn solely from this method is now challenged, and "professional obsolescence" and "continuing education" have become common place terms in most professional organizations. The profession of rehabilitation counseling is not immune to these phenomena.

Reprinted by permission from Volume 10 (1979), *Journal of Applied Rehabilitation Counseling*, pp. 154-157.

Inservice training programs and short-term workshops, the two primary mechanisms for continuing education for rehabilitation counselors, have met with questionable success in improving the skills of employed rehabilitation counselors. Some common limiting factors have been identified: programs vary from state to state, little planning has gone into any of the program, and there has been only a minimal attempt to meet agency goals and counselor needs (Dickerson & Roberts, 1973). Richardson and Obermann (1972) found that counselors and supervisors differed in their perceptions of the helpfulness of inservice training and counselors and supervisors perceived different needs for training. Other concerns in rehabilitation continuing education have been the diverse backgrounds of rehabilitation counselors and the lack of agreement on the training and skills needed by rehabilitation counselors (Pankowski & Pankowski, 1975; Roberts & Engelkes, 1970).

A third dimension to the rehabilitation continuing education program emerged with the development of Regional Rehabilitation Continuing Education Programs (RRCEP). RRCEP's were designed to complement other post-employment training; specifically, one of the RRCEP goals was to provide technical assistance to other postemployment programs, such as training needs assessments (RRCEP Directors, 1975). The methods of identifying training needs have ranged from postcard surveys to an eleven-page Field Research Survey (Sullivan & McFarlane, 1978). As RRCEP's are becoming increasingly sophisticated in assessing training needs, the following questions remain unanswered: Do rehabilitation counselors and supervisors have different perceptions of (a) knowledge areas important for rehabilitation counselors, (b) continuing education needs of rehabilitation counselors, and (c) the preferred method of providing continuing education? In addition, do age, sex, and education impact on counselor and supervisor perceptions?

The preceding questions appear to be pertinent questions in an era of accrediting rehabilitation counselor education programs, certifying rehabilitation counselors and utilizing inservice training to maintain certification, and establishing essential competencies for rehabilitation counselors (Sink, Porter, Rubin & Painter, 1979).

POPULATION AND PROCEDURES

The population for this study consisted of all of the vocational rehabilitation counselors ($N=104$) and supervisors ($N=19$) in three western states with small urban populations (Montana, Wyoming and North Dakota). A Training Needs Survey (TNS) was developed with assistance from state staff development specialists and an RRCEP director. The TNS was field tested on twenty-five rehabilitation counseling graduate students. As a result of the field test, certain instructions were modified, but the format and items remained unchanged. The

Counselor Form of the TNS was divided into eight areas: counseling, behavioral sciences, medical and psychological aspects of disability, assessment, community-related skills, teaching independent living skills, personal competencies, and policy/program information. The eight areas included fifty-five specific items. The TNS was divided into two sections; the first section consisted of three scales: Scale I—Importance, Scale II—Need, and Scale III—Method.

For the first scale, Importance, counselors were asked to rate each of the fifty-five items on a four-point Likert Scale (4—very important, 3—important, 2—of limited importance and 1—not important) on the basis of how important the counselor viewed the knowledge area/skill as necessary for effective functioning as a counselor in a state agency. For the second scale, Needs, counselors rated the same fifty-five items on a similar four-point Likert Scale on the basis of their need for special training on that item to increase their effectiveness as a counselor. The third scale, Method, asked counselors to select their preferred means of training for each of the eight areas. The methods included (a) regular college/university credit, (b) extension classes, (c) correspondence courses, (d) workshops or seminars, and (e) on-the-job training.

The second section of the TNS consisted of a prioritized listing of three inservice training items from the first section, the training method and length of training. Counselors selected their first, second and third choices from the fifty-five items in the preceding section. On the second part of that section counselors were asked how important inservice training activities were for them in their present positions; counselors checked "very important," "important," "not critical" or "unnecessary." Space was also provided for counselors to add additional items or comments.

The Supervisor Form of the TNS was the same as the Counselor Form, however supervisors were asked to respond relative to their staff. For example, "How important are inservice training activities for the counselors you supervise?" Both counselors and supervisors completed demographic information to allow for comparisons by age, sex, and education.

The TNS was mailed to each of the counselors and supervisors by the Staff Development Specialist in Montana and Wyoming and individually mailed by the investigator to each of the counselors and supervisors in North Dakota.

RESULTS

Ninety counselors and eighteen supervisors returned the TNS for an overall return rate of eighty-eight percent, however ten counselors and one supervisor were eliminated for failure to complete the demographic information. Of the counselors ($N=80$), thirty-one percent possessed a master's degree, the mean age was 32.1 years, and seventy percent were males. Of the thirty-one percent with master's degrees, only twenty-one percent had master's degrees in rehabilitation counseling, guidance and counseling, psychology or social work. Twenty-six percent of the counselors had been with the agency less than one year. The mean age of the supervisors was thirty-nine years and fifty-three percent had master's degrees, however thirty-five percent had master's degrees in rehabilitation counseling, guidance and counseling, psychology, social work or rehabilitation administration. Sixty-five percent of the supervisors had been with the state agency over five years and forty-one percent had been supervisors more than five years. All of the supervisors were male.

Since each counselor responded to the questionnaire individually and each supervisor responded for his staff as a whole, counselors and supervisors could only be compared using mean responses, standard deviations and mean differences (counselors' means minus supervisors' means). For example, the counselors' means for the importance of knowledge of interviewing principles was 3.51 and the supervisors' mean was 3.75. Thus the mean difference was minus .25, with the supervisors rating knowledge of interviewing principles higher than the counselors.

Items receiving the highest mean Likert ratings on the first scale, Importance, by counselors were psychological aspects of disability, utilizing community resources and counseling techniques. Items receiving the highest mean ratings by supervisors for the same scale were case management, plan development, and psychological aspects of disability. Group counseling received the lowest rating by supervisors and was the third from the bottom in counselor ratings.

On the second scale, Need, the items receiving the highest mean ratings were (a) psychological aspects of disability, (b) test interpretation, and (c) personality disorders. Supervisors rated case management as the highest need, but followed it with psychological aspects of disability, state/federal regulations, placement techniques, personality tests, test interpretation, and orthopedic impairments. The greatest differences between the means of the counselors and the supervisors were on the following items: case recording, state/federal regulations and case management. Supervisors felt these were needed much more than did the counselors.

On the third scale, Method, supervisors, with one exception, consistently rated the workshop/seminar method as the preferred method of training and consistently rated it higher than did the counselors. (The one exception was in the area of behavioral sciences, where college/university credit was the preferred method.)

The second part of the TNS was designed for counselors and supervisors to prioritize training needs, the preferred method of training and the preferred length of training. Some responded by listing one of the major categories such as "assessment," whereas others listed specific items. Overall the category receiving the highest number of responses (first, second and third choices) of the counselors was Medical and Psychological Aspects of Disability. The categories receiving the most responses from supervisors were categories four and five, Assessment, and Community-related Skills. Both counselors and supervisors selected psychological aspects of disability as the most important item. Regardless of their response to the items or categories, most counselors and supervisors listed the same method and length of training for their first, second and third choices. The workshop/seminar was the preferred length of training ranged from two to four days. Seventy-one percent of the counselors preferred the workshop/seminar. College/university credit was the next most frequently mentioned (19%).

Counselors and supervisors also rated the importance of inservice training activities for counselors. Almost forty-four percent of the counselors and forty-seven percent of the supervisors rated inservice training as "very important." No counselors or supervisors rated inservice training as "unnecessary," however 11.2 percent of the counselors and 5.9 percent of the supervisors indicated that inservice training was "not critical."

Using Chi Square tests of independence and Fisher's exact tests, counselors and supervisors were also compared on the basis of (a) education, (b) sex, and (c) age. Educational backgrounds were classified according to the system utilized by Richardson and Obermann (1972); trained counselors were those counselors with a graduate degree in rehabilitation counseling, guidance and counseling, psychology or social work. Untrained counselors were those lacking a graduate degree or those holding a graduate degree, but not in one of the designated areas. Supervisors were divided on the same basis, however the trained category also included a graduate degree in rehabilitation administration. Counselors were compared on the basis of sex, however since all supervisors were male, no comparisons were made. Counselors and supervisors were also compared on the basis of age. The responses of those over age thirty-five were compared with those age thirty-five and under. Although the null hypothesis was rejected for ten of the fifty-five items on Scale I—Importance comparing trained and untrained counselors, no differences were found between trained and untrained counselors on the second scale, Need. The null hypothesis was rejected for three of the eight categories on the third scale, Method. Virtually no differences were found between trained and untrained supervisors on any of the three scales. Likewise, virtually no differences were found when counselors were compared by sex on the three scales. The age of the counselors also did not account for any differences on the three scales, however significant differences (p < .05) were found between supervisors over thirty-five years of age and those age thirty-five and under for ten of the fifty-five items on the Importance Scale.

Although the number of supervisors was too small to permit additional comparisons by state, counselors were compared by state on each of the three scales. Of the nineteen items which were significant on the basis of state, eleven of those items were on the Importance Scale. Statistical comparisons were also made between each of the investigative areas (education, sex, and age) for counselors and supervisors and the rating of importance of inservice training for counselors. Age was the only investigative area which was significant relative to the importance of inservice training for counselors. Trained supervisors viewed inservice training for counselors as more important than did untrained supervisors.

DISCUSSION

Generalizations of the preceding results should consider the geographic location and the limited number of supervisors and counselors possessing master's degrees in rehabilitation counseling. In addition, knowledge of available training resources may have been a limiting factor relative to counselor perceptions of training needs.

The findings demonstrate the state appears to be as important a variable as education, age or sex relative to perceived important knowledge areas. In contrast to the findings of Richardson and Obermann (1972), trained and untrained counselors did perceive some different important knowledge areas for counselors. Although differences emerged, the differences did not suggest a meaningful pattern nor suggest specific inservice changes for trained and untrained counselors. The differences suggest a need for further research. Consistent with the findings of Richardson and Obermann (1972), however, were the few differences between trained and untrained counselors and supervisors on the other scales and the fact that untrained counselors did not significantly value inservice training more than trained counselors.

It is interesting to note that more differences were obtained on the "Importance" scale than on the "Need" scale. Are these differences a result of philosophical differences arising from different training programs, different state agencies, or referenced by past training activities?

This study also contrasts sharply with that of McFarlane and Sullivan (1979) and Sink, Porter, Rubin and Painter (1979) in that a majority of the counselors and supervisors did not possess a master's degree, nor did they place much value on university/college training, at least as a method for inservice training. Although for this study, trained counselors were those with master's degrees in rehabilitation counseling, counseling and guidance, psychology and social work, only fifteen percent of the counselors had master's degrees in rehabilitation counseling. Only two of the three states has master's degree programs in rehabilitation counseling and the state without a master's level rehabilitation counseling program had no counselors with a master's degree in rehabilitation counseling. One reason university/college training was rated low may be proximity to a rehabilitation counselor education program, since the three states all involve great travel distances. However, it appears that rehabilitation counselor education programs are not meeting the demand or states do not have a priority for hiring master's level graduates.

The results of this study also suggest that state differences should be regarded as positive, rather than negative and support the non-standardization of inservice training programs. It appears increased support should be given the state staff development specialists in designing state programs.

The findings of this study are consistent with McFarlane and Sullivan (1979) in that a frequent training area was administrative/agency structure and organization. This was the area that greatest differences between supervisor perceptions of counselor training needs and counselor perceptions of their training needs was found. Unfortunately, if training in an area is viewed as a low need, participation in the training will be low and the best results cannot be obtained. Supervisor perceptions of counselor training needs and counselor perceptions must be reconciled to maximize training effectiveness.

The fact that both supervisors and counselors rated group counseling as one of the least important items for a counselor to function effectively also raises questions, since group counseling could save counselors time over a long period in working with various clients. It would seem with increased emphasis on time management and on serving severely handicapped clients that group counseling could have an important role in an agency.

RECOMMENDATIONS

The following recommendations were taken directly from, and are representative of, counselors' responses to "If any areas which you feel are important have been omitted in Section A, please list them below, in addition to any other comments you may wish to make."

1. "Inservice training is very important but is nearly completely lacking due to lack of funds on the state level. You can say all you want about the need for training but it is very questionable that things will ever change."
2. "We need to be careful not to over-emphasize the importance of higher education as a necessary element to adequate job function. On the job training with appropriate supervision is unsurpassed in meeting counseling requirements and needs rather than learning strictly from an artificial classroom setting."
3. "It was difficult to assess importance at first and then to self-determine need; this survey has given me a chance to consider priorities."
4. "I returned this week from two weeks in ------- for a training session;

for my case-load it was a complete and total waste of time. I would prefer workshops which were geared to similar caseloads, had counselors get involved, and where lectures dealt with problems of VR counselors."

5. "Our agency tends to have *many* workshops regarding federal regulations — great to be informed, but it is overdone. There is a lack of training for new counselors, especially the B.S. counselors."

6. "Having a special degree in rehabilitation I felt I was well prepared, except in dealing with the bureaucracy of my job. How about a course 'Surviving in a Bureaucracy and Still be Effective with and for your Clients'."

7. "I feel I have been with the agency long enough to have a fairly good knowledge of things in general. My supervisor could probably make recommendations for training I need — better than I could. . . ."

8. "The idea of university extension courses, correspondence study, etc., appeals to me greatly, but because I am so highly involved in community and church activities, besides teaching adult education courses, I feel inservice training is the only realistic way for me to obtain the additional training I would like to have."

REFERENCES

Dickerson, L.R. & Roberts, R.R. Inservice training of rehabilitation counselors in state agencies. *Rehabilitation Counseling Bulletin.* 1973, *17,* 22-28.

McFarlane, F. & Sullivan, M. Educational and training needs of rehabilitation counselors: Implications for training. *Journal of Applied Rehabilitation Counseling.* 1979, *10,* 41-43.

Pankowski, M.L. & Pankowski, J.M. Why a master's degree in rehabilitation counseling? *Journal of Applied Rehabilitation Counseling.* 1974, *5,* 147-152.

Richardson, B.K. & Obermann, C.E. Inservice training and supervision: Meeting the new demand. *Rehabilitation Counseling Bulletin,* 1972, *16,* 46-55.

Roberts, R.R. & Engelkes, J.R. Who is a trained rehabilitation counselor? *Rehabilitation Counseling Bulletin,* 1970, *13,* 295-299.

RRCEP Directors. RRCEP directors discuss continuing education. *Journal of Rehabilitation,* 1975, *41*(6), 23-25; 30; 41; 47.

Sink, J.M., Porter, T.L., Rubin, S.E., and Painter, L. *Competencies related to the work of the rehabilitation counselor and vocational evaluator.* (Vol. 1). Athens, Georgia: The University of Georgia and the University of Georgia Printing Department, 1979.

CHAPTER 26

CLIENT FEEDBACK IN REHABILITATION COUNSELOR EVALUATION: A FIELD-BASED, PROFESSIONAL DEVELOPMENT APPLICATION

WILLIAM G. EMENER, MARY G. MARS, AND JOAN F. SCHMIDT

Abstract

Based on recommendations from current rehabilitation literature, a supervising counselor and four rehabilitation counselors, with the assistance of a student intern, surveyed rehabilitation clients closed "26" (rehabilitated) within a twelve-month period. The thirty-one respondents (39.2% return rate) used the Emener and Placido (1982b) "Counselor Evaluation Form" to evaluate their counselors on fifteen items. Client demographics and the clients' evaluations are presented and discussed. With the assistance of a rehabilitation counselor educator, a professional development seminar with a focus on the utilization of the clients' feedback evaluations in facilitating rehabilitation counselor professional development was conducted. The supervising counselor's, rehabilitation counselors', student intern's, and the rehabilitation counselor educator's evaluations of the seminar are presented as well as recommendations for the field of rehabilitation and the profession of rehabilitation counseling.

T HE CONTINUOUS professional development of the practice of rehabilitation counseling is sine qua non to the quality and quantity of rehabilitation services in America. In the recent past, the preparation of rehabilitation counselors has been scrutinized (Dellario, 1980), the rehabilitation counselor certification process has been criticized (Miller & Roberts, 1979), and the manner by which rehabilitation counselor performance has been evaluated has been questioned (Crisler, 1980; Downes, McFarlane, & Alston, 1974). In their research review, Berven and Scofield (1980) concluded: "Evaluation of professional competence in rehabilitation counseling occurs routinely in professional education programs, certification and licensure, and rehabilitation agencies.

Reprinted by permission from Volume 15 (1984), *Journal of Applied Rehabilitation Counseling*, pp. 33-39.

However, the evaluation procedures used may not be fully adequate." (p. 199) Combining a review of related literature with an investigation of rehabilitation counselor evaluation in a surveyed sample of nineteen state vocational rehabilitation agencies and one private rehabilitation company, Emener and Placido (1982a) concluded:

Current rehabilitation counselor evaluation practice:

1. Focuses on agency/company processes, procedures, and outcome criteria;
2. Relies on: (a) subjective evaluations of supervisory personnel; and, (b) rehabilitation counselor attribute measures tangentially related to client service delivery; and,
3. Does not utilize systematic client feedback in a manner designed to facilitate the professional development of rehabilitation counselors. (p. 75)

The Emener and Placido (1982a) project commensurately stated: "The current age of consumerism, and the potential contributions of systematic client feedback to rehabilitation counselor's professional development, offer a compelling recommendation for each state VR agency and each private rehabilitation company to . . . include systematic client feedback for promoting their rehabilitation counselors' professional development" (p. 75). Based on the supported supposition that systematic client feedback in the evaluation of rehabilitation counselors is a valuable but untapped source of counselor development, Emener and Placido (1982b) proposed, developed, and evaluated prototype alternatives for use and implementation. Utilizing information gathered from a sample of twenty-five rehabilitation clients, a proposed instrument was developed. With regard to the implementation of a client feedback model for rehabilitation counselors, two key questions were considered: (a) should it be mandatory or optional?; and (b) should completed qustionnaires be sent to each client's counselor, the counselor-supervisor, someone else in the agency or company, or all three groups.

At a National Rehabilitation Counseling Association conference program during the 1981 National Rehabilitation Association convention, an audience consisting of twenty-one rehabilitation counselors, eleven supervisors, seven administrators, six educators, and seven others were: (a) presented the basic elements of the use of client feedback in the evaluation of rehabilitation counselors; and (b) surveyed in terms of their opinions/evaluations—its helpfulness, its use, and its implementation alternatives. Based on their analyses of the opinions/ evaluations of the fifty-two professionals in attendance at the NRCA conference program, Emener and Placido (1982b) concluded and recommended that:

Survey Sample

Of the seventy-nine possible respondents, thirty-one surveys were received for a 39.2 percent return rate. While some of the respondents did not rate all of the fourteen counselor information items ($R = 27$-31 responses/item), it is interesting to note that in response to the last statement, "If you would like to make additional comments, you may use the back of this sheet," thirteen (41.9%) wrote additional comments.

Findings

Analyses of the thirty-one responding clients' responses to the fourteen rated "Counselor Information" items are displayed in Table 26-1.

Of the thirteen handwritten additional comments, about half were positive/complimentary and about half were negative/critical. The four following statements, edited for confidentiality, are illustrative of the thirteen additional comments:

Positive/complimentary:
1. "Your service of considering all the aspects of a client's case with his or her best interest in mind was invaluable to me."
2. "------ was so very kind, nice and good to me. She's one of two (good) people in any government office. She really helped me when I needed it. I was so sick, scared, afraid and didn't know where to turn or what to do. She is really great. ------ & ------, Dr. ------ and his nurse ------ are the greatest. Thank you."

Negative/critical:
1. "I am sorry to say that your office wasn't of much help to me. They didn't help me find a job or any help financially. If I did not have some saving and my tax return, we would have been real bad off. I cannot see where those tests at ------ did any good at all. ------ was helpful when I called on her at her office or phoned her."
2. "------ was my counselor. He/she took his/her time about getting me a job and he/she hasn't called me for a full year. I am very dissatisfied with ------'s job in helping me. Thank you. As far as I am concerned I am through with ------. P.S. Do not want your service any longer."

DISCUSSION AND FINDINGS

First of all, it must be remembered that the purpose for which the client evaluation data was collected was for the individual professional development benefit of the four rehabilitation counselors and the supervising counselor. The numerous limitations of the data collection procedures and the low response rate (39.2%) notwithstanding, generalizability beyond the population served by these specific professionals and closed "26" (rehabilitated; $N = 96$) would be totally unwarranted. When the four counselors and the supervising counselor reviewed the data, cautions related to the survey procedures and response rate

Table 26-1
Rehabilitation Clients' (Closed "26"-rehabilitated) Responses
to the Rehabilitation Counselor Evaluation Survey

Survey Items*	N	Response Categories						
		Don't Know	None of the Time	Some of the Time	Most of the Time	All of the Time	All/ Most of the Time	Don't Know/ None of the Time
1. really cared about me as a person: (e.g., listened; wanted to do everything he or she could to help me; etc.)	31	3.2%	—%	16.1%	12.9%	67.7%	80.6%	3.2%
2. would "go the extra mile" in order to help me: (e.g., kept me informed as to what was being done; prepared me for new situations; etc.)	30	6.6	10.0	6.6	20.0	56.7	76.7	16.7
3. would listen to my point of view even though he or she may not have agreed with me (e.g., was understanding; compassionate; etc.)	27	3.7	3.7	11.1	25.9	55.6	81.5	7.4
4. respected me as a unique and valuable person; (e.g., was interested in what I needed and wanted; didn't judge me; etc.)	31	—	—	22.6	16.1	61.3	77.4	—
5. was easy to talk to: (e.g., made me feel like what I had to say was important; was not always interrupting; etc.)	31	—	—	22.6	22.6	54.8	77.4	—
6. gave me useful and helpful information: (e.g., told me about information sources; where to go to get things, etc.)	31	—	12.9	16.1	22.6	48.4	71.0	12.9
7. was knowledgeable regarding jobs: (e.g., knew where job opportunities were; knew what types of skills were needed; etc.)	29	10.3	10.3	17.2	17.2	44.8	62.1	20.7
8. was knowledgeable concerning medical aspects: (e.g., understood my disability; knew what I could do and what my limitations were; etc.)	29	6.9	10.3	20.7	24.1	37.9	62.0	17.2
9. was responsive to me: (e.g., was available; returned my phone calls; saw me when it was important; etc.)	30	—	6.7	13.3	20.0	60.0	80.0	6.7
10. was encouraging: (e.g., I felt less scared; praised me; helped me realize that I was capable of things I thought I couldn't do; etc.)	30	6.7	3.3	20.0	20.0	50.0	70.0	10.0
11. "pushed me" and tried to get me to do as much as I was capable of doing: (e.g., encouraged me to try new things when I wasn't sure of myself; etc.)	28	—	25.0	10.7	21.4	42.9	64.3	25.0
12. actually did things for me: (e.g., provided information; contacted doctors; talked with employers; etc.)	29	10.3	17.2	20.7	17.2	34.5	51.7	27.6
13. helped me see myself and my concerns differently: (e.g., helped me appreciate my importance to others and the meaningful things I can do; etc.)	29	—	17.2	20.7	13.8	48.2	62.1	17.2
14. in an overall sense, was helpful to me: (e.g., helped me make adjustments; etc.)	29	—	17.2	10.3	17.2	55.2	72.8	17.2
15. if you would like to make any additional comments you may use the back of this sheet								

Note: *Suggested by Emener and Placido, 1982b.

were considered at all times. It must also be remembered that specific counselors were not identified or matched with the questionnaires. Moreover, the respondents were not asked to provide any demographic information on themselves; thus, relationships among specific client demographic characteristics and evaluations of counselors could not be investigated.

Observations of the population characteristics suggest that the counselors provided a variety of rehabilitation services to a variety of disabled individuals. Overall, the data reflected what was expected; for example, the relatively high percentages of unskilled (43.7%) and semi-skilled/skilled (25.3%) occupations at time of closure and commensurate with the predominately rural, agrarian geographical area served by the four counselors.

Inspection of the clients' evaluations of their rehabilitation counselors yield interesting observations (Table 26-1). As a group, the four counselors were perceived by the clients who were closed "26" (rehabilitated) as:

1. *Having positive attitudes toward them* — for all/most of the time really cared about them as a person (#1 — 80.6%) and respected them as a unique and valuable person (#4 — 77.4%);
2. *Having demonstrated helpful behaviors toward/with them* — for all/most of the time would "go the extra mile" in order to help (#2 — 76.6%), gave them useful and helpful information (#6 — 71%), were responsive (#9 — 80%), and were encouraging (#10 — 70%);
3. *Having professional counseling skills* — for all/most of the time would listen to the client's point of view even though the counselor may not have agreed (#3 — 81.5%), and were easy to talk to (#5 — 77.4%); and
4. *In an overall sense, having been helpful to them* — for the majority of the time (#14 — most of the time, 17.2%; all of the time, 55.2%).

Taken as a whole, these data were rather complimentary of the four counselors.

1. Client feedback evaluation is a critically important component of rehabilitation counselor development;
2. Within an atmosphere of positive regard, trust, and genuine support, rehabilitation counselor development could be tremendously enhanced with appropriate usage of systematic client feedback evaluations; and,
3. Research and demonstration programs should be conducted to identify critical variables and preferred alternative processes and procedures that would maximize counselor growth and development potentials resulting from the use of the client feedback evaluations.

The purposes of this application experience project were to: (a) collect client follow-up data; (b) collect client evaluations of counselors in a district of a state vocational rehabilitation agency using the Emener and Placido (1982b) instrument; (c) operationalize a feedback process; and (d) glean the users' (viz. counselors' and unit supervisor's) evaluations of, and recommendations from, the experience.

METHOD

Client Identification

In August, 1982, a list of all clients closed "26" (closed-rehabilitated) from July 1, 1981 through June 30, 1982 was compiled. This time frame for client identification, commensurate with Bolton's (1976) suggestion that the preferred time to take client evaluation measurements is a period of six months to one year after closure, produced a list of ninety-six clients. All of them had been served by the district vocational rehabilitation office which had four rehabilitation counselors and one supervising counselor. Three of the cases had been re-opened and six files were not available because of peer review, administrative review, or requests for additional services; thus, the useable survey population contained eighty-seven cases closed "26." Client data from the case files were recorded: age, sex, marital status, children, disability, services rendered, employment information, and length of rehabilitation.

Instrumentation

Along with a cover letter, a one-page survey was developed. With the permission of its developers, it contained the fifteen "Counselor Information" items from the Emener and Placido (1982b) *Rehabilitation Client Feedback Questionnaire* (p. 21-23). The instructions for the first fourteen items asked each client to "Rate your rehabilitation counselor on each of the following items by circling the words which best describe your experiences: 0 = Don't Know; 1 = None of the time; 2 = Some of the time; 3 = Most of the time; and 4 = All of the time" (p. 22). The last item was an open-ended request for any additional information and/or feedback.

Procedures

A cover letter with the one-page survey was mailed with a stamped, self-addressed return envelope to each of the eighty-seven (former) clients. When a survey was returned "address unknown," a more current address was sought and the survey was sent out again. Of the survey population of eighty-seven cases, eight were determined "undeliverable;" the remaining seventy-nine were presumed to have received the survey. One week after the mailing, phone calls encouraging the former clients to respond to the survey were made to forty-eight of the seventy-nine. Calls were only made if a home phone number was listed (eighteen resulted in a no answer, eight phones were disconnected, and nine had wrong numbers).

Data Analysis

Frequencies and measures of central tendency were calculated on the client information data and the clients' responses to the fourteen "Counselor Information" items. Representative examples of the responses to the open-ended item are presented in edited form (for confidentiality).

RESULTS

Population Characteristics

Analyses of the data compiled on the eighty-seven clients (closed "26," July 1, 1981 through June 30, 1982) revealed that: (a) sixty-one percent were male and thirty-nine percent were female; (b) their ages ranged from fifteen to fifty-eight ($\overline{X}=31.5$; mdn $=28$; Mo $=19$, 23, and 28); (c) 43.7 percent were single, 31.1 percent married, 14.9 percent divorced, 6.9 percent separated, and 3.4 percent widowed; (d) 70.1 percent had a single disability (54.1% physical, 15% emotional, and 1% mental) and 29.9 percent had multiple disabilities (6.9% multiple physical, 6.9% multiple emotional, 11.5% physical and emotional, and 4.6% physical and mental); (e) of the rehabilitation services rendered, 65.5 percent received Education/Training (e.g., vocational testing, work evaluation, work adjustment), 11.5 percent received Direct Financial Assistance (e.g., cash—for transportation, maintenance, etc.), and 72.4 percent received Medical Assistance (e.g., medical examinations, surgery, therapy); (f) the Length of Rehabilitation (LR) ranged from three to seventy-two months ($\overline{X}=16.3$, mdn $=13.5$, Mo $=14.0$; LR was twelve months or less for 44.8%); (g) records of "how job was secured" indicated $=34.5$ percent—clients' own efforts; 20.7 percent—assistance from family, friends, and/or former employers; 24.1 percent—assistance from counselor; 10.3 percent—assistance from VR and other agencies; and, 10.3 percent—assistance from other agencies; and (h) of the type of occupation at closure, 43.7 percent were unskilled (e.g., janitor, dishwasher), 25.3 percent semi-skilled/skilled (e.g., cement mason, mechanic), 14.9 percent service (e.g., sales, child care), 12.6 percent clerical (e.g., typist, records clerk), and 3.4 percent professional (e.g., teacher, counselor).

Five of the fourteen counselor evaluation items (Table 26-1) are difficult to interpret (primarily as a result of the limitations of the data collected by the instrument). For example, on items #7 and #8, how would a client really know the extent to which his/her rehabilitation counselor was knowledgeable regarding jobs (note that 10.3% indicated "Don't Know") or medical aspects? It is important for a rehabilitation counselor to be knowledgeable about the world of work and about medical aspects of disability. However, even when a rehabilitation counselor is very knowledgeable in these two areas, the counselor tends to act on such knowledge and take it into account (vis-avis flaunting ones knowledge). It is suggested that these two items be further inspected and possibly modified in the future. Moreover, items #11, #12, and #13 need additional information related to them prior to interpreting their meaning. For example, an individual indication of *need* or *appropriateness* level would appear critical: all clients may not need to be "pushed" (#11) or helped to see themselves and their concerns differently (#13). From a philosophical point of view, rehabilitation counselors "help clients help themselves;" thus, at times it could actually be undesireable and/or less helpful for a counselor to do things for clients (#12) that they are capable of doing for themselves. It is thus suggested that these five items (#7, #8, #11, #12, #13) be given careful review, investigation, and possible modification.

Nonetheless, in conclusion, it was hypothesized that the data would be helpful to the four rehabilitation counselors and their supervising counselor with regard to their professional development. Consequently, the following application experience was planned, conducted, and evaluated.

AN APPLICATION EXPERIENCE OR "LET'S SEE WHAT THE COUNSELORS AND THEIR SUPERVISOR THINK ABOUT THIS?"

Up to this point, permission to conduct the project had been received from the appropriate bureau official,[1] and the data had been collected and analyzed. With the continuing assistance of a student intern[2] and a rehabilitation counselor educator,[3] the counselor supervisor[4] planned and conducted a six-hour seminar program with the four rehabilitation counselors.[5] The overall purposes were to: (a) assist the counselors in enriching their knowledge and awareness of the state-of-the-art of rehabilitation counselor evaluation and the importance of client feedback (the Emener & Placido, 1982a, 1982b articles were used for these purposes); (b) present the data to the counselors; (c) facilitate their interpretations and observation of the data with an emphasis on their professional development; and (d) glean the counselors' and their supervisor's evaluations of, and recommendations from, the experience. A presentation-discussion-seminar format was used with regard to the first three goals of the meeting. At the conclusion, each counselor and the supervising counselor were asked to individually reflect on the experience and anonymously respond to a three part, twelve item open-ended "Follow-up Seminar Evaluation Questionnaire" and confidentially return it the following day. The following selected verbatim statements from the four rehabilitation counselors are representative of their evaluations.

I. Evaluation Project
   A. *This Evaluation Project was* . . .

". . . helpful to us to gain greater insight to our roles as counselors (i.e., it added another dimension)."

". . . a first step in providing vocational rehabilitation counselors in our office with important information on the perceived effectiveness of the VR process."

B. *As a rehabilitation counselor, I would suggest that . . .*

". . . this type of research should continue, and should be incorporated into training programs for new counselors."

". . . this type of solicitation of client feedback be used as a resource for improving client-counselor relationships and counselor effectiveness."

C. *The strength(s) of this Project was . . .*

". . . the cover letter was clear and written in easily understood wording. The questions were, for the most part, clear and pertinent. The statistical summary was meaningful."

". . . it provided counselors and their supervisor valuable information about how our performance is viewed by recipients of our services. We need to be made aware of how we will meet the needs of the clients we try to assist."

D. *The weakness(es) of this Project was . . .*

". . . that the counselors could not identify their specific clients. If some method of identification were available, results would be more meaningful."

". . . how valid were the clients' responses? Only the counselor directly involved can assess the validity of the responses. However, we must also consider counselor bias. In all fairness, each case should be reviewed by the counselor, the supervisor, and an impartial, neutral observer."

E. *It would be more helpful if . . .*

". . . caseloads could be cut so that counselors (whose worst enemy is time) could be more actively involved in such projects and thus deliver more effective services."

". . . future surveys would allow for the clients to indicate the services that were not necessary for their rehabilitation to be successful. Also, the survey should be done with clients closed in the 80 series (unsuccessfully rehabilitated) as well as with those who were successful."

II. Career Development

A. *The data from this Project . . .*

". . . convinces me that my clients are receiving the proper services according to their individual needs. This data can also satisfy other counselors' needs as well—positive feedback, ego satisfaction, etc."

". . . should be sent to the counselor with a copy to the supervisor. All client comments should be shared with the (attending) counselor."

B. *Today's seminar, based on the Project, was . . .*

". . . well organized and presented."

". . . positive. All counselors were able to ventilate intelligently. All professional counselors feel that their expertise can contribute to the rehabilitation process; this seminar was a vehicle for their input."

C. *The strength(s) of this seminar was . . .*

". . . the informality and appropriate amount of time allotted for discussion."

". . . the relaxed atmosphere and openness that encouraged comment."

D. *The weakness(es) of this seminar was . . .*

". . . that the individual clients' disability was not indicated in the data (I would want to know if I am perceived differently by different disability groups)."

". . . nothing."

E. *It would be more helpful if . . .*

". . . the same data had been collected from the 80's series closures (non-rehabilitated)."

". . . we could have included data and counselors from the ------ Unit (another district office)."

III. Overall

A. *For the field of rehabilitation, I would recommend . . .*

". . . much more research in this and similar areas that will lead to meeting the needs of our clients."

". . . that we take more seriously the process of obtaining and using client feedback to improve the quality of services."

B. *For the profession of rehabilitation counseling, I would recommend . . .*

". . . mandatory counselor evaluations by clients at least on a yearly basis. Ideally, the surveys should be sent out three to six months after case closure."

". . . that the results be used to plan for future emphasis in services."

It would appear fitting to conclude that the four counselors experienced this project and the Seminar based on the data as: (a) meaningful to their professional development; (b) being in need of expansion and modification; and, (c) being beneficial to the field of rehabilitation and the profession of rehabilitation counseling. The following verbatim statements were taken from the supervising counselor's evaluation of the Project and Seminar:

- "If I were a counselor, I would want to have this type of feedback on a regular basis . . . It helps counselors in seeing clients' views . . . The counselors may prefer having the evaluations sent directly to themselves; that way they would get direct feedback from the clients with whom they worked."

- "This emphasizes the importance of communications with clients — actually verbalizing things that counselors can come to take for granted

. . . the Seminar was very important in that it helped everyone have a greater appreciation for the data."

- "Overall, this feedback can only serve to improve services and communications between counselors and their clients . . . This should *not* be an agency project; it should be a professional development project to be conducted without fear of reprisal."

Thus, it would appear that the supervising counselor had a positive evaluation of the experience and recommends its continuance. Moreover, specific attributes (e.g., the Seminar part, lack of fear of reprisal) would appear to be very important to its meaningfulness and contributions to professional development. The following verbatim statements were taken from the student intern's evaluation of the Project and the Seminar:

- "This Evaluation Project was an invaluable learning experience for me; I developed much greater respect for the counselors—e.g., their willingness to cooperate in spite of the risk(s) involved . . . they want to improve themselves as professionals."
- "Conducting a preliminary meeting would have helped . . . we could have incorporated the counselor's suggestions and recommendations into the Project."

Thus, it would appear that the student intern learned and benefited from being involved in the Project. It was also observed that in using the student intern the agency personnel did not have to take their time away from their clients to collect the data.

SUMMARY COMMENT

This experience of applying a recommended "counselor evaluation—client feedback" activity sufficiently indicated that experiences such as this: (a) can provide valuable information for rehabilitation counselors and their professional development; (b) can be very beneficial to student interns if they are involved in the experience, and, (c) are recommended for utilization in the field of rehabilitation by professional rehabilitation counselors. The limitations, recommendations for improvement, and cautions regarding implementation, as discussed herein, should receive utmost consideration. Nonetheless, the outcomes justified the effort and energy. For example, Tichener, Thomas, and Kravetz (1975) concluded in their research, "The creation of a warm, permissive counseling atmosphere is seen as one way in which counselors might better facilitate both the expression and resolution of client concerns" (p. 304). This conclusion took on enriched meaning when the counselors in this Project observed that their clients, as a group, reported that for most or all of the time their counselor "really cared about me as a person" (80.6%), "would listen to my point of view" (81.5%), and "was responsive to me" (80%) (Table 26-1).

In his invited "Comment" to Emener and Placido's (1982a) recommended counselor-evaluation-utilizing client feedback model, Bordieri (1982) complimented its potentials but fittingly asked: "How would this 'systematic client feedback model' be implemented in a rehabilitation facility? How will 'systematic client evaluation feedback' affect these already existing concerns of counselors? Simply stated, how will the model serve as the panacea for evaluating rehabilitation counselors as the authors intimate it will? (p. 77)

While this Project was not designed to address panacea potentials, it was a "first step" in the gathering of evidence regarding preferred utilization strategies and outcome benefits. Hopefully, other professional rehabilitation counselors will conduct similar projects and share their experiences with their colleagues. The prediction that the ultimate benefits will be realized by our clients, provides compelling encouragement for all of us to work toward finding better ways of improving ourselves. As one of the four counselors in this Project said, "To my fellow professional counselors: the ball's in your court!"

NOTES

1. For her genuine support of this project, sincerest appreciation is extended to Ms. Sidney F. Tatom, Program Supervisor, Office of Vocational Rehabilitation, Department of Health and Rehabilitation Services, Fort Myers, Florida.
2. At the time this project was conducted, Ms. Joan Schmidt was completing her internship (Psychology Department, Florida Southern College) with the Florida Office of Vocational Rehabilitation — HRS in Lakeland, Florida (Subdistrict A).
3. William G. Emener was a Professor in the Department of Rehabilitation Counseling at the University of South Florida, Tampa, Florida.
4. Ms. Mary G. Mars was the Supervising Counselor in the Lakeland (Subdistrict 8-A) office of the Florida Office of Vocational Rehabilitation — HRS.
5. Much gratitude and a hearty "thanks" is extended to the four rehabilitation counselors for their tremendous assistance throughout the conduct of this project: Raymond A. Bush, Frances G. Davis, Judy A. Dertod, and Althea S. Holmes.

ACKNOWLEDGMENT

Genuine appreciation is extended to Denise Placido, MRC, Kentucky Department for the Blind, Lexington, and to Robert Filbeck, Ed.D., University of Nebraska, Lincoln, for their encouragement of this project and valuable critical reading and constructive suggestions in the development of this manuscript.

REFERENCES

Berven, N.L., & Scofield, M.E. Evaluation of professional competence through standardized simulations: A review. *Rehabilitation Counseling Bulletin*, 1980, *24*,(2), 178-202.

Bolton, B.F. *Handbook of measurement and evaluation in rehabilitation.* Baltimore: University Park Press, 1976.

Bordieri, J.E. Requested comment. *Journal of Rehabilitation Administration,* 1982, *6*(2), 77-78.

Crisler, J.R. Rehabilitation counselors' perception of DRV case closure difficulty based on client outcome criteria. *Journal of Applied Rehabilitation Counseling,* 1980, *11*(3), 156-159.

Dellario, D.J. A point of convergence in the evaluation of rehabilitation counselor education (RCE) programs. *Journal of Applied Rehabilitation Counseling,* 1980, *11*(3), 128-131.

Downes, S.C., McFarlane, F.S., & Alston, P.P. Survey of the NRCA membership regarding the basis for evaluating counselor performance. *Journal of Applied Rehabilitation Counseling,* 1974, *5*(4), 196-200.

Emener, W.G., & Placido, D. Rehabilitation counselor evaluation: An analysis and critique. *Journal of Rehabilitation Administration,* 1982, *6*(2), 72-76. (a)

Emener, W.G., & Placido, D. Client feedback: A valuable source of counselor development. *Journal of Applied Rehabilitation Counseling,* 1982, *13*(1), 18-23. (b)

Miller, L.A., & Roberts, R.R. Unmet counselor needs from ambiguity to the Zeigarnik effect. *Journal of Applied Rehabilitation Counseling,* 1979, *10*(2), 60-65.

Tichenor, D.F., Thomas, K.R., & Kravetz, S.P. Client-counselor congruence in perceiving handicapping problems. *Rehabilitation Counseling Bulletin,* 1975, *19*(1), 300-304.

CHAPTER 27

REHABILITATION COUNSELING
IN THE PRIVATE SECTOR:
A TRAINING NEEDS SURVEY

Ross K. Lynch and Terrence Martin

Abstract

With the increasing growth of the private-for-profit sector in rehabilitation, the need to examine the training requirements of service providers becomes of critical importance for rehabilitation counselor education programs. This research examines the education and experience of individuals in the private sector and, also, what they perceive to be the important skill and knowledge areas for effective service provision. Results indicate that private sector rehabilitationists are highly educated (primarily in the field of rehabilitation counseling), a majority are certified rehabilitation counselors or plan to become such, most have many years of rehabilitation related experience, and a sizable majority work with a physically disabled population. With respect to training needs, of primary importance were tangible skill areas related to assessment, job analysis and placement, communication, and organization. Of least importance were those areas typically associated with generic interpersonal counseling. The authors stress the need for curriculum changes reflective of the employment requirements in the private sector.

I N RECENT YEARS, the profession of rehabilitation counseling has undergone significant changes in practically every facet. One major development has been within the area of private-for-profit rehabilitation. As evidence of the employment surge in this area, many rehabilitation counselor training programs are reporting that, as traditional job markets dry up, sizable numbers of their graduates are taking jobs within the private sector. The question that logically follows is, how well has their graduate training prepared them to function in such "non-traditional" employment settings?

Reprinted by permission from Volume 48 (1982), *Journal of Rehabilitation*, pp. 51-53, 73.

A review of the literature indicates that individuals in the private sector feel rehabilitation counselor education curricula should be modified to more adequately address their needs. Sawyer (1978) noted that only individuals properly trained and sufficiently adept at understanding medical issues, worker's compensation systems, and social and vocational problems will be successful in private rehabilitation. Similarly, McMahon (1979), in discussing training needs, stated that private agency directors have been displeased with the product of rehabilitation counselor training programs, citing the complaint that counseling graduates are "overqualified in matters of counseling and training and underqualified in matters of testing, job placement, and general business skills" (p. 58).

Other authors have pointed out additional areas that are either underemphasized or overlooked in current educational curricula. Such areas include knowledge of worker's compensation; basic concepts of insurance; awareness of the free enterprise system; the intricacies of legal and medical case management; an introduction to business administration, basic accounting, and employee benefits; competence in securing labor market information; performing job analyses, and proficiency in providing vocational expert testimony, to name but a few (Sales, 1979; Scher, 1979; McMahon, 1979; Organist, 1979). As pointed out in a recent review of Matkin (1980), "there has not been a demonstrated effort to systematically collect data to identify the particular needs of the private practitioner which could enhance educational training programs preparing those wishing to enter the 'for-profit' sector" (p. 61). In short, the employment opportunities for rehabilitation counselors (in the private sector) have undergone a multifold increase in recent years, however, there has been relatively little done to examine whether the educational preparation of rehabilitation graduates has kept pace with employment trends.

The purpose of the study presented here was to begin the process of identifying and documenting various skill and knowledge areas considered important for effective provision of rehabilitation services within the private-for-profit sector. A second purpose was to gather background information on the private sector providers in order to better assist those involved with training or curriculum planning.

METHOD

Sample

Subjects for the study were selected from the membership directory of the National Association of Rehabilitation Professionals in the Private Sector (NARPPS). NARPPS membership is comprised of persons practicing or participating in the practice of rehabilitation counseling in the private sector, or having a definite interest in the field (Jenkins, 1979). Two hundred and six individuals were listed on the December, 1980 roster. Each was mailed a letter explaining the study, a blank survey form, and a self-addressed return envelope. After one mailing 147 (71.3%) responses were received. These individuals formed the basis for the study group.

Instrumentation

The survey instrument consisted of two major parts. The first part was intended to gather background information on the private sector rehabilitationist and also, on his or her employment setting. Subjects were asked to indicate their highest educational level, major field of study, current position title, employment setting, years of work experience in rehabilitation, whether they were a certified rehabilitation counselor, whether they planned on becoming certified, and a brief description of the client population served.

The second major part of the survey instrument consisted of forty-one skill or knowledge areas related to rehabilitation counseling in the private sector. Items were primarily developed through a review of the available literature on rehabilitation in the private sector. Each item was grouped under one of the following broad categorical headings: Medical, Business, Legislation, Counseling, Vocational, or Psychological. Under Medical, the following areas were presented: functional limitations of disabilities, medical case management, medical practices and terminology, pharmacology, and pain management techniques. Under Business, the following areas were presented: understanding business and free enterprise systems, effective business practice, budget and financial planning, and insurance industry practices. Under Legislation, the following areas were presented: legislation affecting persons with disabilities, affirmative action requirements, worker's compensation legislation and social security and other benefit systems. Under Counseling, the following areas were presented: rehabilitation counseling philosophy, professional ethics, team approach/roles and functions, personality development and dynamics, counseling techniques, interpersonal communication skills, alcohol and drug abuse counseling, group counseling, family counseling, cross-cultural counseling, employee assistance programs, case management, and writing skills. Under Vocational, the following areas were presented: rehabilitation planning, job placement/job seeking skills techniques, employability and transferable skill assessment, vocational evaluation/work sample techniques, job analysis/modification, occupational information/career development, job development techniques, personnel and employment practices, labor market assessment, understanding employee unions, testifying as a vocational expert, and community organizations and resources. Finally, under Psychological, the following areas were presented: psychosocial aspects of disability, psychological testing and evaluation, and industrial psychology. Each item was presented on a five point Likert scale with 1 representing "very important" and 5 representing "of no consequence." Subjects were asked to rate each item with respect to its importance to them in providing rehabilitation services.

RESULTS

Survey items were examined according to frequency and percentage of response. Data were tabulated and presented according to the survey questionnaire format. The following results were obtained.

Highest Education Level

Results indicated that private sector rehabilitationists are, as a group, quite well educated with ninety-five percent ($N=138$) holding at least a bachelor's degree. Within that group, sixty-four percent ($N=93$) hold at least a master's degree and, an additional fourteen percent ($N=20$) hold doctorates.

Major Field of Study

The three most prevalent fields of study are rehabilitation counseling (53%), psychology (25%), and nursing (11%).

Certification

Sixty-four percent ($N=93$) indicated that they were currently certified by the Commission on Rehabilitation Counselor Certification. An additional fifteen percent ($N=21$) reported that they planned to become certified in the future.

Experience

Eighty-five percent ($N=123$) of the respondents reported having five or more years of rehabilitation experience with the largest percentage (35%) reporting five to eight years of rehabilitation-related experience.

Employment Setting

The most frequent employment setting was in a private-for-profit rehabilitation agency (42%), followed by private consultant (19%) and insurance company (16%).

Client Population

The primary client population served by private sector rehabilitationists was overwhelmingly (89%) individuals with physical disabilities.

Table 27-1

Importance Ratings by Rehabilitation Service Providers with Respect To Skill and Knowledge Areas Required in the Private Sector (N=147)

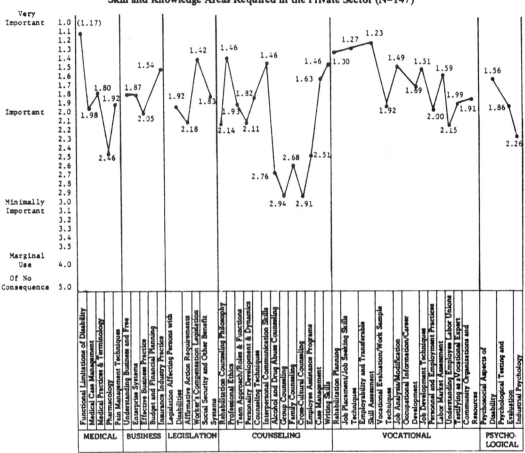

Skill and/or Knowledge Requirements

As can be seen by Table 27-1, many of the knowledge and skill components typically associated with a rehabilitation counselor education curriculum were rated important by private sector rehabilitationists. The ten most critical areas in order of importance were: functional limitations of disability, employability and transferable skill assessment, job placement/job seeking skills techniques, rehabilitation planning, worker's compensation legislation, professional ethics, interpersonal communication skills, writing skills, job analysis/modification, and job development techniques. The ten least critical areas in order of importance were rehabilitation counseling philosophy, understanding employee labor unions, affirmative action requirements, industrial psychology, pharmacology, employee assistance programs, family counseling, alcohol and drug abuse counseling, cross-cultural counseling, and group counseling. The other twenty-one areas were rated between the above two groups with respect to importance.

DISCUSSION

The results of this survey of private sector rehabilitationists provide useful information for rehabilitation counselor education program planners. It appears that, as a group, private sector rehabilitationists are highly educated (primarily in the field of rehabilitation counseling), a majority are certified rehabilitation counselors or plan to become so, most have many years of rehabilitation related experience, and a sizable majority work with a physically disabled population. Such information would indicate that individuals in the private sector should be well aware of standard training curriculum and of issues involving proper professional preparation and credentials. Regarding the areas of skill or knowledge that they perceived to be requisite for effective service delivery, it can be seen that all areas presented were considered at the least, minimally important. This was not surprising as the items were selected from the pertinent literature and their inclusion was based upon their relevance to the private sector. In this respect, the entire list may serve as a resource for curriculum planning. However it is of interest to note which items were rated as most important and those that were considered only marginally important. Of primary importance were tangible skill areas related to assessment, job analysis and placement, communication, and organization. Of least importance were those areas typically associated with generic interpersonal counseling.

The implications of these findings for rehabilitation counselor education curriculums are noteworthy. Changes in traditional course offerings may be warranted. This does not mean to imply that wholesale changes are required, rather a shift in orientation or perhaps a sharpening of definition may achieve the necessary result. Rehabilitation counselor education curriculums have remained basically unchanged since their beginning in the mid-1950s, when individuals with strong clinical or counseling psychology backgrounds laid the foundation for the current educational model. However, since that time, the parameters and the needs of the profession have been both continually refined and increasingly defined. In addition, employment patterns have changed drastically since the state/federal agencies were the primary employer of rehabilitation counselor education graduates. It is time that curricula be modified to reflect these changes. The training needs of the private sector, a large and ever-expanding area of employment, must be incorporated into educational curricula if universities are to be responsive to the changing labor market for rehabilitation counseling graduates. This will require that the training focus must increasingly be upon the development of tangible skills which truly distinguish the domain of rehabilitation counseling graduates from that of other related professions. In this manner, rehabilitation counselors will be able to unquestionably assert their expertise within the free-enterprise system. Lacking in such, rehabilitation counseling graduates may find themselves ill-equipped to function effectively in the highly competitive private sector. As a result, potential employers may find it necessary to search elsewhere for the type of trained employees their company requires.

SUMMARY

This exploratory study of private sector rehabilitation training needs served three basic purposes: (a) it provided information on the background of the service providers; (b) it synthesized knowledge and skill areas cited in the literature as being necessary for successful functioning; and (c) it empirically rated the relative importance of each area with respect to effective service delivery. Findings indicated that private sector rehabilitation counselors are generally well educated and experienced in rehabilitation. The areas rated as most important tended to be of a tangible skill based nature and geared more toward assessment and outcome activities as opposed to those areas that lend themselves more to process activities. This information may be used by rehabilitation counselor educators to modify curriculum content to more adequately reflect the needs of rehabilitation counselors in the private sector.

REFERENCES

Jenkins, W.M. Organizations concerned with the practice of rehabilitation counseling. *Journal of Applied Rehabilitation Counseling*, 1979, *10*(2), 102-106.

Matkin, R.E. The rehabilitation counselor in private practice: Perspectives for education and preparation. *Journal of Rehabilitation*, 1980, *46*(2), 60-62.

McMahon, B.T. Private sector rehabilitation: Benefits, dangers, and implications for education, *Journal of Rehabilitation*, 1979, *45*(3), 56-58.

Organist, J. Private sector rehabilitation practitioners—Organize within NRA. *Journal of Rehabilitation*, 1979, *45*(3), 52-55.

Sales, A. Rehabilitation counseling in the private sector: Implications for graduate education. *Journal of Rehabilitation*, 1979, *45*(3), 59-61.

Sawyer, G. Private insurance company rehabilitation programming. Southeastern Industrial Rehabilitation Institute, Winston-Salem, N.C., April, 1978.

Scher, P.L. NARPPS—Key to survival of rehabilitation in the nineteen-eighties. *Journal of Rehabilitation*, 1979, *45*(3), 50-51.

Selected Abstracts

Attitudes of the NRCA Membership Toward Inservice Training
D.C. McAlees and D.W. Corthell (1972)

Based on questionnaire data received from 2,672 NRCA Members (64% return rate), the authors summarized: (a) while the respondents as a whole believe inservice training is effective and relevant, counselors were less positive in their evaluation; (b) groups of the respondents were about equally effective in their own area of specific knowledge; (c) counselors did not perceive their agency as strongly supporting their inservice training; (d) vocational rehabilitation counselors receive about six inservice training days per year (all respondent sub-groups indicated counselors should receive more than eleven days per year); and (e) NRCA should take a more active role in determining the inservice training needs of its members.

Evaluation of Short-Term Training in Rehabilitation: A Neglected Necessity
S.H. Godley, M.D. Hafer, L. Vieceli, and M.D. Godley (1984, p. 28)

An evaluation of a short-term training program in rehabilitation was conducted using multiple baseline and true experimental design. The training program taught job placement skills to counselors whose clients were legally blind. Results indicated that program participants reported higher mean numbers of total placements, competitive placements, and employer contacts after training, and also had more favorable attitudes toward placement than did members of a control group. This study is discussed as an example of a rigorous methodology in the evaluation of short-term training, which could be followed elsewhere.

Predicting Evaluation Ratings of Rehabilitation Short-Term Training Programs
J.E. Moore (1981, p. 58)

The evaluation responses of four (4) regional rehabilitation short-term training projects were studied in an effort to identify those variables most highly correlated with subjective evaluation ratings. A total of twelve variables were used in the regression analyses including instructional methodologies, personality characteristics, and other selected demographic variables. A number of conclusions and implications are presented with regard to the amelioration of short-term training efforts.

Technology of Rehabilitation Short-Term Training: Revisited
D.E. Ferritor and M. LeLand (1982, p. 52)

This study examines current training and training evaluation attitudes and practices from a national sample of rehabilitation trainers and compares them with similar information collected in the early 1970s.

References and Suggested Additional Readings for Part V

Bennis, W.G. (1966). *Changing organizations: Essays on the development and evolution of human organization.* New York: McGraw-Hill.

Bitter, J.A. (1978). Continuing education for new rehabilitation counselors. *Rehabilitation Counseling Bulletin, 22*(1), 74-77.

Bolton, B. (1978). Methodological issues in the assessment of rehabilitation counselor performance. *Rehabilitation Counseling Bulletin, 21,* 190-193.

Browning, P.L., & McGovern, K.B. (1974). Technology in rehabilitation short-term training. *Rehabilitation Counseling Bulletin, 18,* 117-122.

Brubaker, D.R. (1977). Professionalization and rehabilitation counseling. *Journal of Applied Rehabilitation Counseling, 8*(4), 208-217.

Bruyere, S.M., & Elliot, J.D. (1979). RRCEPs and continuing education for rehabilitation personnel. *Rehabilitation Counseling Bulletin, 23*(2), 131-135.

Downes, S.C., McFarlane, F.S., & Alston, P.P. (1974). Survey of the NRCA membership regarding the basis for evaluating counselor performance. *Journal of Applied Rehabilitation Counseling, 5*(4), 196-200.

Emener, W.G., & Placido, D. (1982). Rehabilitation counselor evaluation: An analysis and critique. *Journal of Rehabilitation Administration, 6*(2), 72-76.

Emener, W.G., Mars, M.G., & Schmidt, J.F. (1984). Client feedback in rehabilitation counselor evaluation: A field-based, professional development application. *Journal of Applied Rehabilitation Counseling, 15*(1), 33-39.

Ferritor, D.E., & Leland, M. (1982). Technology of rehabilitation short-term training: Revisited. *Rehabilitation Counseling Bulletin, 26*(1), 52-54.

Freeman, J.B. (1979). Rehabilitation counselor and supervisor perceptions of counselor training needs and continuing education. *Journal of Applied Rehabilitation Counseling, 10*(3), 154-157.

Gianforte, G. (1976). Certification: A challenge and a choice. *Journal of Rehabilitation, 45*(5), 15-17, 39.

Godley, S.H., Hafer, M.D., Vieceli, L., & Godley, M.D. (1984). Evaluation of short-term training in rehabilitation: A neglected necessity. *Rehabilitation Counseling Bulletin, 28*(1), 28-38.

Hansen, C.E. (1977). The question of rehabilitation counselor certification. *Journal of Rehabilitation, 43*(2), 2.

Hawley, I.D., & Capshaw, T.B. (1981). Professionalism and ethical responsibilities in rehabilitation. In W.G. Emener, R.S. Luck & S.J. Smits (Eds.), *Rehabilitation administration and supervision.* Baltimore: University Park Press.

Hershenson, D.B. (1982). Rehabilitation counseling is a profession. *Rehabilitation Counseling Bulletin, 25*(4), 251-253.

Kirkpatrick, D.L. (1975). Techniques for evaluating training programs. In D.L. Kirkpatrick (Ed.), *Evaluating training programs.* Madison, Wisconsin: American Society for Training and Development.

Lorenz, J.R. (1979). Setting performance objectives and evaluating individual performance in rehabilitation settings. *Journal of Rehabilitation Administration, 3*(1), 5-11.

Luck, R.S., & Lassiter, R.A. (1978). Assertive behavior development for rehabilitation personnel: An approach to training. *Journal of Applied Rehabilitation Counseling, 9*(2), 6-9.

Lynch, R.K., & Martin, T. (1982). Rehabilitation counseling in the private sector: A training needs survey. *Journal of Rehabilitation, 48*(3), 51-53, 73.

Lynch, R.K., & McSweeney, K. (1981). The professional status of rehabilitation counseling in the state/federal vocational rehabilitation agencies. *Journal of Applied Rehabilitation Counseling, 12*(4), 186-190.

McAlees, D.C., & Corthell, D.W. (1972). Attitudes of the NRCA membership toward inservice training. *Rehabilitation Counseling Bulletin, 3*(1), 27-32.

McFarlane, F.R., & Sullivan, M. (1979). Educational and training needs of rehabilitation counselors: Implications for training. *Journal of Applied Rehabilitation Counseling, 10*(1), 41-43.

Moore, J.E. (1981). Predicting evaluation ratings of rehabilitation short-term training programs. *Journal of Rehabilitation, 47*(3), 57-61.

Nadler, L. (1979). *Developing human resources.* 2nd ed. Austin: Learning Concepts.

National Rehabilitation Association, Committee on Training (1951). Personnel standards and training. *Journal of Rehabilitation, 17*(3), 26.

Newman, J. (1979). Certification/licensure: Premature priorities? *Rehabilitation Literature, 40,* 336-339.

Ninth Annual Workshop on Guidance, Training, and Placement (1956). *Utilization of counselors' services in state VR agencies,* Report of Proceedings. Washington, D.C.: Office of Vocational Rehabilitation, United States Department of Health, Education and Welfare.

Parker, R.M., & Thomas, K.R. (1981). Rehabilitation at the crossroads: Is professional rehabilitation experiencing growth pains or death throes? *Journal of Applied Rehabilitation Counseling, 12*(2), 85-86.

Porter, T.L., & Settles, R.B. (1968). *Post-entry training programs for rehabilitation counselors.* Preliminary Report of Workshop Proceedings, Atlanta, April 24-26, 1968.

Richardson, B.K., & Obermann, C.E. (1972). Inservice training and supervision: Meeting a new demand. *Rehabilitation Counseling Bulletin, 16,* 46-55.

RRCEP Directors (1975). RRCEP directors discuss continuing education. *Journal of Rehabilitation, 41*(6), 23-25, 30, 41, 47.

Scofield, M.E., Berven, N.L., & Harrison, R.P. (1981). Competence, credentialing, and the future of rehabilitation. *Journal of Rehabilitation, 47*(1), 31-35.

Shipman, J.H. (1961). Michigan DVR staff training academies. *Journal of Rehabilitation, 17*(2), 20-21.

Smits, S.J., Emener, W.G., & Luck, R.S. (1981). Prologue to the present. In W.G. Emener, R.S. Luck, and S.J. Smits (Eds.), *Rehabilitation administration and supervision.* Baltimore: University Park Press.

Stephens, J.E., & Kniepp, S. (1981). Managing human resource development in rehabilitation. In W.G. Emener, R.S. Luck & S.J. Smits., *Rehabilitation administration and supervision.* Baltimore: University Park Press.

Stretch, J.J. (1978). Increasing accountability for human services administrators. *Social Casework, 59*(6), 323.

Struthers, R.D., & Miller, J.V. (1981). Program planning, program evaluation, and research utilization in state vocational rehabilitation agencies. In W.G. Emener, R.S. Luck, & S.J. Smits (Eds.), *Rehabilitation administration and supervision*. Baltimore, Maryland: University Park Press.

Thomas, K.R. (1982). A critique of trends in rehabilitation counselor education toward specialization. *Journal of Rehabilitation, 48*(1), 49-51.

Wright, G.N., Reagles, K.W., & Scorzelli, J.F. (1973). Measuring the effectiveness and variations of rehabilitation counselor education programs. *Journal of Applied Rehabilitation Counseling, 4*(2), 76-87.

PART VI

ADMINISTRATIVE, SUPERVISORY, AND SETTING-BASED ISSUES

Part IV

ADMINISTRATIVE AND LEGISLATIVE
RESPONSES TO THE ISSUE

PART VI. ADMINISTRATIVE, SUPERVISORY, AND SETTING-BASED ISSUES

Introduction Commentary

RESEARCH SURVEYS of the employment trends of rehabilitation counselor education graduates (reviewed in Part IV of this book), especially those of the 1980s (Geist & McMahon, 1981; Urban Institute, 1980), clearly support McMahon and Matkin's (1983) observation that "the field of rehabilitation has expanded into nontraditional employment settings in recent years" (p. 54). Rehabilitation counselors have and still are working in a variety of work settings within the field of rehabilitation (Feinberg & McFarlane, 1979; Lorenz, 1979; Sussman & Haug, 1967) as well as in a variety of other work settings (e.g., in industry—Dickman & Emener, 1982; Shrey, 1979). Moreover, research evidence has shown that the rehabilitation counselor's roles, functions, and job tasks differ according to the work setting in which they are employed (Emener & Rubin, 1980). Thus, in view of the expanding field of rehabilitation and the expanding and diverse employment settings in which rehabilitation counselor education graduates are being employed, it indeed would appear critical for rehabilitation counselor education graduates to be cognizant and aware of a variety of important, relevant, and somewhat generic issues. These would include:

1. *Cutback Management, Economic, and Relevant Societal Issues* (Baker & Sawyer, 1978; Emener, Lauth, Renick & Smits, 1985; Levine, 1979; Matkin, 1980a; McFarlane & Frost, 1981; Mosher, 1978)
2. *Legislative Development Issues* (Graves, 1979; Ross, 1979)
3. *Agency Structure, Bureaucratic, and Systems Issues* (Downs, 1967; Drucker, 1966, 1980; Emener, 1978b; Smits & Emener, 1980; Smits & Ledbetter, 1979)
4. *Rehabilitation Outcome Issues* (Conley, 1969; Cooper, Harper & Davis, 1980; Crisler, 1980; Emener, 1980; Worrall, 1978)

It would also appear fitting for a rehabilitation counselor education program to offer coursework (e.g., in the form of a seminar) focusing on issues

265

such as these above four as a prerequisite for what could be considered "specialization coursework" or coursework within a "specialty track" (for further discussion of this, see Emener and McFarlane, 1985). Such specialization could be developed in numerous areas (see Thomas, 1982). And while there is a variety of "specializations" a rehabilitation counselor education program can have, such as those addressed in Part V of this book, five examples are highlighted herein: (1) Supervision, (2) Administration, (3) Facilities, (4) Vocational Evaluation, and (5) Private Sector Rehabilitation.

The majority of supervisors of rehabilitation counselors are former rehabilitation counselors (Smits, 1972). It is suggested that rehabilitation counseling students study supervision (e.g., English, Oberle & Byrne, 1979; Good, 1974; Smits, 1972; Winder & Mugford, 1973) and the variety of approaches to supervision (see Emener, 1978a; James, 1973; Luck, 1978), not only because there is a good chance that in their careers they will become supervisors but because: (a) they will be better consumers of supervision and (b) they will be more sophisticated in terms of how to use supervision. It is not uncommon for a rehabilitation counselor education program to conduct inservice training programs for supervisors (see Emener & Hutchinson, 1979), and in such instances it can be beneficial for all concerned if the program's rehabilitation counseling students are involved. Formal academic offerings (e.g., a seminar) can serve this function, as well.

In an article, "Rehabilitation Administration and Supervision: A Critical Component of Rehabilitation Education," published in the *NCRE Report,* Emener (1983), on behalf of the National Rehabilitation Administration Association (NRAA), appealed to members of the National Council on Rehabilitation Education (NCRE) to provide coursework in rehabilitation administration and supervision for students in rehabilitation education programs. His urging was predicated on the rationale that it would be beneficial to students in view of their long-term career development (see Stephens & Kniepp, 1981), and in the more immediate sense it would enhance their awareness of important rehabilitation service delivery phenomena in terms of their being consumers of administrative and supervisor practices (see Patti & Austin, 1977). Among other suggestions such as recommended journals (e.g., the *Journal of Rehabilitation Administration*), book chapters (e.g., Lorenz & Hill, 1984), and textbooks (e.g., Emener, Luck & Smits, 1981), he suggested the use of local NRAA members as curriculum development consultants, guest speakers, and adjunct instructors. "Must reading" would include Matkin, Sawyer, Lorenz and Rubin's (1982) research (see Chapter 28). For example, it would be essential for students to study and discuss the work role categories of rehabilitation administrators (Table 28-2). Moreover, discussions of how it would be as a rehabilitation counselor oriented professional to perform such administrative work roles can be very enlightening for students (see Feindel, 1980; Riggar & Matkin, 1984). Rehabilitation educators and their students might also be interested in knowing the inservice training needs of practicing rehabilitation administrators (see Hutchinson, Luck & Hardy, 1978; Matkin, Sawyer, Lorenz & Rubin, 1982) as they develop their curricular offerings. Moreover, careful study of Matkin, Sawyer, Lorenz and Rubin's (1982) Table 28-6, along with the works of other researchers (e.g., Alonzo & Autry, 1977; Byrd, Lesnik & Byrd, 1981; Sales & Downey, 1981; Schweitzer & Deely, 1981; Young, 1977), can provide valuable information for the development of preservice rehabilitation administration coursework. The experiences of rehabilitation counselor educators who have developed and offered rehabilitation administration and supervision coursework for advanced rehabilitation counseling students and practicing rehabilitation professionals (e.g., Emener, 1983) have reported that such offerings are considered very valuable by the students, practitioners, and the educators who teach the course(s).

Rehabilitation service delivery has always valued the roles of rehabilitation facilities (Carter, Shinnick & McDaniel, 1981; Massie, 1962), and the preparation and continuing development of facility personnel is an important component of rehabilitation education. Fry (1980) reported that thirteen professional training programs for rehabilitation facility administrators exist throughout the United States; there are, however, numerous other programs for other facility personnel. Rehabilitation counselor education programs are encouraged to review such facility oriented education and training programs (see Carter, Shinnick & McDaniel, 1981; Fry, 1980; McDonald, 1976; McDonald & Lorenz, 1977; Salkind, 1974; Shinnick, 1978), and consider alternative ways of availing their students to opportunities to learn about facilities and the roles and functions of the rehabilitation professionals who work in them.

In their classic work, "Convergence and Divergence in Rehabilitation Counseling and Vocational Education," Sink and Porter (1978) identified the similarities, differences, and overlapping attributes of the practices of rehabilitation counseling and vocational evaluation. Baker and Lorenz (1978), Chapter 29 in this book, wrote a requested reaction/comment piece and addressed numerous implications for rehabilitation education. Baker and Lorenz (1978) offer numerous compelling reasons as to why the rehabilitation counseling student should study areas of evaluation; additional rationale and suggestions for study can be found in the works of Anderson (1979), McFarlane and DiPaola (1979), Sink and Porter (1978), and Sink, Porter, Rubin and Painter (1979). Consistent with identified inservice training needs of vocational evaluators (e.g., see Sankovsky, Brolin & Coffey, 1977), critical and important vocational evaluation curricula areas have also been identified (for example, see Baker & Lorenz's Chapter 29; other suggested sources include: Chan & Questad, 1981; Coffey & Ellien, 1979; Gellman, 1968; Lytel, McFarlane & Jones, 1975; Nadolsky, 1975). Rehabilitation counseling students are encouraged to study the roles, functions, and job duties of the vocational evaluator (e.g., see Nadolsky, 1974; Sink & Porter, 1978; Sink, Porter, Rubin & Painter, 1979); not only will such study help students better understand their vocational evaluation colleagues and what they do, but rehabilitation counseling students will also better understand themselves and what they do!

In the past few years, the private-for-profit sector of rehabilitation has mushroomed. To illustrate, Matkin (1982b) reported that approximately 5,300 practitioners represented by about 200 corporate members of the National Association of Rehabilitation Professionals in the Private Sector (NARPPS) were working in private-for-profit rehabilitation. Importantly, nearly one-third of these 5,300 professionals were graduates of rehabilitation counselor education programs. McMahon (1979), in Chapter 30, discusses this emerging "privatization trend" and addresses potential benefits such as increased opportunity, increased responsibility, unrestrained management, placement orientation, and increased exposure. Thorough study of McMahon's (1979) chapter, McMahon and Matkin's (1983) Chapter 31, and other relevant sources regarding private sector rehabilitation (e.g., Matkin, 1980b) reveals numerous critical issues. For example, in Petrangelo, Abeln and Rudrud's (1984) research on "qualified rehabilitation consultants" (QRC's), they concluded: "Most disturbing are the opinions expressed by attorneys, disabled workers, and physicians, that placement of the disabled worker is the QRC's primary concern, rather than the welfare of the client. This is in direct opposition to the opinions expressed by claims adjusters that the results, measured in terms of job placements, are not as good as expected" (p. 8). The question "For whom does the private sector professional work?" raises numerous issues relevant to professional role strain and ethics. Rehabilitation counselor educators and their students indeed should study reported inservice training needs surveys of private sector rehabilitation counselors (e.g., Lynch & Martin, 1982) as well as recommended curricula for pre-service education for private sector rehabilitation (see Matkin, 1980b; McMahon, 1979; McMahon & Matkin, 1983; Sales, 1979). Moreover, rehabilitation counseling students are urged to read the writings of Couch (1979), Diamond and Petkas (1979), Griswold and Scott (1979), Lewin, Ramseur and Sink (1979), McMahon, Matkin, Growick, Mahaffey and Gianforte (1983), and Whittington (1975), and ponder and discuss the numerous critical issues amid the emerging of private sector rehabilitation (for example, its organization and relationship to state-federal rehabilitation programs).

In conclusion, this part of this book raises numerous critical issues relevant to the preparation and development of professional rehabilitation counselors. The areas of supervision, administration, facilities, vocational evaluation, and private sector rehabilitation are addressed directly; nevertheless, many of the critical issues in these areas are also relevant to the numerous other cognate areas within rehabilitation counselor education discussed in Parts II and III of this book. For example, in Chapter 29, Baker and Lorenz (1978) raise a rather generic critical issues: "The major educational issue confronting rehabilitation education is not 'Who can do what?' but 'How should we train whom to do what?' " Practitioners, students, and university professors should individually and collectively continue to address issues such as these. As Emener (1975) suggests in Chapter 20 of this book, rehabilitation counseling students should be "students of life and students for life"; fittingly, rehabilitation counselor education programs should include course content and coursework in the areas suggesting in this Part VI of this book—their commitment is to their students' careers in the field of rehabilitation not just their students' jobs as rehabilitation counselors.

W.G. Emener

CHAPTER 28

REHABILITATION ADMINISTRATORS AND SUPERVISORS: THEIR WORK ASSIGNMENTS, TRAINING NEEDS, AND SUGGESTIONS FOR PREPARATION

Ralph E. Matkin, Horace W. Sawyer, Jerome R. Lorenz, and Stanford E. Rubin

Abstract

A national survey of 426 randomly selected members of the National Rehabilitation Administration Association was conducted to identify respondents' work assignments, inservice training needs, and academic preparation needs as administrators and supervisors. A total of 243 members responded (57% return) to the sixty-four item Rehabilitation Administrator Task Inventory (RATI) which yielded 178 respondents employed in either private not-for-profit rehabilitation facilities ($N=59$) or state-federal rehabilitation agencies ($N=119$). Facility personnel consisted of thirty-nine top level and twenty middle level administrators, while agency personnel included twenty-nine top level administrators, fifty-four middle level administrators, and thirty-six first-line supervisors. Factor analysis of the RATI revealed fifty task items distributed over ten Work Role Categories: (1) General Personnel Management, (2) Professional Management, (3) Fiscal Management, (4) Production Management, (5) Program Planning and Evaluation, (6) Public Relations, (7) Marketing Service (8) Labor Relations, (9) Purchasing, and (10) Research. Data were analyzed for the ten work role categories, as well as on each task item, using one-way analysis of variance and Duncan's multiple comparison test when significant differences occurred at the .05 level. Results and their implications were reported for the roles and functions of rehabilitation administrators and supervisors, continuing education and training needs, and suggestions for rehabilitation administration academic curriculum development.

THERE ARE an estimated 12,000 to 13,000 administrators, managers, and supervisors employed in the field of rehabilitation in the United States (Lorenz, 1977). These individuals primarily work either in state-federal

Reprinted by permission from Volume 6 (1982), *Journal of Rehabilitation Administration*, pp. 170-183.

rehabilitation agencies or in approximately 5,000 private, not-for-profit rehabilitation facilities (Lorenz, Graham, Hashey, & Baker, 1981). While their numbers are sufficiently large to warrant a professional status, that status has not been unquestioned. One challenge relates to the existence of a body of knowledge that is unique to the role and function of the rehabilitation administrator. There appears to be a general agreement that a quantifiable body of knowledge is, at best, in the process of being identified (McDonald & Lorenz, 1977; Alonzo & Autry, 1977). According to Young (1977), while the theory and practice of rehabilitation administration may not be unique, the administrative application requires specialized knowledge and skills to attain rehabilitation specific goals. This is contrary to the position of many schools and colleges of administration that promote the concept of generic management in which a broadly trained administrator is prepared to manage any organization (Suojanen, 1977). Lorenz (1977) has suggested that generic management training programs have failed to respond to the unique management problems of the applied fields and as a result, more specialized areas of administrative training have evolved. Examples of these specialized fields include hospital administration, social work administration, educational administration, and public administration. While rehabilitation administration has recently joined this group, its validity as a specialized field rests on a questionable foundation due to the limited amount of available empirical data regarding management personnel within rehabilitation facilities and agencies. Therefore, it became readily apparent to the current authors that a role delineation study on the rehabilitation administrator was badly needed.

There also appeared to be a pressing need for information on the development and training needs of individuals in rehabilitation administration. The problem of finding qualified individuals to manage the increasing number of rehabilitation facilities and to provide management training for established administrators was not fully realized until the mid-1960s. Prior to that point, a lack of formal preparation and training were not serious problems as many programs were small and accountability was not a major issue (Lorenz & Hill, in press). Since that time, the gap between a rehabilitation administrator's body of knowledge and the amount of information needed to fulfill the management role has continued to widen. This problem has been further exacerbated by a deficiency of management training available and the lack of administrative experience prior to assuming the role (Sawyer & Schumacher, 1980). If the trend to recruit rehabilitation administrators from a pool of direct service practitioners continues, and if these individuals are to have the necessary skills for their new job role, the preservice and inservice training needed by rehabilitation facility and agency administrators must be fully identified and made available.

In recognition of the fact that a basic knowledge gap existed in the field, the authors decided to conduct a national study designed to delineate both the rehabilitation administrator's job role and functions, and the associated preservice and inservice training needs for such positions. This national survey was directed toward practicing administrators in both state agencies and private, not-for-profit rehabilitation facilities. It was recognized that knowledge generated from such a study could be of value to those involved in developing an academic curriculum for the training and education of rehabilitation administrators. It was also recognized that since a role and function study of the rehabilitation administrator did not exist, results of this study could contribute to the definition of that professional role. Furthermore, the potential results from the study could have relevance for current accreditation activities and provide direction for inservice training efforts.

The following specific research questions were addressed by the current study:

1. What are the job functions of rehabilitation administrators?
2. What are the inservice training needs perceived by rehabilitation administrators?
3. What are the recommendations for preparational curricula of rehabilitation administrators?

METHODOLOGY

Sample

Approximately 1,300 members of the National Rehabilitation Administration Association (NRAA) who resided in the United States and Canada constituted the population for this study. A random sample of 426 NRAA members were surveyed whereby, each participant was sent a cover letter explaining the nature and purpose of the study and the Rehabilitation Administrator Task Inventory (RATI).[3] All told, 243 members of the sample (57%) responded yielding a final usable sample of 178 RATI questionnaires.[4] The final sample contained fifty-nine administrators working in non-profit rehabilitation facilities (containing two subsets: thirty-nine top level administrators and twenty middle level administrators) and 119 administrators working in state rehabilitation agencies (containing three subsets: twenty-nine top level administrators, fifty-four level administrators, and thirty-six first-line supervisors).

A brief overview of the demographic characteristics of the respondents are reported in Table 28-1.[5] In total, the majority of rehabilitation administrators and supervisors were white, non-disabled, males who generally had completed graduate degree programs at the master's level.

Instrumentation

The RATI was developed from four sources: (1) a review of duties performed

Table 28–1
Demographic Characteristics of Respondents

Characteristics	Non-Profit Facility		State/Federal Agency		
	Top Level N = 39	Middle Level N = 20	Top Level N = 29	Middle Level N = 54	First-Line N = 36
Sex: Male	31	12	27	40	30
Female	8	8	2	14	6
Age: 25-39	23	14	13	19	11
40-54	13	6	11	28	18
55+	3	-	5	7	7
Formal Rehab. Admin. training:					
None	31	17	21	44	30
Grad. School	5	1	7	6	1
Certificate	3	2	1	4	5
CRC: Yes	6	3	12	27	18
No	33	17	17	27	18
Direct Rehab. Service (years):					
None	10	2	2	4	1
1-10	29	17	24	40	26
11+	-	1	3	10	9
Rehab. Supervisor (years):					
None	4	-	1	-	1
1-10	29	20	15	34	24
11+	6	-	13	20	11
Non-Rehab. Supv. (years):					
None	19	12	16	25	23
1-10	16	7	11	24	13
11+	4	1	2	5	1
Staff Size:	3	1	1	8	
1-15	24	11	12	24	24
16-30	6	6	5	6	12
31+	6	2	11	16	-
Budget Size:					
None	4	8	6	25	15
up to $100,000	1	2	1	3	5
$100,001-500,000	15	5	3	6	13
over $500,000	19	5	19	20	3
Location Size:					
less than 10,000	5	2	1	4	3
10,001-50,000	8	4	3	5	9
50,001-100,000	8	4	7	8	3
over 100,000	18	10	18	37	21
RSA Region:					
I	3	1	-	2	-
II	2	4	-	2	2
III	3	-	5	10	5
IV	8	3	15	22	8
V	11	2	2	6	7
VI	3	4	-	5	4
VII	2	2	5	2	3
VIII	2	2	2	-	3
IX	3	-	-	3	1
X	2	1	-	2	3

Table 28-2
RATI Work Role Categories

Questionnaire section and Item Number		
General Personnel Management		
I-1	Supervisory management of personnel within your agency.	
I-5	Management of employee conflicts.	
I-7	Interview applicants for direct service professional positions.	
I-8	Interview applicants for indirect service positions.	
I-11	Engage in recruitment activities for staff positions vacant.	
I-12	Develop strategies for retaining/promoting employees.	
I-13	Conduct personnel evaluation reports on a periodic basis.	
I-16	Responsible for disciplining personnel under your supervision.	
I-17	Conduct follow-up activities of duties assigned to subordinates.	
Professional Management		
I-3	Supervision of direct service personnel in the office.	
I-4	Supervision of direct service personnel in the field.	
I-9	Coordinate active client caseloads in addition to your supervisory duties.	
I-14	Assist counselors in preparation of individual written rehabilitation plans for clients served.	
I-18	Assign work to counselors.	
II-5	Maintain a system for case finding and procurement.	
Fiscal Management		
III-1	Prepare budgets for your total agency.	
III-3	Manage a bookkeeping and accounting system within your agency.	
III-6	Develop means for identifying financial resources.	
III-7	Prepare financial analysis studies.	
III-8	Responsible for implementing financial decisions.	
III-9	Responsible for cost accounting procedures.	
III-10	Controlling agency expenses.	
Production Management		
V-2	Responsible for contract procurement.	
V-3	Perform contract cost estimating and bidding.	
V-4	Conduct work method (task) analyses in production operations.	
V-5	Conduct time and motion studies for work measurement assessment.	

V-6	Assess work place design and layout (accessibility).	
V-7	Responsible for renovation planning and development.	
Program Planning and Evaluation		
II-1	Develop written goals and policy statements for your agency.	
II-2	Use program evaluation data for public policy formulation or reformulation.	
II-4	Conduct community needs assessment.	
II-6	Study manuals, case reports, and other materials to learn how to apply policies and procedures.	
II-7	Preparation of reports dealing with rehabilitation activities, statistical breakdowns, employee evaluations, and fiscal management (program evaluation).	
II-9	Develop written program objectives.	
II-10	Perform program evaluations on a periodic basis.	
II-11	Develop resource materials related to facility programs.	
Public Relations		
II-3	Prepare grant applications for your agency.	
IV-1	Engage in public speaking activities representing your agency.	
IV-5	Engage in working directly with the Board of Directors of your agency.	
IV-6	Contact media personnel	
IV-7	Establish affiliation agreements with other service agencies.	
IV-8	Involvement in rehabilitation legislative relations.	
IV-9	Provide testimony for rehabilitation issues.	
IV-10	Perform technical writing for presentation on rehabilitation issues.	
IV-11	Develop public education/information strategies for your agency (e.g., brochures).	
Marketing Service		
IV-3	Perform marketing/sales activities for your agency.	
IV-4	Solicitation of volunteer assistance to your agency.	
Labor Relations		
I-10	Engage in labor relations activities within your agency.	
Purchasing		
III-4	Purchase goods and supplies.	
Research		
II-8	Conduct research in the area of rehabilitation.	

by administrators and supervisors found in the rehabilitation literature, (2) descriptions of curricula in graduate rehabilitation administration training programs, and (3) descriptions of inservice training courses offered by Regional Rehabilitation Continuing Education Programs. Finally, tasks were reviewed by several rehabilitation educators familiar with tasks performed by rehabilitation administrators and supervisors such that the final version of the RATI contained fifty-nine items plus five items denoted as "other" for participant input. Thus the RATI was considered to be an accurate reflection of the primary job tasks of rehabilitation administrators and first-line supervisors.

Table 28-3
**Scales for Rehabilitation Administrators in
Non-Profit Facilities and Rehabilitation Administrators/
First-Line Supervisors in State/Federal Agencies**

Scale 1. To what extent is the task a part of your work?
     1 = Definitely not a part
     2 = A minor part
     3 = A moderate part
     4 = A substantial part
     5 = A crucial and most significant part

Scale 2. To what extent do you perceive a need for additional inservice training?
     1 = Definitely not needed
     2 = Minor need for training
     3 = Moderate need for training
     4 = Training need is substantial
     5 = Vital and significant need for training

Scale 3. To what extent is academic preparation necessary for job entry?[a]
     1 = Definitely not needed
     2 = A minor need
     3 = A moderate need
     4 = a substantial need
     5 = A vital and significant need

Each subject was asked to rate each of the sixty-four RATI items found on Table 28-1 using the three scales found in Table 28-1,[6] Scales 1, 2, and 3 represented the relative degree to which subjects perceived: (a) tasks to be part of their present job duties, (b) additional inservice training as necessary to perform those tasks, and (c) academic preparation as necessary to prepare persons to perform the tasks. For purposes of meaningful interpretation of mean item and task category scores on the three scales, the authors pre-established the following criteria based on the 5-point Likert-type scaling (Table 28-3):

2.49   or lower = Scale 1 — minor part of job constituted by the task; Scale 2 — task category without much need for additional inservice training; Scale 3 — task category with minor need for preservice training.

2.50   to 3.49 = Scale 1 — moderate part of job constituted by the task; Scale 2 — task category with a moderate need for additional inservice training, Scale 3 — task category with a moderate need for preservice training.

3.50   or higher = Scale 1 — substantial part of job constituted by the task; Scale 2 — task category with a substantial need for additional inservice training; Scale 3 — task category with a substantial need for preservice training.

Data Analysis

In order to allow for parsimonious analysis and interpretation of the data, the Scale 1 ratings of the 178 usable respondents on the sixty-four item RATI (2.8:1 subject to item ratio) were factor analyzed. The principal components factor solution was used with Varimax rotation (Statistical Analysis System, 1979). A series of one-way analysis of variance (ANOVA), employing the general linear model (Statistical Analysis System, 1979) were used to answer the research questions. The .05 level was used to test for significant differences between groups and where appropriate, Duncan's multiple comparison post hoc analyses following the ANOVA were used.

RESULTS AND DISCUSSION

Factor Analysis of the RATI

The Factor Analysis yielded ten factors accounting for eighty-six percent of the total variance.[7] In order for a RATI item to be retained on a factor, a factor loading criterion of .45 or higher had to be present. As a result of this arbitrary decision rule established by the authors, nine of the original sixty-four items were omitted for failure to meet the criterion level. An additional five items (i.e., RATI items denoted as "other" were omitted because they did not contribute to the inventory in meaningful way). The item composition of each of the ten factors can be observed on Table 28-2.

Definition of Identified Work Role Factors

GENERAL PERSONNEL MANAGEMENT. This factor grouping consisted of nine tasks that represent responsibility for the overall supervisory management of personnel within the facility/agent (see Table 28-2). Examples of the duties performed under this heading include: recruiting, interviewing and selecting applicants for hiring, conducting periodic personnel evaluations, developing strategies for the retention and promotion for existing personnel, managing employee conflicts, disciplining employees, and monitoring the duties assigned to subordinates.

PROFESSIONAL MANAGEMENT. Six task items were contained under this factor heading which consist of duties associated with the supervision of professional direct service personnel (see Table 28-2). Examples of tasks performed by administrators and supervisors within this area include: developing and maintaining an appropriate system for case finding and referral intake, coordination of active client caseloads, assigning work to counselors, and assisting counselors in the preparation of individualized written rehabilitation programs.

FISCAL MANAGEMENT. Seven tasks were grouped under the factor which consists of associated responsibilities of overall budget management and financial analyses within rehabilitation facilities or agencies (see Table 28-2). Tasks represented include: identifying appropriate financial resources, preparing facility/agency budgets, establishing and managing appropriate bookkeeping and financial and cost accounting systems, controlling agency expenses, preparing financial analysis studies, and making and implementing financial decisions.

PROGRAM PLANNING AND EVALUATION. This factor grouping consisted of eight job tasks related to responsibilities for the overall planning implementation, and assessment of facility or agency program goals, policies, and objectives (see Table 28-2). Duties generally performed as part of this area include: conducting needs assessments within the community developing written goals, objectives, and policy statements, developing resource materials, conducting program evaluations and preparing evaluation reports, and using program evaluation outcomes to reformulate facility/agency policies and procedures.

PUBLIC RELATIONS. Nine tasks were identified within this factor grouping which represents development of an overall public education and information strategy of the facility of agency (see Table 28-2). Examples of tasks performed include: working with the Board of Directors, preparing grant applications, establishing affiliation agreements, managing legislative relations and testifying before committees as needed, writing presentations on a variety of rehabilitation issues, performing public speaking activities, and contacting media sources as needed.

MARKETING SERVICE. Two task items formed this grouping which consist of job responsibilities for conducting marketing and sales activities for the facility or agency, and soliciting volunteers for the service program from within the community (see Table 28-2).

LABOR RELATIONS. One task composed this factor heading which represents job responsibility related to establishing, improving, and maintaining appropriate labor relations for the rehabilitation facility or agency with external labor groups (see Table 28-2).

PURCHASING. One task composed this factor which represents activities of purchasing goods and supplies for the facility or agency that are necessary for the day-to-day, as well as long-term operation of the program (see Table 28-2).

RESEARCH. One task item was identified within this factor consisting of the responsibility of administrators and supervisors to conduct research in rehabilitation relative to the activities performed with their employment setting (see Table 28-2).

Rehabilitation Administrator Roles and Functions[8]

Table 28-4 reports the mean, Facility Top Level (FTL) Administrator, Facility Middle Level (FML) Administrator, Agency Top Level (ATL) Administrator, Agency Middle Level (AML) Administrator, and Agency First-Line

Table 28–4
Means, ANOVA F's, and Significant Duncan's for Comparisons of the
Scale 1 Response of Five Groups of Administrators/Supervisors
on the Work Role Categories

Work Role Category	Non-Profit Facility		State/Federal Agency			F Ratio	Significant Duncan's (p <.05)
	1 Top Level $\overline{X}$	2 Middle Level $\overline{X}$	3 Top Level $\overline{X}$	4 Middle Level $\overline{X}$	5 First-Line $\overline{X}$		
General Personnel Management:	3.52	3.28	3.06	2.70	3.20	5.09 +	1,2, vs 4 3 vs 4
Professional Management:	2.16	2.47	2.17	2.05	3.42	16.73 + +	5 vs 1,2,3,&4
Fiscal Management:	3.42	2.32	2.76	2.00	1.75	22.06 + +	1 vs 2,3,4,&5 2 vs 5 3 vs 4 & 5
Production Management:	2.18	1.87	1.82	1.41	1.49	5.95 +	1 vs 3 & 5
Program Planning and Evaluation:	3.24	3.06	3.30	2.90	2.26	9.30 + +	3 vs 4 & 5 1,2,&4 vs 5
Public Relations:	3.07	2.09	2.57	1.89	1.70	23.56 + +	1 vs 2,3,4,&5 3 vs 2,4,&5
Marketing Service:	2.58	1.78	1.84	1.42	1.29	10.90 + +	1 vs 2,3,&4 1 & 3 vs 5
Labor Relations:	2.82	2.15	1.72	1.57	1.54	9.02 + +	1 vs 2,3,4,&5
Purchasing:	2.29	3.05	2.10	1.69	2.00	5.72 + +	2 vs 1,3,&4
Research:	1.82	1.90	2.24	1.87	1.53	2.16	

* <.05   ** <.01   + <.001   + + <.0001

(AFL) Supervisor ratings to the extent that each of ten work roles are a part of their job. Only the General Personnel Management work role was rated by all five groups as constituting more than a minor part of their job. Four groups of administrator/supervisors report the General Personnel Management as a moderate part of their job (Scale 1 mean ≥ 2.50), while FTL administrators rated that work role as a substantial (Scale 1 mean ≥ 3.50) part of their job. However, it should be pointed out that individual item means indicated that AML administrators rated recruiting and interviewing job applicants (Items I-7, I-8, and I-11) as a minor part of their job (see Table 28-2 for description of specific items), while AFL supervisors rated interviewing applicants for in-direct service positions (Items I-8) as a minor part of their job. It should also be noted that Table 28-4 shows that FTL administrators, FML administrators and AFL supervisors reported the General Personnel Management work role as a significantly greater part of their job than did the AML administrators.

As can also be seen on Table 28-4 the work role category of Program Planning and Evaluation was reported as being a moderate part of their job by top and middle level administrators regardless of setting, but as a minor part of the job of the first-line supervisor. However, observation of the individual item means under this work role category showed that (as would be expected) AFL supervisors rated the following two job tasks as a moderate and substantial part of their job respectively:

II-7   Preparation of reports dealing with rehabilitation activities, statistical breakdowns, employee evaluations, and fiscal management (Program Evaluation).

II-6   Study manuals, case reports, and other materials to learn how to apply policies and procedures.

The area of Public Relations generally was perceived as more relevant to the work role of top level administrators in both state agency and facility settings than to middle level administrators or supervisors (see Table 28-4). The results of the multiple comparison tests between groups also indicated a statistically significant difference in the extent this work role was reported as a part of the job of the top level administrators employed in rehabilitation facilities and state agencies. The significantly greater extent that FTL administrators reported this work role as a part of their job than did ATL administrators appeared to be greatly the result of differences on two job tasks contained within the category; (Item II-3) Prepare grant applications for your agency, and (Item IV-5) Engage in working directly with the Board of Directors of your agency). Item II-3 was rated as a substantial part of the job of FTL administrators ($\overline{X}=3.74$), while being a minor part of the job of ATL administrators ($\overline{X}=2.03$). It should also be noted that all five administrator/supervisor groups rated Item IV-9 (Provide testimony for rehabilitation issues) and Item IV-10 (Perform technical writing for presentation on rehabilitation issues) as a minor part of their job.

Similar findings were evident in the work role category of Fiscal Management found in Table 28-4. As was the case for Public Relations, Fiscal Management was perceived as more relevant to the work role of top level administrators in both state agency and facility settings than to middle level administrators and supervisors. In addition FTL administrators rated the Fiscal Management work role as a significantly greater part of their job than did ATL administrators. That difference appeared to be greatly attributed to the following individual task items which were rated by facility top level administrators as a substantial part of their job: (a) preparing budget for their total facility (III-1), (b) developing means to identify financial resources (III-6), (c) implementing financial decisions (III-8), and (d) controlling facility expenses (III-10). Significant differences (in favor of FTL administrators) between facility and agency top level administrators were found on all four of those task items.

As might have been expected, the area of Professional Management appeared to be a minor part of the job of all groups with the exception of the first-line supervisor who rated the category as approaching a substantial part of their work role (see Table 28-4). Inspection of the individual item means revealed three job tasks within this work role category that first-line supervisors rated as a substantial part of their job. These are: (a) supervision of direct service personnel in the office (Item I-3), (b) supervision of direct service personnel in the field, and (c) assigning work to counselor (Item I-18).

Also worthy of note on Table 28-4 were the following:

1. The Production Management and Research work roles were rated by all groups as no more than a minor part of their job.
2. The Marketing Service and Labor Relations work roles were rated by four groups as no more than a minor part of their job. The exception was the FTL administrators who rated those work roles as a moderate part of their job.

Rehabilitation Administrator Inservice Training Needs[8]

Mean ratings, F ratios, and significant Duncan multiple comparisons for the ten work role categories are reported in Table 28-5 as they pertain to the perceived inservice training needs of rehabilitation administrators and supervisors. All levels of administrators in rehabilitation facilities and state agencies reported a moderate need for additional inservice training General Personnel Management (Scale 2 Mean $\geq$ 2.5). An examination of the individual items revealed that regardless of setting or administrative level, respondents reported a moderate need for training on Items I-1, I-5, I-12, I-13, and I-16. This suggests training needs exist across the administrator/supervisor levels in the area of overall supervisory management of personnel, conducting personnel evaluation, management of employee conflicts and discipline, and strategy development for retaining and promoting existing staff members. It should also be recalled from Table 28-4 that General Personnel Management, received mean ratings indicating that it was a moderate or substantial part of the job for all levels of administrators.

Within the work role category of Professional Management, the only group to report at least a moderate need for training in this area was the first-line supervisor groups in state rehabilitation agencies (see Table 28-5) who also rated this work role category as a moderate part of their job (see Table 28-4). As was previously noted, examinations of Scale 1 means on Items I-3, I-4, and I-18 revealed that supervision of direct service personnel in the office and in the field, as well as the assigning of work to counselors, were seen as substantial aspects of their job. However, an examination of the Scale 2 means on Items I-3, I-4, and I-18 showed that a training need area by administrators at all levels was supervision of direct service personnel in the office. Overall, it may be concluded that the data suggest a clear need for inservice training programs focused on

Table 28–5

Means, ANOVA F's and Significant Duncan's for Comparisons of the
Scale 2 Responses of Five Groups of Administrators/Supervisors
on the 10 Work Role Categories

Work Role Category	Non-Profit Facility		State/Federal Agency			F Ratio	Significant Duncan's (p < .05)
	1 Top Level $\overline{X}$	2 Middle Level $\overline{X}$	3 Top Level $\overline{X}$	4 Middle Level $\overline{X}$	5 First-Line $\overline{X}$		
General Personnel Management:	2.90	2.71	2.82	2.52	2.87	1.76	
Professional Management:	2.14	2.49	2.41	2.29	2.76	3.31*	5 vs 1 & 4
Fiscal Management:	2.96	2.68	2.68	2.23	1.98	6.16 + +	1 vs 4 & 5 2 & 3vs5
Production Management:	2.70	2.62	2.08	1.83	1.69	6.36 + +	1 vs 3,4,&5 2 vs 4 & 5
Program Planning and Evaluation:	3.02	2.79	2.93	2.86	2.33	3.55**	1,3,&4 vs 5 2 vs 4 & 5
Public Relations:	2.79	2.49	2.61	2.09	1.85	7.60 + +	1 vs 4 & 5 3 vs 4 2 & 3 vs 5
Marketing Service:	2.80	2.47	2.05	1.78	1.38	9.75 + +	1 vs 3,4, & 5 2 vs. 3,4, & 5
Labor Relations:	3.22	2.89	2.10	2.02	2.22	7.60 + +	1 vs 3,4,&5 2 vs 3,4, & 5
Purchasing:	2.05	2.35	1.76	1.65	1.94	2.16	
Research:	2.32	2.53	2.62	2.43	1.92	1.71	

* < .05 ** < .01 + < .001 + + < .0001

the development of skills for supervising direct service personnel with the group most in need being state agency first-line supervisors.

Program Planning and Evaluation was the second highest rated job task category in both work roles (see Table 28-4) and inservice training needs (see Table 28-5). This indication by administrators may well reflect the emphasis being placed on accountability in both rehabilitation facilities and state rehabilitation agencies. As this administrative responsibility continues to increase in rehabilitation, inservice training efforts in this area will assist administrators in keeping pace with new developments and strategies.

In assessing inservice training needs, top and middle level facility administrators reported a greater variety of training needs than their state agency counterparts. Rehabilitation facility administrators reflected skill deficits in Production Management, Marketing Service and Labor Relations, whereas state agency administrators did not perceive training needs in those areas.

The results in Table 28-5 also suggests a consistency among state rehabilitation agency administrators to perceive training needs in the same areas of administration that they rate as being a moderate or substantial part of their job, the only exception being research (see Table 28-4). These findings are consistent with previous studies suggesting that rehabilitation agency administrators are promoted from practitioner ranks to assume administrative job roles without training (Feindel, 1980). Similar findings were also observed for administrators in non-profit rehabilitation facilities, however, there was not the same degree of consistency (see Tables 28-4 and 28-5). The only job task category that was seen as a moderate part of the job without training being needed was Purchasing (FML administrators). In contrast to this finding, several job task categories (Fiscal Management, Production Management, Labor Relations, and Research) were perceived as areas on which the FML administrators needed training but were not seen as a moderate or substantial part of their work role. FTL administrators had a greater tendency to match work functions with inservice training needs that did FML administrators, that if additional skills could be gained through inservice training, these job task categories would become more integrated into their job role. Another possibility relates to the motivation of middle level administrators gaining additional skills outside of their job role responsibilities in order to become top level administrators.

It is interesting to note from the observations of Tables 28-4 and 28-5 that the closer the administrator group is to the service delivery aspect of the state rehabilitation agency system (i.e., first-line supervision), the narrower the scope of administrative work functions and perceived inservice training needs delineated. Since a majority of administrators are secured from practitioner ranks (Feindel, 1980), the closer they remain to service delivery and practitioner activities, the more they apparently continue to identify with this job role and its function. First-line supervisors are reported to perceive a need for training in all job task areas of General Personnel Management with the exception of interviewing applicants for indirect service positions (Item I-8). A substantial need for training was expressed by this group for managing employee conflicts. Training programs in rehabilitation administration will need to develop a training focus for these individuals as they make the transition from practitioner to administrator.

As can be seen in Table 28-5, a need for training was perceived by various levels of administrators in twenty-two instances (Scale 2 mean ≥ 2.50). This is an interesting finding when compared to mean ratings of work function in which there were seventeen instances where work roles were identified as a moderate or substantial part of their work (see Table 28-4). Administrators in rehabilitation appear to be perceiving a continuing professional development of their job role in which inservice training will be an essential component in acquiring this eventual level of job role and function.

Rehabilitation Administrator Preparational Curriculum Needs[8]

An investigation of the academic preparation necessary for job entry as a rehabilitation administrator was included in this study for two reasons. First, there is a paucity of research on this topic. Second, the question can be clearly differentiated from the question on inservice training since unlike training or continuing education, preservice higher education provides a foundation of knowledge and skills which influence attitudes and behavior in virtually all functions related to a major occupational role. On the other hand, inservice training and continuing education serve to enhance fundamental core knowledge and skills by impacting on attitudes and behavior in discrete areas of occupational funtioning. It is interesting to note that, while the majority of respondents in the study have from one to ten years experience in a rehabilitation administration capacity, the vast majority having no preparatory training for their administrative role.

In order to identify the work role categories and specific job functions perceived by practicing rehabilitation facility and state agency administrators to require preservice training commensurate for job entry, Scale 3 (see Table 28-6) was included.

Mean ratings, F ratios, and significant Duncan multiple comparisons for the ten work role categories are reported in Table 28-6 as they pertain to perceived preservice training needs of rehabilitation administrators and supervisors. A quick observation of the cell means in Table 28-6 shows a consistently greater need (with one exception) perceived by the facility administrators than by agency administrators/supervisors for preservice training. Turning to the individual work role categories, both levels of facility administrators perceived a substantial need for preservice training in General Personnel Management, while all levels of agency administrators reported a moderate need. None of these differences were statistically significant. On the other hand, all levels and types of rehabilitation managers reported a moderate need for preservice training in Professional Management. Again, there were no statistically significant differences among them.

In the area of Fiscal Management, both levels of facility administrators reported a substantial need for preservice training while all levels of agency administrators reported a moderate preservice training need in this area. Statistically significant differences were reported between FTL and FML administrators versus AML administrators and AFL supervisors; and between ATL administrators versus AFL supervisors. However, ATL administrators perceived the importance of this work role category in a similar manner as facility administrators than did other levels of agency administrators. Specific items which played a major role in this outcome included III-1 (Agency budget preparation) and III-7 (Financial analysis). A parallel finding occurred in the Public Relations area, i.e., ATL administrators reported more importance to

Table 28-6
Means, ANOVA F's and Significant Duncan's for Comparisons of the
Scale 3 Responses of Five Groups of Administrators and
Supervisors on the 10 Work Role Categories

Work Role Category	Facility		Agency			F Ratios	Significant Duncan's (p <.05)
	1 Top Level $\bar{X}$	2 Middle Level $\bar{X}$	3 Top Level $\bar{X}$	4 Middle Level $\bar{X}$	5 Supervisor Level $\bar{X}$		
General Personnel Management:	3.50	3.59	3.21	3.22	3.34	1.37	
Professional Management:	3.22	3.38	2.96	3.05	2.92	1.39	
Fiscal Management:	3.58	3.93	3.31	3.14	2.75	4.42*	2vs4,5 1vs4,5 3vs5
Production Management:	3.29	3.22	2.77	2.70	2.49	2.94*	1vs4,5
Program Planning and Evaluation:	3.70	3.78	3.50	3.34	2.95	5.08+	1,2,3,4,vs5
Public Relations:	3.60	3.51	3.24	2.97	2.73	6.19++	1vs4,5 2vs4,5 3vs5
Marketing	3.24	3.10	2.86	2.78	2.42	2.75*	1vs4,5
Labor Relations:	3.21	3.13	2.68	2.56	2.75	2.08	1vs4
Purchasing:	2.62	2.79	2.39	2.59	2.17	1.09	
Research:	2.77	3.27	3.21	3.05	2.52	1.73	

* <.05   ** <.01   + <.001   ++ < .0001

those work functions than did other agency administrators. Specific items which contributed significantly to this difference included IV-5 (Relations with boards of directors), IV-10 (Technical writing in rehabilitation), and IV-11 (Public education/information strategies). Item IV-6 (Media relations) appeared to be the primary province of FTL administrators. In the area of Program Planning and Evaluation the results were similar to the above two findings except that ATL administrators also reported substantial preservice training needs in this work role category as did both levels of facility administrators. Specific items which were primarily involved in the difference between FTL, FML, and ATL administrators versus AML and AFL administrators included II-1 (Establishing goals and policies), and II-2 (Use of program evaluation results).

In the areas of Production Management and Marketing all levels of managers reported moderate preservice training needs except AFL supervisors who reported a minor training need. In both instances the statistically significant differences were between FTL administrators versus AML administrators and

Table 28-7

Means and ANOVA F's for Comparisons of Non-Profit Rehabilitation
Facility Administrators' and State/Federal Rehabilitation Agency
Administrators'/Supervisors' Responses on Scale 3 for the 10 Work
Role Categories

Work Role Category	Non-Profit Facility	State/Federal Agency	F Ratios
	$\overline{X}$	$\overline{X}$	
General Personnel Management:	3.53	3.25	4.84*
Professional Management:	3.26	3.01	4.23*
Fiscal Management:	3.68	3.09	12.40+
Production Management:	3.27	2.67	11.37+
Program Planning and Evaluation:	3.72	3.30	11.89+
Public Relations:	3.57	2.98	19.69++
Marketing Service:	3.20	2.72	8.30**
Labor Relations:	3.19	2.62	8.12**
Purchasing:	2.66	2.45	1.33
Research:	2.91	2.99	.19

*< .05   **< .01   +< .001   ++< .0001

AFL supervisors. Specific items which seemed to play the greatest role in these differences included: V-2 (Contract procurement), V-3 (Contract costing and bidding), V-7 (Renovation planning and development), and V-4 (Work method analysis). Item IV-4 (Solicitation of volunteers) seemed to be the primary province of facility administrators.

No statistically significant differences were found among levels of administrators in Labor Relations and Research with all reporting moderate preservice training needs. In the area of Purchasing there were also no statistically significant differences among the levels of administrators, but ATL administrators and AFL supervisors did report only a minor training need in contrast to all other levels which reported a moderate need.

While it can be argued that important differences in job functions and work roles exist between groups of administration according to both work setting and level of management variables, long-term rehabilitation administration training programs traditionally have been separated in terms of facility versus agency orientation. Thus, it seems logical to see if such a dichotomy was the most efficient method for preservice rehabilitation administration curriculum development. Therefore, it seemed most appropriate to review the data on perceived preservice training needs according to work setting. Table 28-7 provides mean ratings, F ratios, and significant Duncan multiple comparisons for the

Table 28-8
Rank Order of Perceived Preservice Training Needs of
Work Role Categories for
Rehabilitation Facility and Agency Administrators

Facility Administrator	State Agency Administrator
1. Program Planning and Evaluation	1. Program Planning and Evaluation
2. Fiscal Management	2. General Personnel Management
3. Public Relations	3. Fiscal Management
4. General Personnel Management	4. Professional Management
5. Production Management	5. Research
6. Professional Management	6. Public Relations
7. Marketing	7. Marketing
8. Labor Relations	8. Production Management
9. Research	9. Labor Relations
10. Purchasing	10. Purchasing

ten work role categories, comparing facility versus agency administrators. Data contained in Table 28-7 revealed that significant differences occur in eight of ten categories of preservice training needs according to work setting where rehabilitation administrators are employed. When comparing Table 28-7 with Table 28-6, it becomes apparent that AFL supervisors have dissimilar training needs than other agency administrators in work role categories of Fiscal Management, Production Management, Program Planning and Evaluation, Public Relations, and Marketing Services. As a result, statistical differences are highest among those five areas in Table 28-7. A rank ordering of work role categories for which preservice training was perceived to be needed was assembled from Table 28-7 and Table 28-8 according to employment setting.

Based on the results of the entire study, Table 28-9 was developed to reflect a recommended curriculum for preservice rehabilitation administration education (RAE) programs. Curriculum studies in general can benefit greatly from the results of scientific inquiry but in the end, the resulting curriculum must reflect, in large measure, the value judgments of the authors. What follows is a systematic discussion of those value judgments, supported where possible on the basis of the results of this investigation.

The first four work role categories and related items were included as required curriculum content based on the perceived need for preservice training by practicing rehabilitation administrators and supervisors by job site and level. An additional factor was considered to establish the cut off between required content and recommended electives, that being the actual tasks included in the job for which students were being prepared. Two specific value judgments were simultaneously employed, that is (1) students should be prepared for the top level for which they may aspire in the field, not some mid-range, and (2) given the small size of our field and relative limitation of training funds, parsimony of training programs that allow maximum flexibility

Table 28–9
**Recommended Curriculum for Preservice
Rehabilitation Administration Education Programs**

1. Program Planning and Evaluation (Required)
   a. Program evaluation design and implementation
   b. Preparation of program evaluation reports
   c. Utilization of program evaluation results
   d. Development of program objectives
   e. Development of program goals and policies
   f. Needs assessment.

2. Fiscal Management (Required)
   a. Budget preparation
   b. Financial decision making
   c. Controlling agency expenses
   d. Financial resource identification
   e. Financial analysis
   f. Cost accounting
   g. Management of financial accounting and bookkeeping systems.

3. General Personnel Management (Required)
   a. Employee supervision
   b. Management of employee conflicts
   c. Personnel evaluation
   d. Employee discipline
   e. Employee selection
   f. Employee retention and promotion
   g. Delegation of authority

4. Public Relations (Required)
   a. Legislative relations
   b. Public speaking
   c. Grantsmanship
   d. Development of public relations strategies
   e. Relations with board of directors
   f. Technical writing in rehabilitation
   g. Affiliation agreement
   h. Media relations.

5. Professional Management (Recommended General Elective)
   a. Professional supervision in office
   b. Professional supervision in field
   c. IWRP preparation
   d. Case finding and selection
   e. Caseload coordination
   f. Professional work assignment.

6. Production Management (Recommended General Elective)
   a. Work method analysis
   b. Work place design and layout
   c. Renovation planning and development
   d. Contract costing and bidding
   e. Motion and time studies
   f. Contract procurement.

7. Research (Recommended General Elective)
   a. Design and conduct of research in rehabilitation.

8. Marketing (Recommended Elective for Facility Orientation)
   a. Marketing and sales in rehabilitation
   b. Recruitment and utilization of volunteers in rehabilitation.

9. Labor Relations (Recommended Elective for Facility Orientation)
   a. Labor relations in rehabilitation.

for site of placement was considered the most desirable outcome of the effort.

Given these considerations the first four work role categories were included as requirements not only because they were rated highest by the survey respondents in terms of perceived preservice training needs, but also due to the fact that top level administrators, regardless of sector are required to perform work in these categories. The next three categories were included as recommended general electives because all levels and types of administrators recommended them, even though they reported they do not perform these tasks as even a moderate part of the job, with the exception of Professional Management which is a moderate part of the job of AFL supervisors. The remaining two work categories are performed only by FTL administrators and were therefore included as electives recommended for students of facility administration only. Purchasing did not appear to be of enough substance to be included in the curriculum for either setting.

CONCLUSIONS AND RECOMMENDATIONS

Reviewing the findings of this study, the vast majority of rehabilitation administrators and supervisors are white, male, and non-handicapped. While the incidence of female and handicapped administrators and supervisors tends to be higher in the rehabilitation ranks than in the business community generally, there is clearly a need for continued and improved affirmative action efforts in the recruitment and selection of management personnel in rehabilitation. The findings with regard to racial minorities in rehabilitation management positions is far less encouraging and quite consistent with previous findings (Atkins & Wright, 1980).

Clearly only a small percentage of practicing rehabilitation administrators and supervisors have any formal academic preparation for their work role, and most come from the direct service practitioner ranks with little management experience. This heightens the potential for new rehabilitation managers to learn their work role by modeling the behavior of their supervisors who also likely came from the practitioner ranks with no specific management preparation. The result is a group of persons who hold key job assignments who have high risk potential for elevated role strain and subsequent "burnout" (Sawyer & Schumacher, 1980). The key to reducing that risk would seem to lie in more adequate preservice preparation for administrators and supervisors in rehabilitation and more responsive inservice educational opportunities for those already caught in the dilemma.

The work roles of practicing rehabilitation administrators and supervisors seem to be described by the following ten categories: Program Planning and Evaluation, Fiscal Management, General Personnel Management, Public Relations, Professional Management, Production Management, Research,

Marketing, Labor Relations, and Purchasing. General Personnel Management is a moderate to substantial part of all levels of rehabilitation managers' work role. Program Planning and Evaluation is a moderate part of work role for all levels of rehabilitation management except AFL supervisors. Professional Management is a moderate part of the work role for AFL supervisors but not for the others. Top level managers from both settings rate Public Relations and Fiscal Management as at least a moderate portion of their job, while all other levels see these categories as minor parts of their job. All other work role categories were rated as minor parts of the job save Marketing and Labor Relations which was seen as a moderate component for FTL administrators, and Purchasing which was a moderate function for AML administrators. The question which remains is, "Are the work roles which are being performed reflective of what should be performed based on the needs of the agency or facility?"

Rehabilitation managers report moderate inservice training needs, which for the most part, are consistent with their actual work role. This consistency is greatest at the top levels of administration, with middle managers reflecting more inservice training needs in a variety of work role categories than their current work functions would suggest. This phenomena may reflect a desire for job enrichment or upward mobility for middle level rehabilitation managers regardless of sector. AFL supervisors on the other hand, report the narrowest work role and the least number of inservice training needs which are quite consistent with the disabled work role. This finding is quite consistent with the previous work of Feindel (1980).

In short, all levels of rehabilitation managers report moderate inservice training needs in General Personnel Management and Program Planning and Evaluation. Both levels of facility administrators and ATL administrators report moderate training needs in Fiscal Management. Only top level administrators from both sectors report moderate inservice training needs in Public Relations. Specific inservice training needs are also reported for the following groups: Professional Management for AFL supervisors, Research for ATL administrators, and Production Management, Marketing, and Labor Relations for FTL administrators.

While no comparable study has been completed previously, it is interesting to note that Hutchinson, Luck, and Hardy (1978) using an entirely different method and involving only ATL administrators found the following similar inservice training needs to be of the highest order; general personnel management, general framework for rehabilitation administration, fiscal management, and program planning and evaluation. There can be little doubt of the accuracy of Stephens and Kneipp's (1981) admonition of the need to include inservice training considerations for administrators and supervisors when planning an agency or facility's overall staff development efforts. It would seem that the information contained in this study would prove to be of considerable value to National Rehabilitation Administration Association (NRAA), Council of State Administrators of Vocational Rehabilitation (CSAVR), Rehabilitation Service Administration (RSA), National Association of Rehabilitation Facilities (NARF), and the various state agencies and private facilities as each work toward developing more adequate managers of the rehabilitation process.

After reviewing the aforegoing material it is quite clear that we are viewing a separate specialty in rehabilitation administration which is quite distinct from direct service rehabilitation specialties in terms both of work roles and training needs. To deal with its preservice preparation needs, what is needed is a specialized curriculum and not just a course or two on rehabilitation management superimposed over an existing rehabilitation counseling, vocational evaluation, or other direct service curriculum. Such a modification of an existing direct service rehabilitation academic program, that is, the addition of course work in professional and general personnel management, would only be adequate for the preparation of first level supervisor (primarily in agency settings).

The separate specialized curriculum should include at a minimum, course work designed to prepare students in the following areas: Program Planning and Evaluation, Fiscal Management, General Personnel Management, and Public Relations. The most desirable curriculum would also include general electives in Professional Management, Production Management, and Research, as well as electives for those primarily interested in facility administration in Marketing and Labor Relations. When reviewing the first four curricular components, the similarity with the areas of general management described by Kazmier (1974) is amazing, that is, production (Program Planning an Evaluation), financial (Fiscal Management), personnel (General Personnel Management), and sales (Public Relations). These curricular recommendations are remarkably similar to the recommendations of a previous study by McDonald and Lorenz (1977) which recommended a curriculum which would include a general framework for rehabilitation administration, fiscal management, program planning and evaluation, professional management, public relations, and research.

These findings should at a minimum pave the way for the establishment, improvement, and development of accreditation standards for curricula in rehabilitation administration. Such curricula would no doubt contribute greatly to an improved rehabilitation system in this country. Moreover, such preparation opportunities could in the final analysis lead to a certification program in rehabilitation administration and supervision which would help select only those who are best prepared to effectively manage the rehabilitation service delivery program.

The reader is cautioned to recognize that certain limitations of this study should give rise to selected reservations when interpreting its results, that is, restricted generalizability of the findings due to the incomplete nature of the population studied and the limited sample size, and also the questionable meaning of the specific levels of management employed in the study due to the lack of an operational definition. Such limitations give rise to recommendations for further studies which would include replication of the current study with clear operational definitions of the specific management levels, use of a population which more completely reflects the universe of practicing administrators and supervisors in rehabilitation and employment of a larger sample size. Follow-up studies to this survey, one employing direct behavioral observation of the work role of rehabilitation managers, and a second using a delphi technique to determine what the work roles of practicing rehabilitation administrators should be would greatly expand our knowledge in this most important area of inquiry. Finally, a follow-up study of graduates of rehabilitation administration education programs, which use the recommended curriculum, based both on self and supervisory reporting would help considerably to refine and finalize these findings in terms of the efficiency and effectiveness of these training efforts.

In closing, it should be clear that what is needed most, if we are to improve the practice of rehabilitation administration and supervision, is increased inservice and preservice training opportunities in this specific area of specialization. Such training should help to expand the work role of practicing rehabilitation managers and promote greater job flexibility during a period of shrinking economy. In this fashion we will ultimately achieve the goal of producing rehabilitation managers who do what should be accomplished to improve the program rather than simply model what has gone before.

NOTES

1. This research was supported in part by the National Rehabilitation Administration Association, a professional division of the National Rehabilitation Association, and was the recipient of the 1982 American Rehabilitation Counseling Association Research Award.
2. Acknowledgements: Sincerest appreciation is extended to Ronald D. Hickman, Joe Dowd, Patricia Kenny, Steve Magers, Susan McRae and Darnecea Moultrie for their technical assistance with this project. Special thanks are due to Leona Ogbara who orchestrated the word processing necessary to produce this report; without her good work our efforts would have been in vain. Also, appreciation is extended to Brian Bolton for his valuable suggestions during the data analysis phase of the project.
3. The actual RATI sent to members of the sample can be found in the Technical Report, available from the Oklahoma Clearinghouse.
4. Two hundred forty-three questionnaires were returned, of which sixty-five were not used in the final analysis for the following reasons:

   Forty-one respondents indicated their location of employment as Medical Institutions ($N=17$), Educational Institution ($N=20$), or Other ($N=4$). The small Ns in these groups made comparisons with the larger N groups inappropriate.

   Twelve questionnaires had no responses to at least seven consecutive items which constituted at least one major category in the inventory.

Seven questionnaires were returned unanswered.

Five questionnaires include members who either failed to indicate their present level of management or represented a first-line supervisor within a non-profit rehabilitation facility ($N=1$).

5. A comprehensive demographic description of the sample can be found in Table 28-1 in the Technical Report available from the Oklahoma Clearinghouse. The demographic questionnaire can also be found in the Technical Report Information Supplement.

6. When the questionnaire was originally sent to the sample, Scale 3 was worded as follows:

To what extent is academic preparation necessary for job entry?

   1 = not applicable
   2 = strongly disagree
   3 = disagree
   4 = agree
   5 = strongly agree

Immediately following the analysis of this Scale 3 data, current authors realized that the results made little sense and were basically uninterpretable due to the labels (e.g., not applicable) attached to the points of the Scales and the incompatibility of those Scale point labels with those found on Scales 1 and 2. To remedy the situation, Scale 3 was modified to its present form and the original 426 recipients of the first questionnaire were mailed a follow-up questionnaire containing the demographic questions and the RATI with only the modified version of Scale 3 (RATI items were not re-rated on Scales 1 and 2).

The Scale 3 data in this report are based totally on the responses of the follow-up questionnaire. Of the 239 NRAA members who responded (57% return rate), 174 questionnaires (i.e., 40.8% of the total sample) were in usable form for subsequent analyses.

7. Complete statistical results data on the Factor Analysis can be observed in the Technical Report Information Supplement available from the Oklahoma Clearinghouse.

8. The Technical Report Information Supplement available from the Oklahoma Clearinghouse contains group means, standard deviations, Ns, F ratios, and Duncan's (Multiple Comparison) for each Work Role Category and for each of the fifty individual job task items for Scales 1, 2, and 3.

REFERENCES

Alonzo, R., & Autry, L.H. Rehabilitation administration: Creativity and accountability. *Journal of Rehabilitation Administration*, 1977, *1*(4), 4-10.

Atkins, B.J., & Wright, G.N. Three views: vocational rehabilitation of blacks: The statement. *Journal of Rehabilitation*, 1980, *46*(2), 40; 42-46.

Feindel, M. A comparison of occupational values and opportunities of rehabilitation counselors and administrators. *Journal of Rehabilitation Administration*, 1980, *4*, 14-18.

Hutchinson, J.D., Luck, R.S., & Hardy, R.E. Training needs of a group of vocational rehabilitation agency administrators. *Journal of Rehabilitation Administration*, 1978, *2*, 156-159; 178.

Kazmier, L.J. *Principles of management* (3rd ed.). New York: McGraw-Hill, 1974.

Lorenz, J.R. Our roots. In J.R. Lorenz, I.B. Hawley, & A.A. McDonald (Eds.), Rehabilitation administration: Fact or fiction? A symposium. *Journal of Rehabilitation Administration,* 1977, *1,*(4), 24-37.

Lorenz, J.R., & Hill, J. Administration and supervision. In W.G. Emener, A. Patrick, & D.K. Hollingsworth. *Critical issues in rehabilitation counseling.* Baltimore, MD: University Park Press, in press.

Lorenz, J.R., Graham, C.S., Hashey, P.L., & Baker, R.J. *Selected aspects of financial management in rehabilitation facilities: A resource manual.* Washington, DC: National Association of Rehabilitation Facilities, 1981.

McDonald, A.A., & Lorenz, J.R. Graduate curriculum and training delivery preference of practicing rehabilitation facility administrators. *Journal of Rehabilitation Administration,* 1977, *1*(4), 12-22.

Sawyer, H.W., & Schumacher, B. Stress and the rehabilitation administrator. *Journal of Rehabilitation Administration,* 1980, *4,* 49-56.

Statistical Analysis System Institute. *SAS user's guide,* Cary, N.C.: Author, 1979.

Stephens, J.E., & Kneipp, S. Managing human resource-development in rehabilitation. In W.G. Emener, R.S. Luck, & S.J. Smits (Eds.), *Rehabilitation administration and supervision.* Baltimore: University Park Press, 1981.

Suojanen, W.W. Responsibility and professional management in vocational rehabilitation agencies: A reaction to Crawford's research *Journal of Rehabilitation Administration,* 1977, *1*(1), 21-26.

Young, W.M. Rehabilitation administration from the perspective of a rehabilitation counselor turned rehabilitation administrator. In J.R. Lorenz, I.B. Hawley, & A.A. McDonald (Eds.), Rehabilitation administration: Fact or fiction? A symposium. *Journal of Rehabilitation Administration,* 1977, *1*(4), 24-37.

CHAPTER 29

CONVERGENCE AND DIVERGENCE IN REHABILITATION COUNSELING AND VOCATIONAL EVALUATION: IMPLICATIONS FOR REHABILITATION EDUCATION

RICHARD J. BAKER AND JEROME R. LORENZ

IN THEIR DISCUSSION of the unique functions of vocational evaluators and rehabilitation counselors, Sink and Porter have established that the job responsibilities of these two professions are indeed different and require different skills. However, their categorization of certain functions (such as, determining eligibility, assisting clients in the development of the Individual Written Rehabilitation Plan (IWRP), and managing case service funds) as being unique to the counselor suggests that their job analysis was based primarily on the role of state agency counselors. In settings serving clients other than those of state vocational rehabilitation agencies some of these "counselor functions" are often shared by evaluators who may have responsibility for determining eligibility, for developing the rehabilitation plan with/for the client, or for case-finding. They may also serve as program managers, insuring continuity of services and interpreting data to the client; in some cases, as counselor/evaluators they may be involved in a counseling relationship. In fact, depending on the work setting, the job functions of the vocational evaluator may be quite similar to those of the rehabilitation counselor.

Similarly, Sink and Porter's statement that "the ultimate goal of the rehabilitation process is placement" and that "to further the vocational independence of the handicapped should be the goal of all rehabilitation workers" seems to emphasize the program goals of state rehabilitation agencies. However, many severely disabled persons seeking rehabilitation services do not pursue work-

---

Reprinted by permission from Volume 9 (1978), *Journal of Applied Rehabilitation Counseling*, pp. 27-31.

oriented goals (Baker & Sawyer, 1978). Further, deletion, in the Rehabilitation Act of 1973, of the term "vocational" signals that competitive employment is no longer the only goal of the rehabilitation process. In their study of rehabilitation counselor performance and outcome, Bozarth and Rubin (1975) suggested that psychological change per se should be considered a viable rehabilitation goal. If we consider rehabilitation in its broadest sense our goal statements become more and more general, e.g., "to help handicapped people become more independent." This in turn implies curricula in rehabilitation education that reflect a more expanded concept of rehabilitation and hence, a broader range of performance skills.

As long as the similarities and differences between the functions of rehabilitation counselors and vocational evaluators are discussed in relation to specific job settings, fairly clear-cut statements of job functions can be made. For example, in some settings evaluators might, as Sink and Porter suggest, administer and interpret "A" level psychometric tests. In many other settings, however, they may need to administer and interpret "B" level tests and under the supervision of a qualified psychologist, administer "C" level tests such as the WAIS, Stanford Binet, Bender Gestalt, etc. Further, while we would agree that the vocational evaluator's major responsibilities are diagnosis and prescriptive planning, he also has a major responsibility in helping clients learn about themselves on the basis of the information obtained through the evaluation experience. It is this aspect of the evaluator-client relationship that, we feel, most directly bears on the client's recognition of the evaluator and expresses the evaluator's concern for the client's future. We would hesitate to interpret this relationship as an instance of evaluators "commonly demonstrating possessive attitudes towards their clients."

Another point: while some evaluators may become involved with the modification of jobs to meet the needs of the severely handicapped, we feel that job restructuring and job engineering are separate specialties and that evaluators should not be expected to have competence in these areas. Similarly, although some state agency rehabilitation counselors actually do job placement, it is our experience that most placement efforts, at least those related to the severely disabled, are handled by private agencies or by specialists or coordinators hired by state rehabilitation agencies specifically to carry out the placement function.

The major educational issue confronting rehabilitation educators is not "Who can do what?," but "How should we train whom to do what?" Graduates from rehabilitation education programs in areas such as rehabilitation counseling, vocational evaluation, adjustment services, job development and placement, and rehabilitation administration are finding jobs in an expanding number of settings and are working with a variety of client populations. The roles and functions of the vocational evaluator, in many of these settings, seem to be at least as diverse as those of the vocational rehabilitation counselor.

There are many similarities and overlaps in the skills and functions performed by evaluators and counselors.

Given such similarities and overlaps, what are the implications for the development of training programs for either or both of these professions? In the light of projected reductions in federal appropriations for rehabilitation education, this question takes on added urgency.

As Sink and Porter report, the demand for rehabilitation counselors has stabilized, while the demand for trained evaluators far exceeds the number of graduates of the relatively few graduate programs in vocational education.

The imbalance between the demand for evaluators and the supply produced by the various training programs, coupled with a shrinking market in state rehabilitation agencies, has led many rehabilitation counselors with little or no specific preservice preparation to seek, and secure, positions as vocational evaluators. This has created a considerable demand for inservice and short-term training in vocational evaluation. In an attempt to respond to this need, some rehabilitation counselor education programs have added vocational evaluation components to their curricula, and many others are contemplating a similar strategy.

While this approach offers a partial solution, it also generates new problems. With increased competition for fewer rehabilitation education dollars the question arises: What constitutes reasonable standards or guidelines for determining whether a given rehabilitation counseling education program is eligible for funds earmarked for vocational evaluation education? Anticipating this problem, the Vocational Evaluation and Work Adjustment Association (VEWAA) in 1976 established a Curriculum Guidelines Committee to study this issue. Its initial charge was to develop guidelines for rehabilitation counselor education programs wishing to add a vocational evaluation emphasis to their programs; it was felt that, by expanding existing rehabilitation counselor programs to meet manpower needs in vocational evaluation RSA funds could be utilized more efficiently than if new programs had to be established. It was felt that such guidelines would also be of value to the Rehabilitation Services Administration (RSA); Council on Rehabilitation Education (CORE); Association of Educators of Rehabilitation Facility Personnel (AERFP); American Rehabilitation Counseling Association (ARCA); National Rehabilitation Counseling Association (NRCA); Rehabilitation Psychology, Division 22, American Psychological Association, and VEWAA.

The approach used in developing these guidelines was to analyze the two existing major studies dealing with competencies required for rehabilitation counselors and vocational evaluators (Wright & Fraser, 1976, and Coffey, 1977) and to identify areas of overlap and uniqueness. Competencies considered unique to vocational evaluators are being translated into course content areas that can be added to the curriculum of existing rehabilitation counselor programs. These course content areas are being reviewed to ensure compliance with CORE Standards for Rehabilitation Counselor Education (Manual of Accreditation, 1974).

An initial list of course competencies, along with guidelines for additional faculty and clinical resource requirements, was sent, for critique and comments, to all specific vocational evaluation education programs, to selected rehabilitation counselor educators with an interest in vocational evaluation, and to five practicing vocational evaluators with demonstrated interest in this area. Based on the reactions received, a revised set of guidelines was developed.

This preliminary analysis, while providing clear indication of a common rehabilitation core, has yielded an equally clear set of unique competencies for vocational evaluators in the following areas: general background and theory of vocational evaluation; broader skills than required by counselors in the areas of individual assessment, including development of evaluation techniques, report writing, observation, and behavioral recording skills; job requirements and labor market trends; vocational evaluation program development and operations; and skills for the evaluator as a team member.

At present, these guidelines are being reviewed by a second group of rehabilitation educators and practitioners. Based on their input, the guidelines will be revised once more before being submitted to the VEWAA Executive Council for approval and to RSA and CORE for review and adoption.

We believe that guidelines will prove useful to rehabilitation counselor education programs wishing to provide vocational evaluation education. Moreover, this effort should begin to establish a core of information and competencies generic to rehabilitation as well as a mechanism for utilizing existing rehabilitation education resources in the efficient delivery of training/education in other rehabilitation specialties.

REFERENCES

Baker, R.J., & Sawyer, H.W. The development of personal, social and community adjustment programs: A legitimate mandate for rehabilitation professionals. *Journal of Rehabilitation*, 1978, in press.

Bozarth, J.D., & Rubin, S.E. Empirical observations of rehabilitation counselor performance and outcome: Some implications. *Rehabilitation Counseling Bulletin*, 1975, *19*, 294-298.

Coffey, D.D. *Vocational evaluation competencies and their relative importance as perceived by practitioners and educators in vocational evaluation.* Unpublished doctoral dissertation, Auburn University, 1977.

Commission Standards and Accreditation of Rehabilitation Counselor Education, *Manual of Accreditation.* Washington, D.C.: Council Rehabilitation Education, 1974.

Wright, G.N. & Fraser, R.T. Improving manpower utilization: The "Rehabilitation Task Performance Scale," *Wisconsin Studies in Vocational Rehabilitation*, 1976.

CHAPTER 30

PRIVATE SECTOR REHABILITATION: BENEFITS, DANGERS, AND IMPLICATIONS FOR EDUCATION

BRIAN T. McMAHON

PERHAPS WE LIVE in a society which simply does not fare well with so-cial programming and planning, a society which lacks self-corrective measures other than competition, quality control, and consumer choice. If this is true, then vocational rehabilitation (V.R.) is not immune from certain in-herent, refractory problems which can be related to the *public nature* of the exist-ing service delivery system. The following are examples of such problems (Whittington, 1975).

PROBLEMS INHERENT IN PUBLIC SERVICES

Funding

The corrosive effects of government funding are still not clearly related to productivity, efficiency, or consumer satisfaction. The manpower required and the psychological price exacted to obtain and maintain governmental sanctions for funding are extremely high. This situation places a heavy burden upon the delivery of prompt, direct services to clients.

Managerial Restraints

Management is at least somewhat restrained in the proper exercise of its authority by civil service regulations, citizen advisory boards, political exigen-cies, and legislative changes (such as the Rehabilitation Act of 1973) which may suddenly alter the entire course of rehabilitation. Recent civil service

Reprinted by permission from Volume 45 (1979), *Journal of Rehabilitation*, pp. 56-58.

reforms at the federal level notwithstanding, management still appears limited in its power to reward superior performance or discipline the lazy, ineffective employee.

Lack of Consumer Choice

For each practitioner there exists the nagging realization that the client, if provided reasonable alternatives, might well choose to be served elsewhere. At the present time disabled consumers do not control their V.R. dollars and thus lack free choice, which is perhaps the most effective safeguard against exploitation, unfair pricing, and the squandering of resources. This is the most powerful feedback for self correction — personal choice by consumers who have the power to monitor and/or change their treatment (Rosenblum & Rusalem, 1976).

Limited Resources

The need in this country for V.R. services still far exceeds the capabilities of the current public service delivery system alone. While V.R. has expanded in terms of the number and kinds of services provided (comprehensive or "independent living" services), it has retracted sharply in terms of services to potentially needy populations, contrary to the prediction of some (Rusalem, 1976, pp. 42-43). This is particularly true of the older worker, the industrially injured (Ross, 1976), the culturally disadvantaged, and the less than severely disabled. The limitation of resources can be partially traced to the deep, historical entrenchment of V.R. in federal legislation, which may be perceived as a blessing (a form of minimal security) or a curse (vulnerability to legislative whims) for the profession.

THE PRIVATIZATION TREND

These problems and the need for solutions have influenced the development nationally of a network of private providers of V.R. services. Key ingredients in private rehabilitation are *consumerism, quality control,* and *competition*. This is not to suggest that public sector rehabilitation is completely lacking these ingredients. Certainly the element of consumerism has been furthered by the Individually Written Rehabilitation Program. Indeed, quality control has been enhanced by the accreditation procedures of the Commission on Accreditation on Rehabilitation Facilities and the Commission on Rehabilitation Education as well as the certification procedures of the Commission of Rehabilitation Counselor Certification (Bitter, 1979). It is only suggested that public sector service delivery has progressed in recent years to the extent that it has accepted two of these three elements. Evidence of the third ingredient, competition, is very sparse. But all three of these elements—consumerism, quality control, and competition—are part and parcel of private sector rehabilitation. For this reason, the privatization trend is perceived as a healthy movement which merits our attention.

What is the scope of this movement? In the country today there are in excess of 350 private providers of rehabilitation services. They range in size from nationwide firms with hundreds of employees to one person operations. Referrals generally come from clients, insurance carriers, self-insured employers, attorneys, physicians, hearing officers, and the state workers' compensation agency. The services provided generally mirror those of the public sector, although vocational evaluation and job placement are more frequently requested (as they are more profitable), while counseling and training receive significantly less emphasis.

Another gauge of the scope of privatization is the development of professional associations. In September 1977, the National Association of Rehabilitation Professionals in the Private Sector (NARPPS) was formed to represent the interests of those providing V.R. services within the free enterprise system. Current NARPPS membership exceeds 200 individuals representing numerous private firms and a rapidly growing contingent of rehabilitationists working in industry. They have a constitution, a board of directors, and five working committees including Nominations, Membership, Public Relations and Programming, Legislative and Government Affairs, and Ethics and Professional Development. There are four established affiliates and others in various stages of development. It is obvious that the privatization movement is formidable, that it is here to stay, and that it has tremendous potential for both good and evil.

POTENTIAL FOR GOOD

Reasons for optimism concerning privatization include the following:

Increased Opportunity

The private sector represents increasing employment opportunities, higher wages, smaller caseloads, greater freedom to innovate, more and faster advancement, and more variety for capable rehabilitationists.

Increased Responsibility

A corollary to the above is the increased potential for responsibility. Private practitioners generally perform directly a wider range of V.R. services than their public sector counterparts. For the most part they provide rather than coordinate their own vocational testing, counseling, plan development, and placement services. Furthermore, their actions and decisions are open for criticism by the client, supervisor, and many others not trained in rehabilitation, e.g., attorneys, insurance carriers, judges, and physicians. Activities must be thoroughly documented and decisions assertively communicated, often in a litigious environment which provides the "acid test" of each practitioner's convictions (Hesselund, 1978).

Unrestrained Management

In the private sector management is relatively unrestrained. Administrators have more freedom to reward and discipline employees, and may avail themselves of comparatively unlimited capital at psychological and administrative costs far cheaper than those paid for by public tax funds. Managers may choose to limit activities to only those which can be done well and profitably considering staff expertise and resources. In so doing, duplication of services can begin to serve new or currently neglected populations, as is already occurring with the industrially injured; the less than severely disabled (those ineligible or not highly prioritized for public services); and, in some instances, even the nondisabled. This expansion in terms of types of clients served can complement the public sector's expansion in terms of kinds of services provided. In the arena of rehabilitation in industry, the once idealistic notion of preventative rehabilitation is becoming a reality in the form of troubled employee assistance programs.

Placement Orientation

The current private V.R. service delivery system is unequivocally "placement oriented." This emphasis on the importance of placement and post-placement services is something the public sector, still heavily invested in training, is only beginning to realize *in practice*. Private providers place a high value upon on-the-job training and have developed a "place and train" approach which is only in experimental stages in the public sector (Dunn, 1976).

Increased Exposure

The privatization movement has brought to rehabilitation a newfound acceptance and appreciation of the profession by justices, attorneys, physicians, employers, insurance carriers and others heretofore ignorant of the discipline. Ironically, V.R. has "gone public" through the private sector movement. This exposure and awareness is long overdue and can only benefit the profession in the long run.

PROBLEMS INHERENT IN PRIVATE SERVICES

What, then, is the potential for evil in the privatization movement? As in the case of public services there are certain inherent, refractory problems which can be related to the *private nature* of this new network of service providers. Most of these dangers result directly from the relative lack of controls in a free enterprise system — skimming, profiteering, potential for malpractice lawsuits, the "jumping" of competent practitioners to the competition, and scores of unique administrative concerns. Also there exist pressures and ethical conflicts, not encountered in the public sector, brought to bear by nonrehabilitation principals (e.g., attorneys, insurance carriers, etc.) who have differing interests in each case. Another problem is that some firms, by developing an exclusive placement orientation, have abandoned the rehabilitation process and have come to more closely resemble private employment agencies.

None of these is so dangerous, however, as the tendency by some firms to utilize nonprofessionals in the place of professionally trained rehabilitationists, thus deprofessionalizing V.R. as a whole. The private sector V.R. movement is at a crossroads with respect to this issue. Many directors of private firms have openly expressed their disappointment with the product of graduate rehabilitation counselor training programs. The most frequently heard complaint is that the typical graduate is overqualified in matters of counseling and training and underqualified in matters of testing, job placement, and general business skills (Hesselund, 1978). Knowledge of worker compensation legislation and insurance practices, highly desirable in the private sector, is also lacking. Reacting to this situation, some firms have hired "counselors" from the business world whose knowledge of rehabilitation is to be obtained on the job. Other firms have requested that appropriate changes be made in rehabilitation counselor training program curricula. They have offered internship experience, oftentimes paid, to graduate students interested in private sector rehabilitation. These latter firms appreciate the value and adaptability of the graduate trained rehabilitation professional. They actively recruit the better graduates each year.

TRAINING IMPLICATIONS

This, then, is the crucial training issue. Where will the private providers obtain their personnel? Are they going to begin with professional counselors and provide them additional training in business matters relative to private concerns? Or are they going to hire business persons and expect them to learn on-the-job how to be rehabilitation professionals? There have already been instances of highly unprofessional practices, especially in the form of questionable marketing practices, resulting from the latter stance. It should be noted that such violations of good business practices and professional ethics appear to involve the smaller, one person operations more frequently. Nonetheless, as the supply of private providers begins to meet the demand and competition intensifies, these dubious activities have increased and have already begun to reflect poorly upon privatization in some areas. While little is known about the hiring practices and professionalism of private practitioners at this time, this is an area of extremely high interest to such groups as the NARPPS Committee on Ethics and Professional Development and the National Council on Rehabilitation Education.

Given that private sector rehabilitation is here to stay, and recognizing its potential as a positive development, it behooves rehabilitation educators to take the initiative in resolving the professionalization problem in the private sector.

This may be accomplished in the following ways.

1. Educators should learn everything they can about private rehabilitation activities in their communities. This can be achieved by establishing liaison and internship arrangements with reputable firms, and attending local programming related to the concerns of private practitioners.

2. Educators who participate in private rehabilitation activities, or care to, or are interested in the privatization movement should join NARPPS and serve on committees, especially the Committee on Ethics and Professional Development. Whether members of NARPPS or other professional organizations, educators should speak out for stringent standards for all providers of V.R. services.

3. Educators should institute an elective course on private sector rehabilitation. Such a course would include an overview of the field, its opportunities, its dangers; presentations by private practitioners and rehabilitationists in industry; mock trials to simulate the activities of forensic rehabilitationists; and a heavy emphasis on professional ethics.

4. Educators should advise students interested in private sector rehabilitation to take elective courses covering labor market and job analysis, insurance contracts and practices, worker compensation legislation, and the management of ethical conflicts. Such courses may be obtained from other departments in business, public or personnel administration; industrial psychology; occupational sociology; economics; and law.

5. Educators should add and/or improve existing courses dealing with vocational testing emphasizing work samples, job placement, and rehabilitation planning. While such activities are emphasized in the private sector, this does not detract from the importance of knowing counseling, community resources, and the medical and psychosocial aspects of disability.

6. Educators should extend course offerings to private practitioners in need of further professionalization, and recruit and accommodate them in training programs.

7. Educators should research the scope of private sector rehabilitation, its

standards, its impact, and its potential for interface with the existing service delivery system.

In these ways educators can modify (not overhaul) their curricula to accommodate interested students, further professionalize private V.R. service providers, and keep abreast of what may be the most significant development in rehabilitation in the seventies.

REFERENCES

Bitter, J.A. *Introduction to rehabilitation.* St. Louis: Mosby, 1979.

Dunn, D.J. *Placement services in the vocational rehabilitation program.* Report, RT No. 22, Stout Vocational Rehabilitation Institute, Menomonie, WI, 1976.

Hesselund, T.A. *Vocational rehabilitation counseling in the private sector.* Paper presented at the American Personnel and Guidance Association Annual Convention, Washington, D.C., March, 1978.

Rosenblum, L., & Rusalem, H. The consumer and the rehabilitation process. In H. Rusalem & D. Malikin (Eds.), *Contemporary vocational rehabilitation.* New York: New York University Press, 1976, 87-98.

Ross, E.M. *Workmen's compensation rehabilitation: A study of the rehabilitation of injured workers in the United States and member jurisdictions of The International Association of Industrial Accident Boards and Commissions.* Des Moines, IA: IAIABC, 1976.

Rusalem, H. A personalized recent history of vocational rehabilitation in America. In H. Rusalem & D. Malikin (Eds.), *Contemporary vocational rehabilitation.* New York: New York University Press, 1976, 29-45.

Whittington, H.G. A case for private enterprise in mental health. *Administration in Mental Health,* Spring, 1975.

CHAPTER 31

PRESERVICE GRADUATE EDUCATION FOR PRIVATE SECTOR REHABILITATION COUNSELORS

Brian T. McMahon and Ralph E. Matkin

Abstract

The field of rehabilitation has expanded into nontraditional employment settings in recent years. Most notably, there has been a dramatic increase in employment opportunities for rehabilitation counselors in the private (for-profit) sector, while job openings have declined in the state-federal rehabilitation system. Because this trend is expected to continue, attention has been focused recently on the adequacy of graduate level rehabilitation training curricula to prepare graduates for private sector work. This issue was examined by independent task forces formed by the National Council on Rehabilitation Education and the National Association of Rehabilitation Professionals in the Private Sector. The similarity between the two groups' recommendations for rehabilitation counselor education programs were striking and are summarized in this article.

THE DEMAND for graduate trained rehabilitation professionals by the for-profit rehabilitation sector continues to grow in a manner commensurate with the expansion of that industry. *Industry Week* recently estimated that the for-profit rehabilitation business "has grown from nothing in 1970 to nearly 1,000 companies and total annual revenues approaching $250 million" (Lauterbach, 1982, p. 53). Matkin (1982a) reported that approximately 5,300 practitioners, represented by some 200 corporate members of the National Association of Rehabilitation Professionals in the Private Sector (NARPPS), were working in this arena, and that nearly one-third of this total were graduates of accredited rehabilitation counselor education (RCE) programs.

Indeed, there are a number of recent studies that suggest that the current

Reprinted by permission from Volume 27 (1983), *Rehabilitation Counseling Bulletin*, pp. 54-60.

marketplace for RCE graduates is the private for-profit and not-for-profit rehabilitation sectors (Geist & McMahon, 1981; Gutowski, 1979; Hasbrook, 1981; Urban Institute, 1980). The most frequently cited reason for reduced openings in the public sector is the federal funding uncertainty for human service programs (Matkin, 1980a,b; Rule & Wright, 1981). Furthermore, this apparent redirection in the employment of RCE graduates is being reinforced by an awareness that while the majority of private sector rehabilitation professionals are involved primarily with serving industrially injured workers, others are actively practicing in a variety of previously unexplored settings. For example, employee assistance programs, industrial and facility consulting, job placement for a fee, and clinical practice are among the assortment of nontraditional applications of vocational rehabilitation in the private sector (McMahon, Matkin, Growick, Mahaffey, & Gianforte, 1983).

In recognizing this trend toward employment of RCE graduates in the private sector, the National Council on Rehabilitation Education (NCRE) and NARPPS independently established task forces to study the need for curriculum revision. Their recommendations for training modifications to better prepare RCE graduates for private sector employment were sent to the Council on Rehabilitation Education (CORE). Separately, each task force reviewed: (a) the literature on private sector rehabilitation educational needs (e.g., Lynch & Martin, 1982; McMahon, 1979; Organist, 1979; Sales, 1979); (b) research on the roles and functions of private rehabilitation specialists (Matkin, 1982b); (c) suggestions offered by prominent members of the private rehabilitation community; and (d) relevant course materials suggested by various NCRE members. The following represents an attempt to synthesize the final reports submitted by the NARPPS and NCRE task forces.

REHABILITATION PHILOSOPHY

Perhaps the most fundamental difference between the private and public rehabilitation sectors concerns the desired outcome of rehabilitation services. The NARPPS report aptly summarized the issue as follows: "Stated simply, services offered in the private sector . . . have as their goal the maximization of client's potential. On the other hand, services offered in the private for-profit rehabilitation sector have as their goal the eventual return of the injured worker to gainful employment at a level as close as possible to that attained prior to the disability" (Matkin, 1982c, p. 3). Thus, services in the private sector tend to be short in duration and placement-oriented (Matkin, 1982a). This fundamental distinction must be presented, discussed, and appreciated early in the graduate RCE program, perhaps in the introductory rehabilitation course wherein philosophical issues are typically treated.

PLACEMENT TRAINING

The strongest and most persistent suggestion in the NCRE and NARPPS reports is summarized by two words—MORE PLACEMENT. Private sector employers are seeking graduates who have more and better placement skills than those possessed by the typical RCE graduate. Particular areas of emphasis include job development, job analysis, job modification, job restructuring, job-seeking skills training, labor market analyses, union policies and practices, affirmative action, and state and federal worker compensation mandates. Moreover, structured activities that students can perform with close supervision are preferred to lectures, readings, or audiovisual presentations (McMahon, 1982).

MEDICAL AND PSYCHOSOCIAL ASPECTS

Students wishing to enter private sector employment require more exposure to and understanding of the rehabilitation implications associated with orthopedic disabilities (especially injuries to the lower back and joints), neurological disorders, occupationally induced diseases, and pain management. RCE students should become familiar with a variety of medical references (e.g., *Diagnostic and Statistical Manual III* and the *Physician's Desk Reference*). Perhaps most importantly, students must be able to communicate with medical, paramedical, and nonmedical persons about the medical aspects of developing an effective vocational plan.

With regard to psychosocial aspects of disability, students should be familiar with such topical areas as pschosomatic pain and motivational problems (e.g., work disincentives and fear of reinjury). Again, field experiences cannot be overstated as a desirable method for helping students understand these concepts.

VOCATIONAL AND PERSONAL ADJUSTMENT COUNSELING

This area of rehabilitation counselor training, identified only within the NCRE report was divided into two parts: vocational counseling and personal adjustment counseling. From the NARPPS perspective, vocational counseling was taken to be part of the overall rationale underlying the "return-to-work" philosophy. The omission of personal adjustment counseling in the NARPPS report was predicated on earlier research findings that suggested such services were performed by less than half of all NARPPS members (Matkin, 1982a).

The NCRE report (McMahon, 1982) indicated that vocational counseling instructors should expand their treatment of such areas as transferable skills, sources of local occupational information, models of career development applicable to persons with disabilities, short-term and goal-directed counseling strategies, and working with resistive clients. The matter of personal adjustment counseling, its role and significance, is somewhat more controversial. It seems that the increasing attention to placement activity has been accompanied by a decreasing emphasis on counseling activities and associated skills. This can happen in the private sector because referral sources, typically insurance carriers, have little understanding of counseling and its relation to successful vocational outcome. Because counseling activities are not readily measurable, they may be perceived as nonessential services and are therefore neither encouraged nor authorized for payment. This unfortunate occurrence sometimes results in the prescription of rehabilitation "treatment" by nonrehabilitationists.

Educators are not likely to abandon their commitment to training in this area, and justifiably so. Rather, individual private sector rehabilitation practitioners may have to become "educators" in their own right on this issue by confronting and informing referral sources regarding the rationale for counseling intervention. Whether a rehabilitation service delivery system is public or private, placement-oriented or training-oriented, counseling is the lubricant that makes the rehabilitation process work. Therefore, private rehabilitation providers are encouraged to reassess the centrality of counseling and reconstitute this modality in their settings as dictated by client need.

FIELDWORK PLACEMENTS

One result of appropriately modified curricula is the reasonable expectation that increasing numbers of rehabilitation counselors will be employed by corporations. Rehabilitation training is regarded as desirable for employee assistance professionals, affirmative action specialists, training and staff development personnel, personnel representatives, job analysis, in-house rehabilitation specialists, and rehabilitation consultants to industry (Dickman & Emener, 1982; McMahon et al., 1983). Fieldwork experience in industry seems appropriate as a method for training students, not only for the occupations mentioned but for the performance of job placement tasks in general. Certainly, the employer perspective is best understood by firsthand experience in that system. Unique methods are required for educators to develop and evaluate such fieldwork sites so that both the necessary flexibility and rehabilitation relevance are maintained. Presumably, the innovative and successful programs at Boston University, wherein scores of students have been trained in industrial environments, can be studied for guidance (Shrey, 1982).

The duration and type of private sector fieldwork in preservice RCE training are matters of disagreement in the NARPPS and NCRE reports. On the one hand, NARPPS recommends two practica and one full-time, six-month internship, all in the private sector (Matkin, 1982c). The NCRE report, on the other hand, contends that such a recommendation is overly restrictive insofar as it assumes that students are prepared to commit to the private sector from the beginning of their program (McMahon, 1982). Perhaps a more flexible approach, suggested in the NCRE report and currently in effect in a number of RCE programs, involves the careful prescription of practica in neutral settings (e.g., pain clinics, industry, or placement programs) followed by internships with private sector firms. In this way RCE students can acquire practicum experience relevant to both the public and private sectors without prematurely committing to either.

CONTENT AREAS

Both the NARPPS and NCRE task forces identified a variety of specific curriculum topics that may be introduced or given greater emphasis in RCE programs. These include but are not limited to the following areas:

1. Full scope of private sector settings and activities beyond rehabilitation of the industrially injured worker;
2. Worker compensation issues, such as history and philosophy, insurance matters in the rehabilitation process, claims handling, and the specialized needs of self-insured employers;
3. Program planning and evaluation methodologies;
4. Medical case management as related and contrasted to vocational management and medical/psychosocial aspects of disability;
5. Case management, service coordination, and follow-up;
6. Vocational evaluation methods;
7. Gathering, synthesizing, and reporting information to different audiences;
8. Identification and utilization of short-term vocational training programs;
9. Casefinding methods and techniques for private sector rehabilitation; and
10. Legal and ethical issues, such as vocational expert testimony, malpractice issues, privacy and confidentiality, and credentialing.

Additionally, several areas of elective coursework are appropriate for RCE students bound for private sector employment. These include business or rehabilitation administration, fiscal management and budgeting, and employee selection and supervision. Accordingly, faculty must become familiar with the full range of university or college electives available and applicable to private sector work. Measures other than prescribed electives (e.g., interdependent co-taught courses, special sections for existing courses, or invited speakers and non-RCE university programs and industry) should also be considered.

VEHICLES OF CURRICULUM REVISION

Both NARPPS and NCRE task force members were aware of the different needs, organizational structures, and methods and philosophies of RCE programs throughout the country. Accordingly, task force recommendations did not include specific mechanisms for creating the curriculum modifications described in this article. Among the many possible methods of revision are developing new lectures to fit into current courses, use of guest speakers and audiovisual materials, broadening the base of fieldwork sites, developing new courses when appropriate, incorporating elective courses, and developing specialization tracks. Those fifty RCE programs that also offer an undergraduate rehabilitation degree have the option of expanding the curriculum downward (i.e., fitting a number of aforementioned training components into an undergraduate curriculum). Such is the vehicle of choice in other professions, in which we regard prelaw, premedical, and presocial work majors as commonplace. The deployment of a particular change strategy is a matter of individual RCE program discretion. It is strongly recommended, however, that local private sector rehabilitation providers and their referral sources participate in the revision process.

FUNDING

RCE programs that have experienced funding reduction, graduate successful private sector rehabilitation counselors, or made some or all of the suggested curriculum modifications should not hesitate to approach industry and private sector rehabilitation firms for support. A commitment to the investment in properly trained rehabilitation counselors for private sector employment can be demonstrated by such firms in the form of paid internships, grants-in-aid, work-study programs, fellowships, or training grants. It can be surmised that successful acquisition of such funds will be directly related to the extent of curriculum modification undertaken by RCE programs.

FACULTY INVOLVEMENT

If the aforementioned measures for implementation are to be effective, there should be evidence of a faculty attitude supportive for or open to private sector rehabilitation. A faculty member who specializes in private sector issues or is involved in private sector activities is helpful. Additionally, faculty members should become familiar with reputable private sector rehabilitation companies and professionals as one method for maintaining up-to-date knowledge of the applied practices within the rehabilitation counseling discipline.

In the final analysis, the reports submitted by both NARPPS and NCRE task forces revealed substantial overlap and agreement on the key issues of RCE program revision, despite the differing opinions concerning the extent and nature of private sector fieldwork experiences. Certainly, the goals of both reports were similar, such that independently derived recommendations were very consistent and highly compatible. Indeed, the revision of RCE programs would seem attainable for those interested in change. It is hoped that the suggestions contained herein will expedite that process.

REFERENCES

Dickman, F., & Emener, W.G. Employee assistance programs: An emerging vista for rehabilitation counseling. *Journal of Applied Rehabilitation Counseling,* 1982, *13*(3), 18-20.

Geist, G.O., & McMahon, B.T. Preservice rehabilitation education: Where graduates are employed. *Journal of Rehabilitation,* 1981, *47*(3), 45-47.

Gutowski, M. *Rehabilitation in the private sector: Changing the structure of the rehabilitation industry.* Washington, D.C.: The Urban Institute, 1979.

Hasbrook, R.F. Editorial: If you have it — flaunt it. *Journal of Applied Rehabilitation Counseling,* 1981, *12,* 143-145.

Lauterback, J.R. Coaching the disabled back to work. *Industry Week,* April 5, 1982, pp. 52-55.

Lynch, R.K., & Martin, T. Rehabilitation counseling in the private sector: A training needs survey. *Journal of Rehabilitation,* 1982, *48*(3), 51-53; 73.

Matkin, R.E. Public/private rehabilitation during economic recession: A cooperative partnership. *Journal of Rehabilitation,* 1980, *46*(4), 58-61. (a)

Matkin, R.E. Vocational rehabilitation during economic recession. *Journal of Applied Rehabilitation Counseling,* 1980, *11,* 124-127. (b)

Matkin, R.E. Rehabilitation services offered in the private sector: A pilot investigation. *Journal of Rehabilitation,* 1982, *48*(4), 31-33. (a)

Matkin, R.E. The roles and functions of rehabilitation specialists in the private sector (Doctoral dissertation, Southern Illinois University, 1982). *Dissertation Abstracts International,* 1982, *43,* 05A. (b)

Matkin, R.E. *Rehabilitation education curricula: Preparing counselors to enter the private for-profit sector.* Report of the Training and Research Committee, National Association of Rehabilitation Professionals in the Private Sector, 1982. (c)

McMahon, B.T. Private sector rehabilitation: Benefits, dangers, and implications for education. *Journal of Rehabilitation,* 1979, *45*(3), 56-58.

McMahon, B., Matkin, R., Growick, B., Mahaffey, D., & Gianforte, G. Recent trends in private sector rehabilitation. *Rehabilitation Counseling Bulletin,* 1983, *27.*

Organist, J. Private sector rehabilitation practitioners organize within NRA. *Journal of Applied Rehabilitation Counseling,* 1981, *12,* 208-211.

Sales, A. Rehabilitation counseling in the private sector: Implications for graduate education. *Journal of Rehabilitation,* 1979, *45*(3), 59-61; 72.

Shrey, E.D. (Ed.) *Rehabilitation in industry — state of the art: Proceedings of a national conference.* Boston: Boston University, 1982.

The Urban Institute. *Forecasting manpower requirements in the rehabilitation industry.* Washington, D.C.: Author, 1980.

Selected Abstracts

Rehabilitation Counselors Working as Administrators: A Pilot Investigation

T.F. Riggar and R.E. Matkin (1984, p. 9)

A pilot investigation was conducted among 100 randomly selected RCE graduates from four programs offered in three universities. The purpose of the study was to identify the percentage of those RCE graduates receiving their master's degrees between 1978 through 1982 who were performing administrative or supervisory duties, how soon after graduation those activities became part of their job, and how much time during a forty-hour workweek they performed those functions. Based on a 72.5 percent return rate of an eleven-item questionnaire, results indicated: (a) currently 74.2 percent are performing administrative/supervisory duties, whereas at the time of graduation only 36.4 percent were engaged in such activities; (b) the average length of time post-graduation before RCE graduates begin fulfilling managerial roles was 14.25 months; and (c) 54.6 percent of those performing such activities did so for twenty or more hours per week. Results of this study revealed a need for CORE to investigate further the need to include a rehabilitation administration and supervision curriculum content area within RCE program accreditation standards.

Training Needs of a Group of Vocational Rehabilitation Agency Administrators

J.D. Hutchinson, R.S. Luck, and R.E. Hardy (1978, p. 156)

A selected group of top level vocational rehabilitation agency administrators from Region III was convened to participate in the Nominal Group Process to identify administrators' training needs. A prioritized list of ten and then five major concerns of this group was developed. The top two broad concerns with indications for training were in the areas of personnel management and in resource allocation and utilization. Additional information relative to the best training format was also identified. The administrators believe that training should be short in duration, approximately two days in the middle of the week, pragmatic with high impact and tailored to meet their specific needs. The conclusion was reached that administrators do have some very important training needs and that they are committed to participating in training that will afford them new knowledge and skills.

A Pilot Long-Term In-Service Training Project in Rehabilitation Administration

A. Sales and W.T. Downey (1981, p. 150)

The need for supervisors and administrators in the State-Federal Vocational Rehabilitation program has grown as the program has become larger and more complex. While the training needs of most rehabilitation practitioners have been adequately addressed, such has not been the case for supervisors and administrators on the state-federal vocational rehabilitation program. The authors present a pilot, long-term inservice training project for state agency administrators and supervisors that is experiential in nature and which addresses the basic training needs of such rehabilitation practitioners as described in the rehabilitation literature.

Graduate Curriculum and Training Delivery Preferences of Practicing Rehabilitation Facility Administrators
A.A. McDonald and J.R. Lorenz (1977, p. 12)

Some 4,000 rehabilitation facilities exist in this country today to serve the handicapped—more specifically, the severely and most severely handicapped. The large majority of such facilities do not have individuals specifically trained to manage and administer them. In order to gear up for the challenges of the Rehabilitation Act of 1973, curricula in rehabilitation administration and specialized training delivery systems are needed. This study uses a literature review of five related subject areas, a survey of directors of graduate training programs in rehabilitation/workshop administration, a survey of practicing rehabilitation facility/workshop administrators, and a review by experts in the field, to develop a model curriculum and specialized delivery system which, it is hoped, may provide a basis for the development of academic program accreditation standards, criteria for funding decisions, certification of professional administrators, and future research topics, among others.

The Impact of In-Service Training in Rehabilitation Administration
J. Carter, M. Shinnick, and R.S. McDaniel (1981, p. 144)

The objective of the study was to assess the impact of a one-week training program on personnel management for facility administrators. A quasi-experimental approach with three non-equivalent groups was used to assess the impact of inservice training. The major difference between the two groups who received essentially the same training was that they received it at a different time in a different setting. Specifically, the nineteen subjects in group one, who resided in several southeastern states, attended the training program at Auburn University. By contrast, the second treatment group received the training in the one state in which they all resided. Finally, the control group received no training. A questionnaire was administered to participants in each of the three groups prior to training and six months after training. The control group received the pre-posttest during the same period as treatment group one. The results of this study indicate that the one-week facility training program reflected increased participant performance on the post training questionnaire. The relationship between training and increased performance was not found to be a function of prior training in management skills, nor a function of experience in management positions.

The Status of Vocational Evaluation in Rehabilitation Counselor Education Curricula

R. Lytel, Jr., F.R. McFarlane, and R.D. Jones (1975, p. 236)

A survey on the Status of Vocational Evaluation in Rehabilitation Counselor Education Programs was mailed to ninety-one universities and colleges. Responses were received from eighty-nine percent of those polled. Analysis of the nine-question survey revealed wide acceptance of Vocational Evaluation as a component of Rehabilitation Counseling Curricula but a generally low number of specific course offerings. Interest in Vocational Evaluation by graduates was at a moderately high level of interest, and most programs indicated a willingness to participate in a joint venture to explore educational linkages between vocational evaluation and rehabilitation counseling.

Rehabilitation Counseling in the Private Sector: Implications for Graduate Education

A. Sales (1979)

The current impact of private sector rehabilitation counseling on rehabilitation education is presented with a focus on the present master's training model. Recommended curricula area in need of enrichment include: (a) knowledge of workers compensation, (b) basic concepts of insurance, (c) understanding of law, (d) the free enterprise system, and (e) legal and medical management.

The Rehabilitation Counselor in Private Practice: Perspectives for Education and Preparation

R.E. Matkin (1980, p. 60)

An increasing number of rehabilitation counselors and soon-to-be graduates are looking toward the private-for-profit sector for job opportunities in counseling. Assessments of the current graduate rehabilitation counseling educational model have generally concluded that the programs offered are adequately preparing counselors entering the private sector. However, deficit areas in the training programs exist which include functional aspects of rehabilitation in the private sector. There is a need to collect systematic data regarding the makeup, professional qualifications, and needs of those in private-for-profit rehabilitation in order for educational programs to structure relevant curricula for this sector. Mutual cooperation will be necessary between educational institutions and the private rehabilitation organizations in order to satisfy the academic and professional needs of both.

References and Suggested Additional
Readings for Part VI

Alonzo, R., & Autry, L.H. (1977). Rehabilitation administration: Creativity and accountability. *Journal of Rehabilitation Administration, 1*(4), 4-10.

Andersen, R.H. (1979). Vocational expert testimony: the new frontier for the rehabilitation professional. *Journal of Rehabilitation, 45*(3), 38-40, 74.

Baker, R.J., & Lorenz, J.R. (1978). Convergence and divergence in rehabilitation counseling and vocational evaluation: Implications for rehabilitation education. *Journal of Applied Rehabilitation Counseling, 9*(1), 27-31.

Baker, R.J., & Sawyer, H.W. (1978). The development of personal, social and community adjustment programs: A legitimate mandate for rehabilitation professionals. *Journal of Rehabilitation, 44*(1), 35-38; *44*(2), 32.

Byrd, E.K., Lesnik, M.J., & Byrd, P.D. (1981). A role play model for teaching supervision in rehabilitation settings. *Journal of Rehabilitation Administration, 5*(4), 137-141.

Carter, J., Shinnick, M., & McDaniel, R.S. (1981). The impact of inservice training in rehabilitation facility administration. *Journal of Rehabilitation Administration, 5*(4), 144-147.

Chan, F., & Questad, K. (1981). Microcomputers in vocational evaluation: An application for staff training. *Vocational Evaluation and Work Adjustment Bulletin, 14*(4), 153-158.

Coffey, D., & Ellien, V. (1979). *Work adjustment curriculum development project: A summary.* Menomonie, WI: University of Wisconsin — Vocational Rehabilitation Institute, Research and Training Center.

Conley, R. (1969). Benefit-cost analysis of the vocational rehabilitation program. *Journal of Human Resources, 4*(2), 226-252.

Cooper, P.G., Harper, J.N., & Davis, S. (1980). Perceived outcome priorities in a state vocational agency. *Journal of Applied Rehabilitation Counseling, 11*(1), 14-17.

Couch, R.H. (1979). Keeping score and looking good: The dilemma of certification in the private rehabilitation sector. *Journal of Rehabilitation, 45*(3), 62-64.

Crisler, J.R. (1980). Rehabilitation counselors' perception of DVR case closure difficulty based on client outcome criteria. *Journal of Applied Rehabilitation Counseling, 11*(3), 156-159.

Diamond, C.R., & Petkas, E. (1979). A state agency's view of private-for-profit rehabilitation. *Journal of Rehabilitation, 45*(3), 30-31.

Dickman, F., & Emener, W.G. (1982). Employee assistance programs: An emerging vista for rehabilitation counseling. *Journal of Applied Rehabilitation Counseling, 13*(3), 18-20.

Downs, A. (1967). *Inside bureaucracy.* Boston: Little, Brown.

Drucker, P.F. (1966). *The effective executive.* New York: Harper & Row.

Drucker, P.F. (1980). The deadly sins in public administration. *Public Administration Review, 40,* 103-106.

Emener, W.G. (1978). Clinical supervision in rehabilitation settings. *Journal of Rehabilitation Administration, 2*(2), 44-53. (a)

Emener, W.G. (1978). Reconciling personal and professional values with agency goals and processes. *Journal of Rehabilitation Administration, 2*(4), 166-173. (b)

Emener, W.G. (1980). Relationships among rehabilitation counselor characteristics and rehabilitation client outcomes. *Rehabilitation Counseling Bulletin, 23,* 183-192.

Emener, W.G. (1983). Rehabilitation administrtion and supervision: A critical component of rehabilitation education. National Council on Rehabilitation Education, *NCRE Report, 9*(4), 2, 4.

Emener, W.G., & Hutchinson, J.H. (1979). Inservice training in clinical supervision in the rehabilitation counseling process. *Rehabilitation Counseling Bulletin, 22,* 427-430.

Emener, W.G., & McFarlane, F.R. (in press). A futuristic model of rehabilitation education. *Journal of Applied Rehabilitation Counseling.*

Emener, W.G., & Rubin, S.E. (1980). Rehabilitation counselor roles and functions and sources of role strain. *Journal of Applied Rehabilitation Counseling, 11*(2), 57-69.

Emener, W.G., Lauth, T.P., Renick, J.C., & Smits, S.J. (in press). Impact of government retrenchment on professionalism: The cases of rehabilitation counseling and social work. *Journal of Rehabilitation Administration.*

Emener, W.G., Luck, R.S., & Smits, S.J. (1981). *Rehabilitation administration and supervision.* Baltimore: University Park Press.

English, R.W., Oberle, J.G., & Byrne, A.R. (1979). Rehabilitation counselor supervision: A national perspective. *Rehabilitation Counseling Bulletin, 22,* 183-304.

Feinberg, L.B., & McFarlane, F.R. (1979). Setting-based factors in rehabilitation counselor role variability. *Journal of Applied Rehabilitation Counseling, 10*(2), 95-101.

Feindel, M. (1980). A comparison of occupational values and opportunities of rehabilitation counselors and administrators. *Journal of Rehabilitation Administration, 4,* 14-18.

Fry, R. (1980). *Training Programs in work evaluation, adjustment, and facility management.* Material Development Center, University of Wisconsin-Stout, Menomonie, Wisconsin.

Geist, G.O., & McMahon, B.T. (1981). Preservice rehabilitation education: Where graduates are employed. *Journal of Rehabilitation, 47*(3), 45-47.

Gellman, W. (1968). The principles of vocational evaluation. *Rehabilitation Literature, 24,* 98-102.

Good, A.W. (1974). Supervision: The key to good management. *Journal of Rehabilitation, 40,* 13-14, 30-31, 42.

Graves, W. (1979). The impact of federal legislation for handicapped people on the rehabilitation counselor. *Journal of Applied Rehabilitation Counseling, 10*(2), 67-71.

Griswold, P.P., & Scott, J.W. (1979). The state rehabilitation agency and private rehabilitation: A partnership long overdue. *Journal of Rehabilitation, 45*(3), 32-33, 74.

Hutchinson, J.D., Luck, R.S., & Hardy, R.E. (1978). Training needs of a group of vocational rehabilitation agency administrators. *Journal of Rehabilitation Administration, 2*(4), 156-159, 178.

James, D.T. (1973). The supervisor as a counselor-facilitator. *Journal of Rehabilitation, 39,* 18-22.

Levine, C.H. (1979). More on cutback management: Hard questions for hard times. *Public Administration Review, 39,* 179-183.

Lewin, S.S. Ramseur, J.H., & Sink, J.M. (1979). The role of private rehabilitation: founder, catalyst, competitor. *Journal of Rehabilitation, 45*(3), 16-19.

Lorenz, J.R., & Hill, J. (1984). Administration and supervision. In W.G. Emener, A. Patrick, & D.K. Hollingsworth (Eds.), *Critical issues in rehabilitation counseling.* Springfield, IL: Charles C Thomas.

Lorenz, J.R. (1979). Setting performance objectives and evaluating individual performance in rehabilitation settings. *Journal of Rehabilitation Administration, 3*(1), 5-11.

Luck, R.S. (1978). The rehabilitation supervisor: Technical expert and trainer. *Journal of Rehabilitation Administration, 2*(2), 66-72.

Lynch, R.K., & Martin, T. (1982). Rehabilitation counseling in the private sector: A training needs survey. *Journal of Rehabilitation, 48*(3), 51-53, 73.

Lytel, R., Jr., McFarlane, F.R., & Jones, R.D. (1975). The status of vocational evaluation in rehabilitation counselor education curricula. *Journal of Applied Rehabilitation Counseling, 6*(4), 236-243.

Massie, W. (1962). Sheltered workshops: A 1962 portrait. *Journal of Rehabilitation, 28*(5), 17, 20.

Matkin, R.E. (1980). Public/private rehabilitation during recession. *Journal of Rehabilitation, 46*(4), 58-61. (a)

Matkin, R.E. (1980). The rehabilitation counselor in private practice: Perspectives for education and preparation. *Journal of Rehabilitation, 46*(2), 60-62. (b)

Matkin, R.E. (1982). Rehabilitation services offered in the private sector: A pilot investigation. *Journal of Rehabilitation, 48*(4), 31-33.

Matkin, R.E., Sawyer, H.W., Lorenz, J.R., & Rubin, S.E. (1982). Rehabilitation administrators and supervisors: Their work assignments, training needs, and suggestions for preparation. *Journal of Rehabilitation Administration, 6*(4) 170-183.

McDonald, A.A. (1976). *A rationale and design of a graduate program in rehabilitation facility administration for employed personnel.* Doctoral dissertation, University of Wisconsin, Milwaukee.

McDonald, A.A., & Lorenz, J.R. (1977). Graduate curriculum and training delivery preferences of practicing rehabilitation facility administrators. *Journal of Rehabilitation Administration, 1*(4), 12-22.

McFarlane, F.R., & DiPaola, S.M. (1979). Rehabilitation counselor, vocational evaluator and work adjustment specialist: Are these professionals different? *Journal of Applied Rehabilitation Counseling, 10*(3), 142-147.

McFarlane, F.R., & Frost, D.E. (1981). Rehabilitation directions: Feast, famine, or extinction in the 1980's. *Journal of Rehabilitation, 47*(3), 20-23.

McMahon, B.T. (1979). Private sector rehabilitation: Benefits, dangers, and implications for education. *Journal of Rehabilitation, 45*(3), 56-58.

McMahon, B.T., & Matkin, R.E. (1983). Preservice graduate education for private sector rehabilitation counselors. *Rehabilitation Counseling Bulletin, 27*(1), 54-60.

McMahon, B.T., Matkin, R.E., Growick, B., Mahaffey, D., & Gianforte, G. (1983). Recent trends in private sector rehabilitation. *Rehabilitation Counseling Bulletin, 27*(1), 32-47.

Mosher, F.C. (1978). The public service in a temporary society. In J.M. Shafritz & A.C. Hyde (Eds.), *Classics in public administration.* Oak Park, IL: Moore.

Nadolsky, J. (1974). Guidelines for the classification and utilization of vocational evaluation personnel. *Rehabilitation Literature, 35,* 162-173.

Nadolsky, J.M. (1975). Establishment of a basis for the development of a simulation training program for vocational evaluators. *Vocational Evaluation and Work Adjustment Bulletin, 8*(2), 29-41.

Organist, J. (1981). Private sector rehabilitation practitioners organize within NRA. *Journal of Applied Rehabilitation Counseling, 12,* 208-211.

Patti, R.J., & Austin, M.J. (1977). Socializing the direct service practitioner in the ways of management. *Administration in Social Work, 1,* 267-280.

Petrangelo, G.J., Abeln, K.E., & Rudrud, E.H. (1984). Qualified rehabilitation consultants: How are they doing? *Vocational Evaluation and Work Adjustment Bulletin, 17*(1), 5-8.

Riggar, T.F., & Matkin, R.E. (1984). Rehabilitation counselors working as administrators: A pilot investigation. *Journal of Applied Rehabilitation Counseling, 15*(1), 9-13.

Ross, E.M. (1979). Legislative trends in workers' compensation rehabilitation. *Journal of Rehabilitation, 45*(3), 20-23, 70.

Rubin, S.E., & Emener, W.G. (1979). Recent rehabilitation counselor role changes and role strain: A pilot investigation. *Journal of Applied Rehabilitation Counseling, 10*(3), 142-147.

Sales, A. (1979). Rehabilitation counseling in the private sector: Implications for graduate education. *Journal of Rehabilitation, 45*(3), 59-61, 72.

Sales, A., & Downey, W.T. (1981). A pilot long-term inservice training program in rehabilitation administration. *Journal of Rehabilitation Administration, 5*(4), 150-153.

Salkind, I. (1974). The training of workshop directors. In J.G. Cull & R.E. Hardy (Eds.), *Administrative techniques of rehabilitation facility operations.* Springfield, IL: Charles C Thomas.

Sankovsky, R., Brolin, J., & Coffey, D. (1977). Vocational evaluators identify training needs: Report of a national survey. *Vocational Evaluation and Work Adjustment Bulletin, 10*(1), 15-19.

Schweitzer, N.J., & Deely, J. (1981). The awareness factor: A management skills seminar. *Journal of Rehabilitation, 47*(1), 45-50.

Shinnick, M.D. (1978). The follow-up evaluation of rehabilitation facility short-term training. *Vocational Evaluation and Work Adjustment Bulletin, 11*(2), 31-37.

Shrey, D.E. (1979). The rehabilitation counselor in industry: A new frontier. *Journal of Applied Rehabilitation Counseling, 9*(4), 168-172.

Sink, J.M., & Porter, T.L. (1978). Convergence and divergence in rehabilitation counseling and vocational evaluation. *Journal of Applied Rehabilitation Counseling, 9*(1), 5-20.

Sink, J.M., Porter, T.L., Rubin, S.E., & Painter, L.C. (1979). Competencies related to the work of the rehabilitation counselor and vocational evaluator, Volume I. Athens, Georgia: The University of Georgia and the University of Georgia Printing Department.

Smits, S.J. (1972). The rehabilitation supervisor: Within or beyond our reach? *Journal of Rehabilitation, 38,* 22-25.

Smits, S.J., & Emener, W.G. (1980). Insufficient/ineffective counselor involvement in job placement activities: A system failure. *Journal of Rehabilitation Administration, 4,* 147-155.

Smits, S.J., & Ledbetter, J.G. (1979). The practice of rehabilitation counseling within the administrative structure of the state-federal program. *Journal of Applied Rehabilitation Counseling, 10*(2), 78-84.

Stephens, J.E., & Kniepp, S. (1981). Managing human resource development in rehabilitation. In W.G. Emener, R.S. Luck & S.J. Smits. *Rehabilitation administration and supervision.* Baltimore: University Park Press.

Suojanen, W.W., & Spates, J.M. (1979). Motivation and career development of state vocational rehabilitation personnel. *Journal of Rehabilitation Administration, 3,* 119-125.

Sussman, M.B., & Haug, M.R. (1967). *The practitioners: Rehabilitation counselors in three work settings.* Cleveland, Ohio: Western Reserve University.

The Urban Institute (1980). *Forecasting manpower requirements in the rehabilitation industry.* Washington, D.C.: Author.

Thomas, K.R. (1982). A critique of trends in rehabilitation counselor education toward specialization. *Journal of Rehabilitation, 48*(1), 49-51.

Whittington, H.G. (1975). A case for private enterprise in mental health. *Administration in Mental Health,* Spring.

Winder, A.E., & Mugford, T.L. (1973). The autonomous supervisor. *Journal of Rehabilitation, 39,* 28-30.

Worrall, J.D. (1978). Weighted case closure and counselor performance. *Rehabilitation Counseling Bulletin, 21,* 325-334.

Young, W.M. (1977). Rehabilitation administration from the perspective of a rehabilitation counselor turned rehabilitation administrator. In J.R. Lorenz, I.B. Hawley, & A.A. McDonald (Eds.), Rehabilitation administration: Fact or fiction? A symposium. *Journal of Rehabilitation Administration, 1*(4), 24-37.

AUTHOR INDEX

Note to the Reader: Each number refers to the page in the book upon which the author's name as a reference appears. In addition, the **NUMBERS IN BOLD TYPE** indicate the first page of an author's chapter in the book, and the *NUMBERS IN ITALICS* indicate the page of an author's Selected Abstract in the book.

Abeln, K.E. 268, 321

Abood, R.R. 174, *211*, 214

Abramson, M. 148, 157

Alcorn, J.D. 7, 17, 56, 61

Allen, C.M. *164*, 169

Allen, H.A. 7, *16*, 18, 116

Alonzo, R. 267, 272, 293, 318

Alston, P.P. 24, 110, 220, 237, 249, 259

Amer. Assoc. for Coun. & Dev. xxi

Amer. Personnel & Guid. Assoc. 30, 35, 46, 51

Amer. Rehab. Counseling Assoc. 6, 17, 46, 52, 138, 140, 142

Ames, T.R. 26, 109, 117, 167

Andersen, R.H. 267, 318

Andrews, W. 174, 214

Anthony, W.A. 24, 37, 39, 40, 42, 60, 61, *106*, 107, 109, 120, 123, 173, 214

ARCA Research Committee 199, 203

Arkansas Rehab. Rsrch. & Train Ctr. 25, *107*, 109

Arnold, C.K. 7, 17, 56, 61

Ashley, J.M. 32, 36, 77, 83

Atkins, B.J. ix, 116, 117, **137**, 138, 142, 143, 167, 170, 289, 293

Atkinson, D.A. 26, 109, 167

Austin, M.J. 266, 321

Autry, L.H. 267, 272, 293, 318

Avner, A. 162, 163

Ayer, M.J. 119, 123

Baer, D.N. 148, 157

Bailey, J.S. 148, 156

Backer, T.E. 17, 167

Baker, R.J. ix, 55, 61, 118, **159**, 167, 265, 267, 268, 272, 294, **295**, 296, 298, 318

Ballou, M. ix, 115, 168, 175, **205**, 215

Beardsley, M.M. 32, 36, 77, 81, 82, 83

Belcher, S.A. 24, 109

Bendix, L. 37, 42, 173, 214

Bennis, W.G. 55, 61, 219, 259

Bergan, J.R. 149, 156

Bergin, A. 215

Berry, D.J. 23, 111

Berven, N.L. 6, 7, *16*, 17, 18, 25, 59, 64, 65, 72, 109, 115, 116, **165**, 167, 220, 237, 248, 260

Bitter, J.A. 5, 17, 24, 53, 61, 109, 175, **205**, 215

Blum, C.R. ix, 115, 168, 175, **205**, 215

Board, M. 96, 99

Bolton, B. 17, 143, 220, 242, 249, 259

Bordieri, J.E. 248, 249

Borow, H. 197

Bowe, F. 96, 99

Bowen, H.R. 56, 60, 61

Boyle, P.S. 26, 109, 117, 167

Bozarth, J.D. 148, 156, 174, 215, 296, 298

Britton, J.O. ix, 174, **193**, 197, 216

Brolin, D. 96, 99

Brolin, J. 267, 321

Brown, W.H. 199, 203

Browne, J.A. 18

Browning, P.L. 26, 55, 63, *108*, 109, 118, *166*, 169, 219, 259

Brubaker, D.R. 6, 17, 220, 259

Bruyere, S.M. 24, 57, 61, 109, 219, 259

Buckhalt, J.A. 26, 56, 63, 111

Butler, A.J. 90, 91, 119, 123, 203

Byrd, E.K. 267, 318

Byrd, P.D. 267, 318

Byrne, A.R. 266, 319
Cantrell, D. 29, 35
Capshaw, T.B. 117, 168, 220, 259
Carkhuff, R.R. 48, 52, 173, 188, 191, 214
Carter, J. 267, 318
Carter, S.A. ix, 174, **193**, 216, *316*
Cassatt-Dunn, M. 96, 100
Chan, F. 55, 61, 118, *166*, 167, 267, 318
Cherniss, C. 175, 214
Chiko, C.H. 24, 109
Clark, R.P. 117, *165*, 170
Clark, W.D. 174, 214
Clowers, M.R. 6, 18, 24, 81, 82, 109, 123, 135
Cobb, B. 82
Coffey, D. 59, 61, 117, 167, 267, 297, 298, 318, 321
Cogan, F. 26, 111, 117, 168
Cohen, J. 152, 156
Cole, J. 96, 99
Combs, A.W. 140, 143
Commission on Standards and Accreditation 127
Cone, J.D. 149, 156
Conley, R. 265, 318
Conover, W.J. 79, 82
Cook, D. 174, 215
Cooper, P.G. 265, 318
Corthell, D.W. 220, *258*, 260
Couch, R.H. 268, 318
Council on Rehabilitation Education, 6, 7, 17, 23, 57, 59, 61, 65, 66, 72, 109, 115, 117, 120, 123, 135, 148, 156, 167, 298
Crimando, W. ix, 55, 61, 118, **159**, 167
Crisler, J.R. 175, *211*, *213*, 214, 237, 249, 265, 318
Criteria for CRE Eligibility 32, 35
Crystal, R.M. ix, 24, **45**, 60, 61, 109
Culberson, J.O. 7, 17, 56, 57, 60, 61, 175, 214
Cull, J.G. 18, 63, 82, 191, 321
Cuvo, A.J. 148, 156
Daniels, J.L. 7, 17, 56, 61
Darley, J.G. 31, 36
Davis, S. 265, 318
Dawis, R.V. 205, 210
Dayton, C.M. 79, 83
Dayton, C.W. 111
Dean, P.M. 162, 163
Deely, J. 267, 321
Deignan, G.M. 159, 163
DeJong, G. 96, 99
Dell Orto, A.E. 24, 60, 61, *106*, 109, 123
Dellario, D.J. 24, *107*, 109, 237, 249
Deloach, C. 58, 61
Diamond, C.R. 268, 318
Diamonti, M.C. ix, 24, **37**, 60, 62, *106*, *107*, 110
Dickerson, L.R. 230, 236
Dickman, F. 265, 310, 313, 318

DiMichael, S.G. 192, 193, 197
DiPaola, S.M. 23, 33, 36, 111, 117, 168, 267, 320
Division of Counseling Psychology, 8, 17, 24, 46, 52, 110
Dodenhoff, J.T. 141, 143
Doran, E.A. 25, 109, 115, 116, *165*, 167
Dowd, E.T. 26, 54, 62, 110, 117, 167, 174, 214
Downes, S.C. 24, 55, 62, 110, 116, 167, 220, 237, 249, 259, 265, *315*, 318
Downey, W.T. 267, 321
Drucker, P.F. 55, 62, 265, 318
Dublin, S.S. 223, 227
Duncan, J.G. 56, 62
Dunn, D.J. 302, 305
Eaton, M.W. 175, *211*, 214
Eighty-Third Congress 5, 7, 17
Ellien, V. 59, 61, 117, 167, 267, 318
Elliot, J.K. 24, 57, 61, 109, 219, 259
Ellul, J. 38, 42
Emener, W.G. ix, 5, 6, 7, 8, *16*, 17, 18, 19, 20, 24, 25, 26, **53**, 54, 55, 56, 57, 58, 60, 62, 64, **65**, 72, 77, 78, 81, 82, 83, 90, 91, *108*, 110, 112, 115, 116, 117, **125**, 126, 135, 136, 164, 167, 168, 169, 174, 175, **187**, 214, 215, 219, 220, 221, **237**, 238, 240, 241, 242, 244, 248, 249, 259, 260, 261, 265, 266, 267, 269, 294, 310, 313, 318, 319, 320, 321
Engelkes, J.R. 230, 236
English, R.W. 266, 319
Engram, B.E. 26, 110, 117, 168
Fairweather 148, 155
Feinberg, L.B. 7, 17, 23, 26, 55, 56, 57, 62, 110, 134, 135, 265, 319
Feindel, M. 266, 283, 290, 293, 319
Felton, J.S. 117, 168
Ferrandino, J.A. 26, 58, 62, 110, 117, 167
Ferritor, D.E. 155, 156, 221, *258*, 259
Filer, S.P. 174, *211*, 214
Finch, F.H. 5, 17
Finn, D.D. 210
Finn, J.D. 210
Fowler, N.L. 175, *213*, 214
Fraser, R.T. 6, 18, 46, 52, 81, 82, 123, 135, 297, 298
Freeman, J.B. x, 115, 168, 221, **229**, 259
Frieden, L. 96, 99
Frost, D.E. 60, 63, 265, 320
Fry, R. 267, 319
Gagne, R.M. 162, 163
Gandy, G.L. 7, 18, 60, 62, 175, 214
Gaomi, B. 140, 143
Garfield, S. 215
Garrett, J.F. 5, 18, 53, 62, 193, 197
Geist, C.S. 23, 110, 111

Geist, G.O. x, 7, 8, 18, 23, 24, 25, 26, *107*, 110, 111, 116, **145**, 168, 175, *212*, 214, 265, 308, 313, 319
Gellman, W. 267, 319
Gianforte, G. 220, 259, 268, 308, 313, 320
Gilbert, L.D. 117, 168, 174, 214
Glaser, E.M. 148, 156
Glass, G.V. 79, 82
Glick, L.J. 7, 17, 56, 57, 62, 134, 135
Godley, M.D. 219, 221, *258*, 259
Godley, S.H. 148, 156, 219, 221, *258*, 259
Gohs, F.X. 175, 214
Goldston, L.J. 148, 157
Good, A.W. 266, 319
Goodale, J.G. 194, 197
Graham, C.S. 272, 294
Graves, W. xiii, xvii, 7, 18, 265, 319
Greene, B.F. 148, 156
Greenwald, M. 60, 64, 117, *165*, 170
Greenwood, R. 148, 155, 156
Greer, B.G. 58, 61
Greever, K.B. 175, 215
Griswold, P.P. 268, 319
Gross, B.M. 54, 62
Gross, P. 175, *211*, 215
Growick, B. 268, 308, 313, 320
Gualtieri, J.J. x, 115, 168, 175, **205**, 215
Gutowski, M. 308, 313
Hafer, M.D. 24, *107*, 110, 219, 221, *258*, 259
Hahn, M.E. 28, 36
Hall, J.H. 7, 18, 46, 52, 119, 123, 191
Hamberg, J. 18
Hamilton, K. 5, 6, 18, 191
Hanna, C. 26, 111
Hansen, J.C. 139, 143
Hansen, C.E. 5, 6, 7, 18, 19, 220, 259
Hansen, C.L. 117, 169
Hardy, R.E. 18, 63, 82, 191, 267, 290, 293, *315*, 319, 321
Harper, J.N. 265, 318
Harris 148
Harris, W.M. 6, 19, 123, 136
Harrison, D.K. 25, 46, 52, 59, 64, 65, 66, 72, 111, 126, 135, 220, 260
Hasbrook, R.F. 308, 313
Hashey, P.L. 272, 294
Haug, M.R. 23, 112, 199, 203, 265, 322
Havelock, R.G. 148, 156
Hawkins, R.P. 149, 156
Hawley, I.D. 117, 168, 220, 259, 294, 322
Henderson, H.L. 116, 168
Hershenson, D.B. 6, 18, 24, *107*, 110, 220, 259
Hesselund, T.A. 302, 303, 305
Hill, J. 266, 272, 294, 320
Hinman, S. x, 117, **147**, 155, 156, 168
Holbert, W.M. 24, 60, 62, 91, *106*, 111

Hollingsworth, D.K. x, 25, 111, 174, **183**, 216, 294, 320
Hollis, J.W. 148, 157
Horowitz, N.S. 159, 163
Hosie, T.W. 6, *15*, 18
Hull, C.H. 79, 83
Hull, K. 96, 99
Hutchinson, J.H. 26, 111, 117, 168, 267, 290, 293, *315*, 319
Hutchinson, J.D. 266, 319
Hyde, A.C. 63, 111, 320
Hylbert, K.W. 6, 7, *15*, 18, 57, 62
Institute on Rehabilitation Issues, 96, 99, 100
Iovacchini, E.V. 174, *211*, 214
Jacobs, A. 192
James, L.F. 81, 83, 117, 123, 136, 170, 266, 319
Janes, M.W. 60, 62, 115, *164*, 168, 175, 215
Jaques, M.E. x, 7, 17, 18, 39, 42, 115, 143, 168, 175, **205**, 207, 210, 215
Jarrell, A.P. 54, 62
Jellinek, H.M. 25, 109, 115, 167
Jenkins, W.M. 253, 257
Johnston, S.A. 159, 163
Joiner, J. 115, *164*, 168
Joint Liaison Committee 29, 30, 46, 52, 116, 119, 123, 138, 139, 143, 168
Jones, G.B. 111
Jones, L.K. 72
Jones, P. 156, 157
Jones, R.D. 267, *317*, 320
Jordaan, J.P. 192
Jourard, S.M. 191
Kahn, S.E. 24, 109
Kaplan, A. 38, 42
Kaplan, S.P. 116, *165*, 167, 174, 215
Katz, R. 206, 210
Kauppi, D.W. x, 7, 18, 115, 168, 175, **205**, 207, 210, 215
Kazdin, A. 148, 155, 156
Kazmier, L.J. 291, 294
Kell, B.L. 138, 143
Kelley, E.J. 223, 227
Kelz, J.K. 18
Kelz, J.W. 6, *15*, 18
Kimball, M. 159, 163
Kirkpatrick, D.L. 221, 259
Kivlin, B.A. 18
Klein, M.A. 117, *165*, 168
Kniepp, S. 24, 59, 64, 112, 219, 221, 260, 266, 290, 294, 322
Koonce, G.B. 25, 110, 117, 167
Krauft, C. 174, 215
Kravetz, S. 174, 193, 197, 216, 247, 249
Kult, D.A. 116, 138, 142, 143, 170
Kumar, U. 194, 197

Kunce, J.T. x, 26, 111, 173, 175, **199**, 206, 210, 215

Lafaro, G.A. 7, 18, *106*

Lamb, H.R. 39, 43

Lanning, W.L. 116, 138, 139, 140, 143, 168

Laski, F. 54, 62

Lasky, R.G. 24, 60, 61, *106*, 109, 123

Lassiter, R.A. 5, 18, 53, 62, 219, 260

Lauterback, J.R. 307, 313

Lauth, T.P. 7, *16*, 17, 56, 62, 265, 319

Lawler, E.E., III 205, 210

Ledbetter, J.G. 169, 265, 322

Lee, C.C. 46, 52, 65, 66, 72, 126, 135

Leitenberg, H. 149, 156

Leland, M. 221, *258*, 259

Lesnik, M.J. 267, 318

Levine, C.H. 265, 319

Levine, L.S. 29, 36

Levy, R. 148, 156

Lewin, S.S. 268, 320

Lindsay, C.A. 223, 227

Livingston, R. 23, 111

Livneh, H. 82, 83

Lofaro, G.A. 24, 111

Lofquist, L.H. 205, 210

Lorenz, J.R. x, 33, 36, 59, 63, 117, 147, 148, 156, 168, 220, 259, 265, 266, 267, 268, **271**, 272, 291, 294, **295**, *316*, 318, 320, 322

Luck, R.S. 5, 6, 19, 20, 54, 55, 57, 64, 112, 117, 167, 168, 169, 175, 214, 219, 259, 260, 261, 266, 267, 290, 293, 294, *315*, 319, 320

Lutzker, J.R. 147, 148, 156, 157

Lynch, R.K. x, 6, 18, 61, 63, 219, 220, 221, **251**, 260, 268, 308, 313, 320

Lytel, Jr., R. 267, *317*, 320

MacGuffie, R.A. 116, 168

Mackota, C. 39, 43

Magarrell, J. 56, 63

Mahaffey, D. 268, 308, 313, 320

Majumber, R.K. 175, 215

Maki, D.R. 7, *16*, 18, 46, 52

Malamuth, N.M. 159, 163

Malikin, D. 18, 19, 20, 39, 43, 62, 63, 305

Marinelli, R.P. 24, 60, 61, *106*, 109, 123

Marks, J.B. 148, 156

Marks, S.E. 109

Marr, J.N. x, 117, **147**, 148, 149, 155, 156, 168

Mars, M.G. x, 221, **237**, 259

Martin, J.A. 156

Martin, R.D. 148, 175, 215, 221

Martin, T. x, 61, 63, 219, **251**, 260, 268, 308, 313, 320

Massie, W. 267, 320

Matkin, R.E. xi, 23, 32, 33, 36, 59, 60, 63, 77, 81, 82, 83, 111, 117, 168, 169, 252, 257, 265, 266, 267, 268, **271**, **307**, 308, 309, 310, 311, 313, *315*, *317*, 320, 321

Matteson, I. 210

May, V.R. 32, 36, 77, 83

McAlees, D.C. 220, *258*, 260

McCauley, W.A. 120, 123

McCracken, N. 25, 46, 52, 109, 115, 167

McDaniel, R.S. 267, *316*, 318

McDonald, A.A. 267, 272, 291, 294, *316*, 320, 322

McDonald, A.P. 175, 215

McFarlane, F.R. xi, 23, 24, 26, 33, 36, **53**, 55, 59, 60, 62, 63, 110, 111, 115, 117, 167, 168, 220, 221, **223**, 224, 227, 230, 234, 235, 236, 237, 249, 259, 260, 265, 266, 267, *317*, 319, 320

McGovern, K.B. 219, 259

McGowan, J.F. 5, 6, 18, 23, 46, 52, 173, 187, 188, 191, 215

McIntire, R.W. 156

McMahon, B.T. xi, 7, 18, 23, 25, 60, 63, 110, 111, 175, *212*, 214, 252, 257, 265, 268, **299**, **307**, 308, 309, 310, 311, 313, 319, 320

McRae, S. 147, 148, 157

McSweeney, K. 6, 18, 220, 260

Means, B. 96, 100, 149, 156

Melia, R.P. 149, 157

Merrill, H.D. 26, 56, 63, 111

Meyer, A.B. xvii

Michael, G.A. 190

Miller, A.R. 55, 63

Miller, G.A. xiv, xvii

Miller, J.H. 24, 60, 62, *106*, 111, 116, 168

Miller, J.V. 117, 169, 221, 261

Miller, L.A. 175, 199, 203, 215, 237, 249

Mirels, W.S. 193, 197

Moore, C. 162, 163

Moore, J.E. 221, *258*, 260

Morgan, C.A. 56, 59, 63, 117, 168, 190, 191

Morris, J.D. 215

Morrison, J. 223, 227

Mosher, F.C. 23, 55, 63, 111, 265, 320

Moses, H.A. 30, 35, 52, 143

Moyer, W.T. 148, 155, 156

Mueller, W.J. 138, 143

Mugford, T.L. 266, 322

Mulhern, J.R.' 117, 169

Mulkey, S.W. 116, 168

Mullinax, J. 26, 111

Munro, J.A. 148, 157

Murphy, S.T. xi, 24, **37**, 60, 62, 106, *107*, 110

Muthard, J.E. 6, 19, 39, 43, 46, 52, 77, 78, 83, 90, 91, 119, 123, 148, 157, 199, 203, 206,

210, 215
Nadler, L. 34, 36, 59, 63, *163*, 219, 260
Nadolsky, J.M. xi, 173, **177**, 215, 267, 320, 321
National Council on Rehab. Education 136
National Rehab. Counseling Assoc. 46, 52
National Rehabilitation Association, 6, 19, 219, 260
Nave, G. 55, 63, 118, *166*, 169
Neff, W.S. 157, 192, 193, 197
Neumann, M. 140, 143
Newman, J. 220, 260
Nie, N.H. 79, 83
Ninth Annual Workshop on Guidance 6, 19, 219, 260
Nord, W.R. 55, 63
Norman, C. 148, 157
Nunokawa, W.D. 203
Oberle, J.G. 266, 319
Obermann, C.E. 5, 19, 220, 230, 233, 234, 236, 260
Olshansky, S. 6, 19, 24, 111, 173, 215
Onstott, K. 32, 36, 77, 83
Organist, J. 252, 257, 308, 314, 321
Osipow, S.H. 188, 191
Ostby, S.S. 116, *165*, 167
Painter, L.C. 230, 234, 236, 267, 321
Pan, E. 17, 167
Pankowski, J.M. xi, 8, **9**, 19, 230, 236
Pankowski, M.L. xi, 8, **9**, 19, 230, 236
Parham, J.D. 6, 19, 123, 136
Parker, R.M. xi, 5, 6, 7, 19, 174, 175, **199**, 206, 210, 215, 220, 260
Parloff, M. 173, 174, 215
Patrick, A. 294, 320
Patterson, C.H. 6, 19, 23, 26, 28, 29, 30, 31, 35, 36, 39, 43, 52, 63, 85, 89, 91, 111, 116, 138, 140, 142, 143, 169, 174, 192, 215
Patti, R.J. 266, 321
Pence, J.W. 29, 36
Pepinsky, H.B. 192, 194, 197
Pepinsky, H.F. 192
Petkas, E. 268, 318
Petrangelo, G.J. 268, 321
Pfeffer, J. 55, 64
Pflueger, S. 96, 100
Phillips, J.S. 117, 169
Pinkard, C.M. 175, *211*, 215
Pipes, R.B. 26, 56, 63, 111
Placido, D. 25, 110, 219, 220, 238, 240, 241, 242, 244, 248, 249, 259
Polanyi, M. 38, 39, 43
Pollack, R.A. 148, 157
Pope, D.A. 46, 52
Porter, T.L. 5, 6, 8, 18, 19, 23, 46, 52, 65, 72, 112, 117, 126, 136, 169, 173, 187, 188, 191, 215, 219, 230, 234, 236, 260, 267,

295, 296, 297, 321
Possi, M.E. 116, *165*, 167
Power, P.W. 24, 60, 61, *106*, 109, 123
Prather, H. 53, 54, 63
Puckett, F.D. xi, 25, 32, 36, **77**, 78, 83, 112
Questad, K. 55, 61, 118, *166*, 167, 268, 318
Ramseur, J.H. 268, 320
Rasch, J.D. xi, 25, 60, 62, **65**, *108*, 110, 116, 117, **125**, 164, 167, 174, **183**, 216
Reagles, K.W. 23, 25, 111, 112, 115, 170, 221, 261
Redkey, H. 7, *15*, 19
Renick, J.C. 7, *16*, 17, 56, 62, 265, 319
Richardson, B.K. 220, 230, 233, 234, 236, 260
Riggar, T.F. 33, 36, 117, 169, 266, *315*, 321
Rimmer, S.M. 24, 59, 63, 112
Roberts, D. 115, *164*, 168
Roberts, R.R. 175, 215, 230, 236, 237, 249
Roessler, R.T. xi, 5, 19, 23, 26, 53, 60, 63, 77, 83, **93**, 96, 100, 112, 117, 169
Rogers, C. 188
Rogers, E.M. 148, 157
Rojas, A. 162, 163
Rosenblum, L. 300, 305
Ross, E.M. 265, 300, 305, 321
Ross, S.M. 162, 163
RRCEP Directors 219, 236, 260
Rubin, S.E. xi, 5, 6, 17, 19, 23, 25, 32, 33, 36, 53, 59, 63, 65, 72, **77**, 78, 81, 82, 83, 90, 91, 112, 117, 125, 126, 135, 136, 168, 169, 174, 215, 230, 234, 236, 265, 266, 267, **271**, 296, 298, 319, 320, 321
Rudrud, E.H. 268, 321
Rule, 308
Rusalem, H. 5, 18, 19, 20, 39, 43, 53, 62, 63, 300, 305
Sachs, M.B. 117, 169
Sadler, V. 26, 111
Salancik, G.R. 55, 64
Sales, A. 60, 64, 252, 257, 267, 268, 308, 314, *315*, *317*, 321
Salkind, I. 267, 321
Salomone, P.R. 6, 19, 39, 43, 46, 52, 77, 78, 83, 90, 91, 119, 123, 199, 203, 206, 210
Sanders, 148
Sankovsky, R. 267, 321
SAS Institute, Inc. 157
Sawyer, H.W. xi, 33, 36, 59, 63, 116, 117, *164*, *165*, 168, 169, 170, 252, 257, 265, 266, 267, **271**, 272, 289, 294, 296, 298, 318, 320
Saxon, J.P. xi, 24, 60, 64, 112, 174, **183**, 216
Scalia, V.A. xii, 23, 24, **27**, 54, 64, 112
Schafer, W.D. 79, 83
Scher, P.L. 252, 257

Scherman, A. 148, 157
Schinnick, M. *316*, 321
Schmidt, J.F. xi, **237**, 259
Schoen, S. 207, 210
Schofield, W.A. 203
Schontz, F.C. 188, 192
Schumacher, B. 272, 289, 294
Schwab, L. 96, 100
Schweitzer, N.J. 267, 321
Scofield, B.J. 116, 117, 142, 143, 169
Scofield, M.E. 25, 46, 52, 59, 64, 65, 72, 109, 116, 117, 142, 143, *165*, 168, 169, 220, 237, 248, 260
Scorzelli, J.F. xii, 25, 46, 52, 60, 64, 112, 115, **119**, 120, 123, 169, 170, 221, 261
Scott, J.W. 268, 319
Seager, B.R. 159, 163
Sec. 504, Rehabilitation Act/1973 216
Seidenfeld, M.A. 6, *15*, 19
Settles, R.B. 8, 19
Shafritz, J.M. 63, 111, 320
Shepel, L.F. 175, 215
Shinnick, M.D. 267, 318
Shipman, J.H. 219, 260
Shontz, F.C. 87, 91
Shorts, J.G. 139, 140, 142, 143
Shrey, D.E. 24, *106*, 109, 265, 310, 314, 321
Shure, G.H. 159, 163
Sink, J.M. 24, 65, 72, 112, 117, 127, 136, 169, 230, 234, 236, 267, 268, 295, 296, 297, 320, 321
Slowkowski, P. 37, 42, 173, 214
Smith, P.C. 194, 197
Smith, S. 162, 163
Smits, S.J. 5, 6, 7, *16*, 17, 19, 20, 26, 54, 55, 56, 57, 62, 64, 90, 91, 112, 117, 167, 168, 169, 219, 259, 260, 261, 265, 266, 294, 319, 321, 322
Soloff, A. 148, 157
Spaniol, L.J. 24, 60, 61, *106*, 109, 123
Spates, J.M. 322
Spears, M. 55, 60, 64
Spector, P.E. xii, 25, **65**, 110
Spencer, W.A. 192
Sperry, J. 96, 99
Standke, L. 156, 157
Stanley, J.C. 79, 82
Statistical Analysis System Institute 294
Stefflre, B. 193, 197
Steger, J.M. 7, 18, 120, 123
Stephens, J.E. 24, 59, 64, 112, 219, 221, 260, 266, 290, 294, 322
Stokes, T.F. 148, 157
Stoltenberg, C. 141, 143
Stretch, J.J. 219, 260
Struthers, R.D. 117, 169, 221, 261

Sullivan, M. xii, 59, 63, 115, 168, 169, 175, *212*, 216, 220, 221, **223**, 224, 227, 230, 234, 235, 236, 260
Sunblad, L.M. 7, 17, 56, 57, 62, 134, 135
Suojanen, W.W. 272, 294, 322
Super, D.E. 192, 205, 210
Super, D.W. 140, 143
Sussman, M.B. 23, 112, 199, 203, 265, 322
Switzer, M.E. 28, 36
Szuhay, J.A. xv, xvi, xvii, 169
Thomas, K.R. xii, 6, 19, 23, 26, 60, 64, **85**, 112, 174, **183**, **193**, 194, 196, 197, 215, 216, 219, 220, 247, 249, 260, 261, 322
Thomason, B. 24, 60, 64, 112
Thoreson, R.W. xii, 90, 91, 174, 175, 193, 197, **199**, 203, 206, 210, 215, 216, 266
Tichenor, D.F. 247, 249
Tira, D.E. 159, 163
Tobia, P.M. 156, 157
Tolsma, R.J. 24, 109
Tornatzky 148
Townsend, O.H. 26, 112
Traux, C.B. 48, 52
Tripp, J.E. 46, 52
Trotter, A.B. 116, 138, 142, 143, 170
Tyler, L. 192
Urban Institute, The 265, 308, 314, 322
Urmson, J.O. 38, 43
Usdane, W.M. xii, 26, 59, 64, **101**, 112, 117, 170
Vales, L.F. 26, 111
Van Maanen, J. 206, 210
Varella, R. 96, 100
Vash, C.L. 17, 167
Vieceli, L. 219, 221, *258*, 259
Vineberg, S.E. 193, 197
Wagner, W. 162, 163
Walker, M.L. 117, *165*, 170
Walton, K. 96, 100
Wanous, J.P. 205, 210
Wantz, R.A. 148, 157
Warner, R.W. 139, 143
Warren, S.H. 7, 18, 46, 52, 116, 119, 123, 170, 191
Wasicsko, M. 162, 163
Waskow, I. 173, 174, 215
Watt, S. 18
Weber, M. 193, 197
Wehman, P. 148, 157
Weinberger, J. 60, 64, 117, *165*, 170
Whitehouse, F.A. 20, 39, 43
Whittington, H.G. 268, 299, 305, 322
Wijting, J.P. 194, 197
Williams, J. 96, 99
Willis, B.S. 148, 156
Winder, A.E. 266, 322

Witten, B.J. 7, 20, 56, 64, 134, 136, 175, 216
Wolfe, B. 173, 174, 215
Wolfe, R.R. xii, 23, 24, **27**, 54, 64, 112
Wollack, S. 194, 195, 197
Worrall, J.D. 265, 322
Wrenn, C.G. 31, 36
Wrenn, G.C. 173, 216
Wresch, W. 159, 163
Wright, G.N. xii, 5, 6, 7, 8, 20, 23, 25, 46, 52,
    53, 56, 64, **73**, 85, 90, 91, 109, 112, 115,
    117, 119, 123, 140, 142, 143, 170, 173,
    203, 216, 221, 261, 289, 293, 297, 298,
    308
Wright, V. 96, 100
Yen, S. 156
Young, W.M. 267, 272, 294, 322
Zadny, J.J. 81, 83, 117, 123, 136, 170
Zelle, J.A. 117, 170
Zemke, B. 155, 157
Zimmerman, J.W. 156, 157

SUBJECT INDEX

Note to the Reader: Each number refers to the page of the book on which the subject is addressed. In addition, the **NUMBERS IN BOLD TYPE** identify the first page of a chapter in the book that focuses on the subject, and the *NUMBERS IN ITALICS* identify the page of a Selected Abstract in the book that focuses on the subject.

Abbreviated Task Inventory 78

American Association for Counseling and Development (AACD) 185

American Personnel and Guidance Association (APGA) xiv, 30

American Rehabilitation Counseling Association (ARCA) xiv, 6, 30, 138, 199, 297

Association of Educators of Rehabilitation Facility Personnel (AERFP) 297

Bowling Green University Survey of Work Values (SWV) 194-197

Caseload management 50, 134

Change 6
  government 54
  humanitarianism 54
  natural resources 55, 299
  rehabilitation counselor education 51
  rehab. coun. roles and functions 25, 77, 79-81, 85, 126, 219
  society and rehabilitation 219, 265, 299-300
  technology 38, 54
  times 102, 178
  values, attitudes and beliefs 54, 55, 173

Client needs 47

Commission of Accreditation of Rehabilitation Facilities (CARF) xvi

Commission on Rehabilitation Counselor Certification (CRCC) xvi, 32

Community adjustment 95

Community organization, 49, 94

Computers 165

Conceptual narrow-mindedness 39

Continuing education 33, 219-222, 229-230
  attitudes toward *258*

evaluation of *258*
for rehabilitation administration *316*
recommendations 225-227, 235-236, 256-257

Council of Rehabilitation Counselor Educators (CRCE) xv

Council of State Administrators of Vocational Rehabilitation (CSAVR) xiv

Council on Rehabilitation Education (CORE) xvi, 6-7, 23, 31, 61, 65, 66, 117, 122, 127, 297, 298, 308

Counselor education *106*
  models of 106

Counselor Education and Supervision (CES) xxi

Counselor Input *164*

Curriculum 115
  for facility administrators *316*
  for vocational evaluation *317*
  independent living 94
  placement **101**, 103-105
  rehabilitation administration 284-289
  revision 312

Disability group specialization 87

Futurism 53, 57, *107*, *166*, 301-302

Graduate Record Examination (GRE) 200-203

Graduates 175-176, **199**
  employment *212-213*, 265
  follow-up of 211-212
  job satisfaction **205**

Historical perspectives 28

Independent living specialist **93**

Individualized Written Center Plan (IWCP) 149-151, 155

Individualized Written Rehabilitation Program (IRWP) 149, 295

Internship **145**
Job Placement Division (JPD) 105
Job Task Inventory (JTI) 78
Joint Liaison Committee (JLC) 29, 30, 119
Journal of Applied Rehabilitation Counseling (JARC) xvi, xxi
Journal of Rehabilitation (JR) xvi
Journal of Rehabilitation Administration (JRA) xxi, 266
Learning modules 57
Miller Analogy Test (MAT) 200-203
National Association for Rehabilitation Professionals in the Private Sector (NARPPS) 185, 252, 268, 307-308, 310, 311
National Council on Rehabilitation Education (NCRE) xiii, xv, xvii, 66, 126, 128, 138, 183, 308, 310, 311
 NCRE Directory 66, 133
National Rehabilitation Administration Association (NRAA) 266, 273
National Rehabilitation Association (NRA) xiv, 6, 29, 32, 185
National Rehabilitation Counseling Association (NRCA) 185, 238, 297
Placement 102
 training 309
Pre-service education 31
 Nature and limitations 33
Private sector rehabilitation **299**
 problems 302-303
Prioritization trend 300-301
Professionalism *108*, 145-146, 219-220
Projects with Industry (PWI) 102
Qualified rehabilitation consultants 268
Recreation 94
Regional Rehabilitation Continuing Education Programs (RRCEP's) 28, 34, 230, 275
Rehabilitation Administrator Task Inventory (RATI) **271**
Rehabilitation administrators **271**
 roles and functions 278-281
 training needs *315*
 work factors 277
Rehabilitation counseling 51
 evaluation 50
 need orientation *15*
 private sector 23, *317*
 professionalism 6, 7, 27
 public sector 23, **251**
 recommendations for practice 247-248
 specific life areas 89, 190-191
 work setting 88
Rehabilitation Counseling Bulletin xvi, xxi
Rehabilitation Counselor(s)
 as administrators *315*
 career development 245-246, 266-268
 certification 32

competencies 48, **147**, **295**
education and training needs **223**, **229**
evaluation 221, **237**
expertise 89-90, 309-310
generalist *vs* specialist 26, 75
knowledge 7, **9**
philosophy **187**, 308
responsibilities **177**
roles and functions 77
standards 179-180
uniqueness 187
Rehabilitation counselor education **27**
accreditation 23
behavioral objectives **37**, 147-149
clinical practice **137**
contemporary issues 73, *108*, 115
evaluation of 25, 40, *107*, 162, *164*, 211
faculty involvement 312-313
fieldwork placement 310
funding 7, *16*, 180-181, 312
historical perspectives **5**, 28, 73
masters level **9**
models of 24, *106*, *107*, 147
private sector **307**
program contents 116, 117, **119**, *165*, 311-312
science, role of 37
specialization 26, **85**
Rehabilitation education
bachelors level 7, *15*
computer assisted instruction **159**
continuing education 7
doctoral level 7, *16*
education approaches 57
graduate level 8, 101, **307**
instructional areas **125**, 129-133
masters level 7, **9**, 75
models of **53**, 57, *106*, *107*
placement 101
private sector **299**, *317*
training materials *108*
trends *107*
Rehabilitation Education Survey 66, 126-128
Rehabilitation educators'
knowledge adequacies **65**, 76
training needs **65**, 76
Rehabilitation Psychology 297
Rehabilitation supervisors **271**
selection, motivation and evaluation 140-142
training of *165*
Rehabilitation training 160, *164*
for administrators **271**, 281-283, 315
for supervisors **271**
independent living 97
inservice 220
models of **45**
placement 309

private sector **251**, 303-305
Students
  attitudes *211*
  attributes 211
  characteristics 174-175
  recruitment and selection 173-174, **183**, **199**
  student passivity 41
  work ethic **193**
Supervision 142, 266
  defined 138-139
  purposes of 139-140
Training Needs Survey (TNS) 230-234
Undergraduate education *15*
Universities
  Florida State University xxi

Michigan State University xiv
New York University 7
Northeastern University 119-123
Pennsylvania State University 7
Seattle University xxi
State University of New York at Buffalo 207
University of Arkansas xxi
University of Georgia 211
University of Illinois 86
University of South Florida xix, xxi
University of Wisconsin-Madison 75
University of Wisconsin-Milwaukee xvii
Vocational evaluator **295**
Vocational Evaluation and Work Adjustment Association (VEWAA) 297